Difficult Diabetes

Difficult Diabetes

EDITED BY

Geoffrey V. Gill
Reader and Honorary Consultant Physician
Diabetes and Endocrinology Clinical Research Group
University Hospital Aintree
Liverpool
UK

John C. Pickup
Reader and Consultant
Department of Chemical Pathology
Guy's, King's and St Thomas's Hospitals School of Medicine
Guy's Hospital
London
UK

Gareth Williams
Professor of Medicine and Honorary Consultant Physician
Diabetes and Endocrinology Clinical Research Group
University Hospital Aintree
Liverpool
UK

Blackwell
Science

© 2001
Blackwell Science Ltd
Editorial Offices:
Osney Mead, Oxford OX2 0EL
25 John Street, London WC1N 2BS
23 Ainslie Place, Edinburgh EH3 6AJ
350 Main Street, Malden
    MA 02148-5018, USA
54 University Street, Carlton
    Victoria 3053, Australia
10, rue Casimir Delavigne
    75006 Paris, France

Other Editorial Offices:
Blackwell Wissenschafts-Verlag GmbH
Kurfürstendamm 57
10707 Berlin, Germany

Blackwell Science KK
MG Kodenmacho Building
7–10 Kodenmacho Nihombashi
Chuo-ku, Tokyo 104, Japan

The right of the Authors to be identified
as the Authors of this Work has been
asserted in accordance with the
Copyright, Designs and Patents Act 1988.

First published 2001

Set by Graphicraft Limited, Hong Kong
Printed and bound in Great Britain at
MPG Books Ltd, Bodmin, Cornwall

The Blackwell Science logo is a
trade mark of Blackwell Science Ltd,
registered at the United Kingdom
Trade Marks Registry

DISTRIBUTORS

Marston Book Services Ltd
PO Box 269
Abingdon, Oxon OX14 4YN
(*Orders*: Tel: 01235 465500
        Fax: 01235 465555)

USA
Blackwell Science, Inc.
Commerce Place
350 Main Street
Malden, MA 02148-5018
(*Orders*: Tel: 800 759 6102
            781 388 8250
        Fax: 781 388 8255)

Canada
Login Brothers Book Company
324 Saulteaux Crescent
Winnipeg, Manitoba R3J 3T2
(*Orders*: Tel: 204 837 2987)

Australia
Blackwell Science Pty Ltd
54 University Street
Carlton, Victoria 3053
(*Orders*: Tel: 3 9347 0300
        Fax: 3 9347 5001)

A catalogue record for this title
is available from the British Library

ISBN 0-632-05324-0

Library of Congress
Cataloging-in-publication Data

Difficult diabetes/edited by Geoff Gill,
John Pickup, Gareth Williams.
    p. cm.
    Includes bibliographical references
    and index.
    ISBN 0-632-05324-0
    1 Diabetes. I Gill, Geoffrey V.
    II. Pickup, John C. III. Williams, Gareth,
    MD.
    [DNLM: 1. Diabetes Mellitus. WK 810 D569
    2000]
    RC660 .D58 2000
    616.4′62—dc21
                                00-056419

For further information on
Blackwell Science, visit our website:
www.blackwell-science.com

Contents

List of contributors

Michael Berger MD, *Professor of Medicine, Head of Department, Department of Metabolic Diseases and Nutrition (WHO Collaborating Centre for Diabetes Treatment and Prevention), Heinrich-Heine University, Düsseldorf, Moorenstraße 5, D-40225 Düsseldorf, Germany*

Andrew J. M. Boulton MD, FRCP, *Professor of Medicine and Consultant Physician, University Department of Medicine, Manchester Royal Infirmary, Oxford Road, Manchester M13 9WL, UK*

Geoffrey V. Gill MA, MSc, MD, FRCP, *Reader and Honorary Consultant Physician, Diabetes and Endocrinology Clinical Research Group, University Hospital Aintree, Liverpool L9 1AE, UK*

Stephen A. Greene MBBS, FRCPCH, *Senior Lecturer in Child Health, Tayside Institute of Child Health, University of Dundee, Ninewells Hospital and Medical School, Dundee DD1 9SY, UK*

Robert J. Heine MD, PhD, *Professor of Diabetology, Department of Endocrinology, Vrije Universiteit University Hospital, PO Box 7057, 1007 MB, Amsterdam, The Netherlands*

Simon R. Heller DM, FRCP, *Senior Lecturer in Medicine, University of Sheffield, Clincial Sciences Centre, Northern General Hospital, Herries Road, Sheffield S5 7AU, UK*

Maureen M. J. Janssen MD, PhD, *Department of Endocrinology, Vrije Universiteit University Hospital, PO Box 7057, 1007 MB, Amsterdam, The Netherlands*

Raymond V. Johnston *Head of Aeromedical Centre and Occupational Health, Civil Aviation Authority, Gatwick, West Sussex RH6 0YR, UK*

Lois Jovanovic MD, *Clinical Professor of Medicine, University of Southern California and Director and Chief Scientific Officer, Sansum Medical Research Institute, 2219 Bath Street, Santa Barbara, CA 93105, USA*

E. Ann Knowles BSc, RN, ONC, *Senior Diabetes Research Nurse, Manchester Diabetes Centre, Manchester Royal Infirmary, Oxford Road, Manchester M13 9WL, UK*

Kenneth M. MacLeod *Consultant Physician and Senior Lecturer, Department of Diabetes and Vascular Medicine, Royal Devon and Exeter NHS Trust, Postgraduate Medical School, University of Exeter, Exeter EX1 3EF, UK*

Ingrid Mühlhauser MD, PhD, *Professor of Health Sciences, Department of Metabolic Diseases and Nutrition (WHO Collaborating Centre for Diabetes Treatment and Prevention), Heinrich-Heine University, Düsseldorf, Moorenstraße 5, D-40225 Düsseldorf and the Unit of Health Sciences and Education, University of Hamburg, Martin-Luther-King Platz 6, 20146 Hamburg, Germany*

Elaine Murphy MB, MSc, *Metabolic Research Unit, Department of Endocrinology, St James's Hospital and Trinity College Dublin, James's Street, Dublin 8, Ireland*

Peter M. Nilsson MD, PhD, *Senior Lecturer, Department of Internal Medicine, University Hospital, S-20502, Malmö, Sweden*

John J. Nolan MB, FRCPI, *Consultant Endocrinologist, Metabolic Research Unit, Department of Endocrinology, St James's Hospital and Trinity College Dublin, James's Street, Dublin 8, Ireland*

David J. Pettitt MD, *Senior Scientist, Sansum Medical Research Institute, 2219 Bath Street, Santa Barbara, CA 93105, USA*

John C. Pickup MA, BM, BCh, DPhil, FRCPath, *Reader and Consultant, Department of Chemical Pathology, Guy's, King's and St. Thomas's Hospitals School of Medicine, Guy's Hospital, London SE1 9RT, UK*

David E. Price MA, MD, FRCP, *Consultant Physician and Senior Lecturer, Morriston Hospital, Swansea SA6 6NL, UK*

Matthew C. Riddle MD, *Professor of Medicine, Division of Endocrinology, Diabetes and Nutrition, Section of Diabetes L-345, Oregon Health Sciences University, 3181 SW Sam Jackson Park Road, Portland, OR 97201-3098, USA*

Robert A. Sells *Professor and Consultant Transplant Surgeon, Royal Liverpool University Hospital, Prescot Street, Liverpool L7 8XP, UK*

Jonathan E. Shaw MRCP, *Specialist Registrar, Department of Diabetes and Endocrinology, Hope Hospital, Stott Lane, Salford M6 8HD, UK*

David E. R. Sutherland MD, PhD, *Professor of Surgery, University of Minnesota, Department of Surgery, Box 280, 420 Delaware Street SE, Minneapolis, MN 55455, USA*

Stephen M. Thomas MD, MRCP, *Consultant Physician, King's College Hospital, London SE5 9RS, UK*

John Wilding DM, FRCP, *Senior Lecturer in Medicine, University Hospital Aintree, Longmoor Lane, Liverpool L9 7AL, UK*

Gareth Williams MA, MD, FRCP(Edin), *Professor of Medicine, Diabetes and Endocrinology Clinical Research Group, University Hospital Aintree, Longmoor Lane, Liverpool L9 7AL, UK*

Paul Zimmet PhD, FRACP, *International Diabetes Institute, 260 Kooyong Road, Melbourne, Australia 3162*

Preface

The prevalence of diabetes mellitus is increasing in many parts of the world, and the clinical practice of diabetology is becoming more time-consuming and complex. Perhaps for these reasons, books on the subject of diabetes are appearing more and more frequently. Nevertheless, 'yet another book on diabetes' needs some justification by its editors. Our title, we hope, suitably describes what is different about this book. It is emphatically *not* a textbook of diabetes, nor a collection of reviews and updates on important areas of the subject. Rather, we have deliberately chosen difficult and controversial aspects of current diabetes practice, where there is no consensus of opinion. We have also chosen forthright and opinionated experts to present their own view of these 'difficult' areas. Many readers may disagree with aspects of the topics reviewed, but our aim is to encourage debate, rather than to deliver information passively.

The title of each chapter is in the form of a question—emphasizing, we believe, the considerable doubts and uncertainty that pervade clinical diabetology, despite significant scientific advances in our understanding of the disease. It is interesting that even how to diagnose diabetes remains controversial, and the first chapters discuss such issues, including the problems of impaired glucose tolerance (IGT) and gestational diabetes. We have, however, given the most space to management issues, both in type 1 and type 2 diabetes. A strong case for considering surgical options in obesity is presented. A view of oral agent usage is given which is contrary to much routine clinical practice, but which is, the authors argue, based on available evidence. Other hot topics covered in the management sections include hypoglycaemia unawareness, insulin regimens, brittle diabetes, glycaemic control in adolescence, and the evidence base for foot ulcer management. Surgeons from both sides of the Atlantic debate whether sole pancreatic transplantation (without kidney) can be justified in certain sub-groups of type 1 diabetes. In the last section of the book we deal with miscellaneous issues such as erectile dysfunction and hypertension, which affect diabetic patients of both types. A particularly important (and under-discussed) issue here is the impact of diabetes on driving and employment restrictions.

We expect that readers of *Difficult Diabetes* may find at least a little to disagree with, but a great deal to be stimulated by. We welcome feedback on what we believe is a novel presentation of diabetes practice today.

Geoffrey Gill
John Pickup
Gareth Williams
Liverpool and London
September 2000

Diagnostic and screening issues

1: Do we know how to diagnose diabetes and do we need to screen for the disease?

Jonathan E. Shaw and Paul Zimmet

Introduction

Diabetes mellitus comprises a heterogeneous group of complex metabolic disorders of varying aetiology, which leads to a variety of complications. Hyperglycaemia is a common feature of these conditions and has therefore been used to define diabetes. The difficulty in determining accurate and rational diagnostic criteria is evident from the wide range of criteria that have been recommended over the last few decades. This results, in part, from the fact that blood glucose has a continuous distribution in the population. Screening also remains a controversial area. It carries the hope of preventing major disease and its complications by identifying at-risk people at an early stage and intervening successfully. However, evidence for the benefit of screening remains circumstantial, and the ideal approach is yet to be determined. Recent changes in the diagnostic thresholds have sharpened the debate over diagnosis and screening, both of which will be considered in this chapter.

Diagnosis

The basis of the diagnosis of diabetes

There are a number of ways in which diagnostic thresholds for diabetes could be derived. Broadly, diabetes could be seen as a condition in which blood glucose is outside a defined limit for normal healthy people, or a blood glucose which is associated with clinical and diabetes-related pathology. The latter option is the preferred one, but immediately begs the question of which pathology to use as the 'gold standard'. Traditionally, retinopathy has been used. It has the advantage over the other specific diabetic complications of

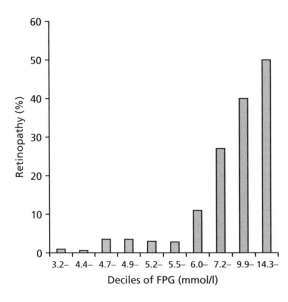

Fig. 1.1 Prevalence of retinopathy according to blood glucose. Data are adapted from the American Diabetes Association [12].

being both relatively easy to identify, and being specific to diabetes, unlike nephropathy or neuropathy, which without sophisticated investigations, can be hard to attribute with confidence to diabetes.

A number of studies have determined the prevalence of retinopathy across a range of glucose values within large (approximately 1000 subjects) population-based samples [1,2]. Figure 1.1 shows an example of such data, and demonstrates both the advantages and limitations of this approach. A clear threshold can be seen, so that below a certain glucose value retinopathy is rare. It then starts to appear above this value. This threshold effect is convenient, because it suggests a single, precise diagnostic value. However, close inspection of the x-axis of Fig. 1.1 reveals that precision is limited. Retinopathy prevalence starts to rise in the group defined by glucose values between 6.0 and 7.1 mmol/l. It cannot be determined exactly where the threshold lies; greater accuracy could only be achieved by including much larger numbers of people, and no such studies have been carried out.

In type 2 diabetes, cardiovascular disease (CVD) is a much greater source of morbidity and mortality than are the specific diabetic complications. It is logical therefore to argue that diabetes should be defined on the basis of the relationships between blood glucose and subsequent CVD outcomes rather than by the relationship with retinopathy. Figure 1.2 shows just such a relationship as illustrated by findings from the Paris Prospective study [3]. It is apparent that the nature of the relationship is very different. Risk starts to

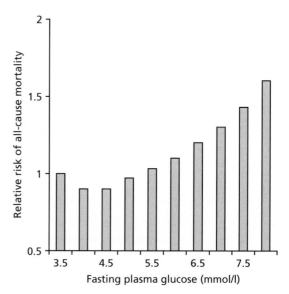

Fig. 1.2 Relationship of all-cause mortality to fasting plasma glucose. Data shown are the relative risks of mortality over 23 years, according to the baseline fasting glucose. Data are adapted from Balkau *et al.* [3].

rise at levels well below those at which diabetes is conventionally diagnosed, with no consistent evidence of a threshold effect [3–5]. The selection of a diagnostic value from these data would be relatively arbitrary (almost any glucose value could be used to identify two groups with higher and lower CVD risk) and probably lower than that derived from associations with retinopathy.

It is hard to resolve the differences between the use of retinopathy and CVD, although it is clear that no single glucose value can be used to determine both macrovascular and microvascular risk and outcomes. It is probably valuable to consider that current diagnostic thresholds for diabetes are useful for microvascular disease, while lower values (perhaps those currently adopted for impaired glucose tolerance (IGT)) and impaired fasting glucose (IFG) signal the risk of hyperglycaemia-related CVD.

What's wrong with previous diagnostic criteria?

Prior to 1979, numerous diagnostic criteria were in use for diabetes. There was variation in glucose loads, timing of blood sampling and values of diagnostic thresholds. This rather chaotic and unsatisfactory state was resolved by the National Diabetes Data Group (NDDG) [6] in 1979 and the World Health Organization (WHO) with the publication of their reports in 1980 and 1985 [7,8]. These documents standardized the diagnosis of diabetes (apart from gestational diabetes) around the world, and based it on a 75-g oral glucose tolerance test (OGTT). Plasma glucose values of ≥7.8 mmol/l in the fasting state, and ≥11.1 mmol/l 2 hours after the glucose load, were instituted as the diagnostic thresholds. These values were based on cross-sectional data, which indicated that they represented thresholds above which diabetic retinopathy started to occur. Furthermore, within high-prevalence communities (such as Pima Indians and Nauruans), they separated the two populations within the bimodal glucose distribution. In addition to defining diabetes, IGT was introduced as an intermediate state between normality and diabetes, since it had been shown that people within this category had a higher risk of developing both diabetes and cardiovascular disease than did people with lower blood glucose values [8,9].

The widespread institution and subsequent acceptance of these diagnostic procedures was a significant aid to both clinical care and research. However, it soon became apparent that there were problems with the recommended diagnostic values. A consistent finding in epidemiological studies was that there were far fewer people with a diagnostic fasting value than there were with a diagnostic 2-hour value [10]. Typically, only 25% of those with a 2-hour plasma glucose (2hPG) ≥11.1 mmol/l also had a fasting plasma glucose (FPG) ≥7.8 mmol/l, while over 90% of those with an FPG ≥7.8 mmol/l had a 2hPG ≥11.1 mmol/l. This evidence that the fasting threshold of 7.8 mmol/l represented a more severe degree of hyperglycaemia than did a 2hPG of 11.1 mmol/l was complemented by a study from a range of Southern Hemisphere populations [11]. This showed that across 13 populations, 7.0 mmol/l was the fasting value that gave a prevalence of diabetes with the closest match to that produced by a 2hPG of 11.1 mmol/l. This methodology when applied to two American populations gave a similar FPG threshold of 6.7 mmol/l [2,12]. Data from South-East Asian populations have suggested that the FPG equivalent (in terms of prevalence) to a 2hPG of 11.1 mmol/l may, in these populations, be even lower than 6.0 mmol/l [13].

In a further comparison with the 'gold standard' 2hPG threshold of 11.1 mmol/l, McCance et al. [2,12] found that a FPG threshold of 6.8 mmol/l was the closest match with regard to its sensitivity and specificity for retinopathy. Similar findings were reported from Egypt, where the FPG equivalent of the 2hPG threshold was found to be 6.9–7.2 mmol/l [1]. Three studies [1,2,12] have also suggested that the FPG threshold for the presence of retinopathy may be lower than 7.8 mmol/l, although the precision in identifying the exact glucose threshold is relatively poor in each of these studies. Importantly, it was also apparent from each of these reports that FPG, 2hPG and HbA$_{1c}$ were all very similar in their associations with retinopathy, and that any single test would be just as good as any other in identifying people at risk of retinopathy.

Finally, the risk of macrovascular disease was noted to be considerably elevated at FPG $\geq$6.9 mmol/l [14], although, as noted above, this risk appears to rise continuously across a wide range of glucose values. Indeed in the same study, cardiovascular mortality was found to be modestly though significantly increased at FPG values between 5.8 and 6.9 mmol/l.

Thus, there was very clear evidence that there was a mismatch between the two glycaemic thresholds, and some suggestion that it was the FPG value that was too high, rather than the 2hPG value that was too low. In the years since the adoption of the NDDG and WHO criteria, diabetes had effectively been defined by the 2hPG value, because it represented a lesser degree of hyperglycaemia. As a result, a large body of evidence had built up around diabetes defined by the 2hPG threshold of 11.1 mmol/l. Furthermore, the 2-hour value has been favoured as the gold standard, since it is not dependent on the fasting status (despite the fact that it is well known that the fasting glucose is much more reproducible than is the 2-hour glucose [15]). Taking all of these arguments into account, the 2hPG threshold was retained, and the fasting threshold fell.

New criteria

In 1997 and 1998, the American Diabetes Association (ADA) and WHO recommended the following changes to the diagnostic criteria [12,16]:
1 The FPG threshold was lowered from 7.8 to 7.0 mmol/l.
2 IFG (FPG 6.1–6.9 mmol/l) was introduced as a new category of intermediate glucose metabolism. (Named impaired fasting glycaemia by the WHO.)

Consequent on these amendments to the fasting criteria, the ADA (but not the WHO) indicated that the FPG rather than the OGTT should be the diagnostic test of choice both for clinical and for epidemiological purposes. FPG has the advantage that it is considerably more reproducible than the 2hPG, and is simpler to perform than the OGTT. Furthermore, it was argued that it was just as closely associated with retinopathy as was the 2hPG. The impact of the changes is complex. They affect both diabetes and the intermediate states of carbohydrate metabolism—IGT and IFG.

Diabetes

What difference will these changes make to the prevalence of diabetes and to

Table 1.1 Numbers of people identified as having diabetes in different studies, according to diagnostic classification.

| | Diabetes diagnosed according to | | | | |
| | ADA fasting criterion* | | WHO (1985) criteria | | |
	Number with diabetes	% of ADA diabetes with 2hPG ≥11.1 mmol/l	Number with diabetes	% of WHO diabetes with FPG ≥7.0 mmol/l
Population-based				
Hoorn† [17]	120	61	118	62
NHANES III† [20]	4 100 000	77	6 000 000	53
Taiwan† [22]	220	79	453	39
Japanese–Brazilians† [23]	124	91	131	86
DECODE‡ [18]	1044	41	904	48
S Hemisphere‡ [19]	1298	70	1319	68
Newcastle (UK)‡ [21]	136	48	96	69
Referral-based				
Hong Kong† [24]	394	91	627	57
Mexico† [26]	78	85	222	30
Manchester (UK)‡ [25]	166	84	178	78

*FPG ≥7.0 mmol/l irrespective of 2hPG.

†WHO diagnosis based on FPG ≥7.8 mmol/l or 2hPG ≥11.1 mmol/l.

‡WHO diagnosis based on 2hPG ≥11.1 mmol/l alone.

the individuals identified as having diabetes? A number of studies have now been published comparing the old and new criteria [17–26]. These are summarized in Table 1.1, and reveal that the changes may have a rather variable impact. As expected, the degree of agreement over the prevalence of diabetes is improved by using the lower fasting threshold. However, compared with the old OGTT-based criteria (which are heavily dependent on the 2hPG threshold of 11.1 mmol/l), and excluding people already known to have diabetes, the new fasting criterion still identifies between 65% fewer (Mexico) and 42% more (Newcastle) people as having newly-diagnosed diabetes. Since in most populations, a significant proportion (at least 50% in developed nations [27], but lower in developing nations) of all those with diabetes are already known to have the disease, the impact of these changes on the total prevalence will be somewhat less than these figures indicate, though how much less is unknown.

Furthermore, even when the total prevalence is similar by the two methods, the actual people identified by screening may be different. The percentage of individuals classified as having diabetes by the new FPG cut-off who also have diabetes on the old OGTT criteria varies from only 41% (DECODE) to 91% (Japanese–Brazilians, Hong Kong). This is worrying, since it indicates that the two diagnostic thresholds (FPG 7.0 mmol/l and 2hPG 11.1 mmol/l) can identify quite different individuals. It is not clear what factors underlie this classification disagreement, but in the DECODE study of 16 different European populations [19], obese diabetic individuals were more likely to satisfy the fasting criterion, and non-obese diabetic individuals were more likely to satisfy the 2-hour criterion. We have reported similar findings in a range of other non-European populations [19]. It is possible that ethnicity is also important, but there are not yet enough data to assess this.

This change in the individuals who are identified raises the further question of whether changing to the new fasting threshold will alter the phenotype of diabetes, or the associations between risk factors such as obesity and the subsequent development of diabetes. The association of hyperglycaemia and cardiovascular disease is a crucial one on which to test the validity of the new criteria. The Hoorn study has shown that people with a FPG ≥7.0 mmol/l (i.e. diabetic), but a non-diabetic 2hPG have an abnormal cardiovascular risk profile [17], and data from two large cohorts of men with a nondiabetic 2-hour glucose value at baseline showed an increased 20-year mortality when the baseline FPG was above 7.0 mmol/l [28]. Similarly, evidence would now indicate that people whose only abnormality is in the postload state have elevated blood pressure and lipids [17], and have a higher

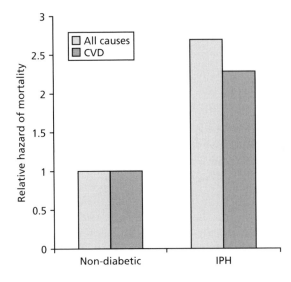

Fig. 1.3 Mortality risk over 5–12 years in people with isolated post-challenge hyperglycaemia (IPH). Data are adapted from Shaw *et al.* [30].

mortality than their non-diabetic counterparts [29]. Three recent studies [30–32] have demonstrated that in isolated postchallenge hyperglycaemia (FPG <7.0 mmol/l with 2hPG ≥11.1 mmol/l), both total and cardiovascular mortality (after adjustment for other relevant risk factors) are significantly elevated in comparison to the non-diabetic population (Fig. 1.3). The mortality risk in isolated postchallenge hyperglycaemia is similar to that observed in people with more severe degrees of hyperglycaemia, while the risk in isolated fasting hyperglycaemia appears to be smaller [30]. It is noteworthy that over 50% of people with isolated postchallenge hyperglycaemia have a completely normal FPG that would not even put them in the IFG category [30]. Amongst older Americans, the ADA (FPG only) criteria were less sensitive than the 1985 WHO OGTT criteria in predicting cardiovascular disease (sensitivity 28% vs 54%) [31]. In the DECODE study, fasting glucose was not independently associated with mortality after adjustment had been made for 2-hour glucose, whereas 2-hour glucose remained independently associated with mortality after adjustment for fasting glucose [32].

IFG and IGT

Table 1.2 shows studies that compare the prevalence of IFG and IGT. In seven out of nine studies, IGT was more common than IFG. Only 22–46%

Table 1.2 Numbers of people identified as having IGT and IFG in different studies.

	IFG		IGT	
	n	% with IGT	*n*	% with IFG
Population-based				
Hoorn* [17]	285	22	252	25
Mauritius* [34]	327	36	631	19
NHANES III* [20]	9 600 000	39	14 900 000	25
Taiwan* [22]	467	38	1 047	17
Japanese–Brazilians* [23]	48	46	95	23
Sweden† [35]	319	44	515	27
Newcastle (UK)† [21]	339	30	275	37
Referral-based				
Mexico* [26]	187	37	407	17
Manchester (UK)† [25]	70	39	94	29

*IGT defined as FPG < 7.8 mmol/l and 2hPG 7.8–11.0 mmol/l.
† IGT defined as 2hPG 7.8–11.0 mmol/l, irrespective of FPG.

(mean 37%) of people with IFG also had IGT, and 19–37% (mean 24%) of those with IGT were classified as having IFG. One of the original reasons for introducing IGT was that as well as increasing the risk of CVD, it carried a high risk of progressing to diabetes, and this has been confirmed in a number of different studies [33].

Can IFG perform a similar role? We recently reported data from a prospective population-based study in Mauritius [34] which addressed this issue. From a baseline population of 3229 subjects, 609 had IGT and 267 had IFG, with only 118 of these subjects having both IFG and IGT. After 5 years of follow-up, 297 subjects had progressed to diabetes, of whom 148 had IGT at baseline, but only 77 had IFG at baseline. Therefore, the ability of IFG to identify those who would progress to diabetes (sensitivity) was considerably less than that of IGT. However, for those people with IFG, the risk of progression (positive predictive value) was slightly higher for IFG than for IGT (29% vs 24%). This difference between IFG and IGT should not be seen as necessarily indicating an absolute difference between the predictive properties of FPG and 2hPG, merely between the two categories as currently defined. Further work in other populations will be needed to assess the prognostic implications of IFG, and to determine what advantage if any can be gained from changing the diagnostic limits of IFG.

Summary

What has become increasingly clear is that fasting hyperglycaemia and post-load hyperglycaemia represent distinct, though overlapping, entities—the one cannot ever entirely substitute for the other. Fasting and 2hPG (as well as HbA_{1c}) have similar relationships with retinopathy, but the 2hPG seems to be more closely related to CVD than is the fasting glucose. At the very least, the 2hPG identifies people at risk of CVD who are not identified by the fasting glucose, even when 6.0 mmol/l is taken as the upper limit of normal FPG. While lowering of the fasting threshold will help to identify one group, abandonment of the OGTT may prevent or delay diagnosis in the other group.

Glycated haemoglobin

Glycated haemoglobin would seem to offer a number of potential advantages over blood glucose for diagnosis of diabetes. It does not require the subject to be fasted or to wait 2 hours for an OGTT, and its relationship with retinopathy is just as strong as are those for fasting or 2hPG [12]. Since it reflects both fasting and postprandial glucose, it may have advantages over either one. Furthermore, given its current role in the management of diabetes, its use in diagnosis would provide a valuable link between diagnostic thresholds and treatment targets. However, the difficulties that have been described above in trying to identify equivalent values of fasting and 2-hour blood glucose are likely to be repeated for HbA_{1c}, which inevitably will classify some individuals in a different way to that in which they are classified by blood glucose. These issues would need addressing, and detailed evidence-based studies relating HbA_{1c} to hard outcomes (including CVD) would be needed to assess its value as a diagnostic tool. Other practical problems exist. Assays for HbA_{1c} are not yet all standardized, and it is therefore not currently possible to produce diagnostic values that could be used universally. In addition, access to HbA_{1c} assays is limited in many parts of the developing world, and if HbA_{1c} was adopted instead of blood glucose, diagnosis could become difficult.

Screening

Should we screen for type 2 diabetes?

Screening for a disease can only be justified if that disease represents an important health problem, is present at a high enough prevalence (within the total or a specific target population) to make screening cost-effective, has a relatively long asymptomatic phase during which cases can be identified by screening that would not normally come to light, and if interventions are available which have a proven beneficial effect on clinically meaningful outcomes. Furthermore, the test for the disease must be safe, acceptable to the target population, and have adequate sensitivity and specificity. Ideally, any screening programme should be assessed in controlled trials measuring health outcomes and costs in screened and unscreened populations. In the absence of such information, screening may be thought to be worthwhile if all or most of the above requirements are fulfilled. Some of the relevant data for type 2 diabetes are outlined below.

1 Type 2 diabetes affects up to 14% [20] of the adult population (aged 40–74) in the developed world, with higher rates seen in parts of the developing world. Approximately 50% of these individuals are undiagnosed.

2 Diabetic complications are common at the time of clinical diagnosis, and less frequent among people diagnosed during screening surveys. It has been calculated that type 2 diabetes begins 4–7 years before the time of clinical diagnosis [36].

3 The UK Prospective Diabetes Study (UKPDS) has shown that aggressive glucose and blood-pressure lowering therapy in newly-diagnosed (after clinical presentation) diabetic people reduces the risk of long-term complications [37,38].

4 Hyperglycaemia is an important CVD risk factor. The risk is apparent amongst people with diabetes, IGT, IFG [9,14,28–32], and even high normal glucose levels (FPG 4.7–6.0 mmol/l) [3,4], and the absolute risk of cardiovascular disease is significantly increased by the presence of diabetes. The recent Heart Outcomes Prevention Evaluation (HOPE) study [39] demonstrated a significant reduction in CVD and mortality when ramipril was given to people with diabetes and one other cardiovascular risk factor. This indicates that knowledge of an individual's diabetes status is important in being able to institute treatment (with an ACE inhibitor) that will prevent CVD.

5 Computer modelling studies have indicated that a small improvement in overall health can be achieved by screening for diabetes, and that the cost per unit of health gained by screening high-risk populations (e.g. African Americans) is comparable to that for screening for other diseases, such as breast cancer [40].

There is much persuasive evidence to indicate that screening for diabetes would be beneficial to both individuals and communities. However, it should be noted that most of the relevant data have been derived from people with clinically diagnosed diabetes (e.g. UKPDS and HOPE). As a group, such people have more advanced disease, and carry a greater risk of further complications than do people identified by screening. The risk reduction (especially the absolute risk reduction) may be considerably smaller in screened individuals than has been shown in intervention trials in clinically diagnosed individuals. Conversely, one might argue that earlier intervention would ultimately have a greater potential to reduce risk, as it can be started before significant complications have developed. Additional concerns about screening relate to the nature of the relationship of hyperglycaemia with cardiovascular disease. It is unclear whether it is truly independent of other risk factors (such as dyslipidaemia and hypertension). Some studies have indicated that it is an independent risk factor while others have not [41].

If hyperglycaemia is not an independent CVD risk factor, screening for diabetes may not offer any advantages over screening for hypertension and dyslipidaemia. In this scenario, diabetes screening could only be effective in reducing the risk of serious microvascular disease (e.g. blindness)—numerically a much smaller problem than cardiovascular disease.

The question of screening can only be answered by randomized trials comparing outcomes in screened and unscreened populations. Such studies would need to be very large, and carefully designed. The cost would necessarily be high, but the evidence is needed to support the adoption of screening programmes. Similar studies have been performed in other areas such as breast and colorectal cancer, and should now be started in diabetes.

Who should be screened?

The prevalence of diabetes is not high enough in most countries to justify mass screening of the whole population. Moreover, most people with undiagnosed diabetes have easily identifiable risk factors [42], indicating that targetted screening of high-risk groups is likely to identify most cases of undiagnosed diabetes. Three studies [42–44] have assessed methods of combining simple clinical risk factors as a means of identifying people with undiagnosed diabetes (defined by OGTT in the whole population irrespective of risk status). When a selection method is derived from one population and tested on another, the sensitivity for the detection of diabetes is 72–78%, the specificity is 55–56%, and the positive predictive value is 6–8%. The selection methods are shown in Table 1.3 and confirm that simple clinical parameters can be used to select people for screening.

Table 1.3 Results of three studies showing optimal combinations of risk factors for diabetes screening.

1 *Any of these pairs* [42]:
Sedentary and obese (self-report weight >120% ideal body weight)
Age 45+ and obese
Age 45+ and treated hypertension
Age 45+ and history of 'borderline diabetes'

2 *Obesity (BMI >30) in a male, or any two of* [43]:
Age 60+
Male
Obesity (BMI >29 for women, >30 for men)
Parent or sibling with diabetes
Chest pain or breathlessness on walking

3 *Any two of* [44]:
Age 60+
Male
Obesity (BMI >30)
1st degree relative with diabetes
Treated hypertension

120% ideal body weight corresponds to a BMI of 26–28 for men and 25–28 for women.
Studies 2 and 3 only included people over the age of 50.

Interestingly, ethnicity was not selected as an important risk factor. Only the North American study [42] included high-risk ethnic groups, and although blacks and Hispanics had a high prevalence of diabetes, other risk factors, such as obesity, were also present in those with diabetes. Gestational diabetes, IGT and IFG all carry a high risk of future diabetes, but were not selected as significant risk factors. The studies relied on clinically available information, and underdiagnosis of these states (especially in the older adults included in these studies) probably accounts for their exclusion. Delivering a large baby appears not to be an independent risk factor for diabetes [45]. Based on these findings on risk factors, Table 1.4 shows suggested target groups for diabetes screening.

Virtually none of the data contributing to the above has been collected on people over the age of 75. However, the elderly are at high risk of diabetes and its complications. UKPDS data showed that the benefits of intensive therapy for diabetes took approximately 10 years to become apparent [37]. These facts should be considered when deciding to screen an elderly person.

Symptoms of hyperglycaemia (such as thirst and polyuria) have a poor sensitivity and specificity for diabetes [46]. Therefore, symptoms are unlikely

Table 1.4 Suggested high-risk groups for targetting of screening.

Screening is recommended in the following groups:
IGT or IFG (current or previous)
Previous gestational diabetes
Any two of:
Age ≥50 (30 in high-risk ethnic groups)
Obesity (BMI >28)
1st degree relative with diabetes
Hypertension
Other clinical macrovascular disease

to be a useful part of a formal screening programme; however, it remains good clinical practice to look for diabetes in someone presenting with typical symptoms of hyperglycaemia.

How to screen and diagnose

Having selected people who are at risk of diabetes, two steps remain—the initial screening test and the final diagnostic test. The screening and diagnostic tests often overlap, but it is useful to consider them separately in order to adopt a logical series of assessments for both the diagnosis and exclusion of diabetes. The first screening test may in fact turn out to be diagnostic (e.g. FPG of 10 mmol/l), but amongst those who do not have a diagnostic first screening test, it is important to set limits to indicate the need to progress to a definitive diagnostic test.

The first screening test

Urine glucose testing is cheap, simple to perform, non-invasive, and can even be self-administered via a postal system [47]. However, its sensitivity for the detection of diabetes is rather low at under 50%, and in most circumstances this means that it is not suitable for diabetes screening. The first screening test should therefore be either a random or fasting blood glucose. Either of these can be used to divide people into three groups—those in whom diabetes can be confidently excluded, those with a result that is diagnostic of diabetes, and an intermediary group who need further investigation. The properties of fasting plasma glucose (at a threshold of ≥6.1 mmol/l) as a screening tool for diabetes have recently been reported in a number of studies using the new diagnostic thresholds for diabetes (Table 1.5). From these data, the median sensitivity was 81%, and the median specificity was 92%. Thus, it is clear

Table 1.5 The performance of a fasting plasma glucose of 6.1 mmol/l as a screen for diabetes.

	n	Sensitivity	Specificity
Population-based			
NHANES III [20]	2844	81	90
Hoorn [17]	2378	88	88
Elderly US [51]	4515	71	87
Hong Kong [52]	1513	58	98
Taiwan [22]*	5303	73	93
Japanese–Brazilians [23]	647	87	92
Mauritius [34]	3528	82	92
Referral-based			
Manchester, UK [25]	401	91	34
Mexico [26]†	1706	33	92

Note: Diabetes is defined using the OGTT (FPG ≥7.0 mmol/l or 2hPG ≥11.1 mmol/l) in the same way in all the studies.
*FPG ≥6.0 mmol/l used as cut-off, instead of 6.1 mmol/l.
†Only included subjects with FPG 3.3–8.9 mmol/l, i.e. true sensitivity would be higher.
Overall, median sensitivity was 81% and median specificity was 92%.

that using the FPG threshold of 6.1 mmol/l will result in approximately 20% of those with undiagnosed diabetes being missed. In order to improve this, a lower threshold (e.g. 5.5 mmol/l) could be used to select people who should be assessed further with an OGTT.

Only two studies [48,49] have examined the properties of random blood glucose (measured by reflectance meter in both studies) as a screening tool for diabetes (Table 1.6). On the basis of these two studies, in order to achieve a sensitivity of 80–90%, the specificity of a random glucose is likely to be significantly lower than that of a fasting glucose. Furthermore, since WHO 1985 criteria were used as the gold standard for both studies, the performance of the test is likely to be slightly worse with current criteria, as people who are diabetic only on the new, lower fasting value are more likely to have normal random blood glucose values. It has been suggested that a random plasma glucose (RPG) of 5.6–11.0 mmol/l should be followed by an OGTT or fasting glucose [16,50], although the lower limit of 5.6 mmol/l has been selected rather arbitrarily.

The available evidence indicates that the FPG has superior screening properties over random samples. However, in practical terms, using the fasting glucose as the first screening test will often mean an additional visit, which is likely to result in a significant non-attendance rate. This would not

Table 1.6 The performance of a random whole blood glucose as a screen for diabetes.		
Engelgau et al. [48]		
At sensitivity of 90%:*	median specificity 48–52% (according to age group)	
At specificity of 90%:	median sensitivity 49–52%	
Optimal:	median sensitivity 73–76% median specificity 76–78%	
Qiao et al. [49]		
Cut-off 5.8 mmol/l:	sensitivity 63%, specificity 85%†	
Cut-off 5.2 mmol/l:	sensitivity 78%, specificity 62%†	

*The cut-off value of random whole blood glucose for a sensitivity of 90% was 4.4–6.7, depending on age and postprandial period.
†Sensitivities and specificities were worse in women than men at all thresholds.

usually apply to RPG, which can be done immediately. It should therefore be an individual decision about which test to use.

The diagnostic test

In population studies, approximately 30% of people with newly diagnosed diabetes have a non-diabetic fasting glucose, and 30% have a non-diabetic 2-hour value (see Table 1.1). It is likely that all of these people are at risk of diabetes-related complications (i.e. are genuinely diabetic), and therefore the OGTT is necessary to exclude diabetes in anyone with a positive screening blood test (FPG 5.5–6.9 mmol/l or RPG 5.6–11.0 mmol/l). An alternative to immediate further investigation in all people with borderline results is a plan to reassess a year later. The recent European Guidelines [50] suggest an OGTT for all those with FPG 6.1–6.9 mmol/l, and a repeat fasting glucose 12 months later in those with FPG 5.0–6.0 mmol/l [50]. This approach assumes that those people in this latter group who actually have diabetes will show a deterioration over time in the fasting glucose.

It should be noted that in the absence of acute metabolic upset, the diagnosis of diabetes cannot rely on a single test, and requires confirmation on another day [16].

All of the above discussion about how to screen could become redundant if current trials into the prevention of diabetes in people with IGT [51] are successful. If that were the case, then the focus would switch to one that allowed IGT to be diagnosed. The fasting glucose is poor at this, and the OGTT would need to be used more widely.

Summary

The diagnosis of diabetes relies on identifying blood glucose values which separate people according to their risk of microvascular and macrovascular disease. This process has been refined recently by the lowering of the FPG threshold to 7.0 mmol/l, and the introduction of IFG. However, the precision of the diagnostic cut-points remains limited. Furthermore, fasting and post-load glucose values are complementary to each other, and neither should be dispensed with in the diagnostic process.

Population screening for diabetes is an attractive means of preventing complications. Much circumstantial evidence is available to support the use of targetted screening, but long-term screening trials are needed to accurately define its role.

References

1 Engelgau MM, Thompson TJ, Herman WH *et al.* Comparison of fasting and 2-hour glucose and HbA$_{1c}$ levels for diagnosing diabetes: diagnostic criteria and performance revisited. *Diabetes Care* 1997; 20: 785–91.

2 McCance DR, Hanson RL, Charles MA *et al.* Comparison of tests for glycated haemoglobin and fasting and 2-hour glucose concentrations as diagnostic methods for diabetes. *BMJ* 1994; 308: 1323–8.

3 Balkau B, Bertrais S, Ducimetiere P, Eschwège E. Is there a glycaemic threshold for mortality risk? *Diabetes Care* 1999; 22: 696–9.

4 Bjornholt JV, Erikssen G, Aaser E *et al.* Fasting blood glucose: an underestimated risk factor for cardiovascular death. Results from a 22-year follow-up of healthy nondiabetic men. *Diabetes Care* 1999; 22: 45–9.

5 Shaw JE, Zimmet PZ, Hodge AM *et al.* Impaired fasting glucose: how low should it go? *Diabetes Care* 2000; 23: 34–9.

6 National Diabetes Data Group. Classification and diagnosis of diabetes mellitus and other categories of glucose intolerance. *Diabetes* 1979; 28: 1039–57.

7 World Health Organization. Diabetes Mellitus: Report of a WHO Study Group. Technical Report series 727. Geneva: WHO, 1985.

8 Harris MI. Impaired glucose tolerance-prevalence and conversion to NIDDM. *Diabet Med* 1996; 13 (Suppl 2): S9–S11.

9 Fuller JH, Shipley MJ, Rose G *et al.* Mortality from coronary heart disease and stroke in relation to degree of glycaemia: the Whitehall Study. *BMJ* 1983; 287: 867–70.

10 Harris MI, Hadden WC, Knowler WC, Bennett PH. Prevalence of diabetes and impaired glucose tolerance and plasma glucose levels in US population aged 20–74. *Diabetes* 1987; 36: 523–34.

11 Finch CF, Zimmet PZ, Alberti KGMM. Determining diabetes prevalence: a rational basis for the use of fasting plasma glucose concentrations? *Diabet Med* 1990; 7: 603–10.

12 American Diabetes Association. Report of the expert committee on the diagnosis and classification of diabetes mellitus. *Diabetes Care* 1997; 20: 1183–97.

13 Cockram CS, Lau JTF, Chan AYW, Woo J, Swaminathan R. Assessment of glucose tolerance test criteria for diagnosis of diabetes in Chinese subjects. *Diabetes Care* 1992; 15: 988–90.

14 Charles MA, Balkau B. Revision of diagnostic criteria for diabetes [letter]. *Lancet* 1996; 348: 1657–8.

15 Mooy JM, Gootenhuis PA, deVries H *et al.* Intra-individual variation of glucose,

specific insulin and proinsulin concentrations measured in two oral glucose tolerance tests in general Caucasian population: the Hoorn study. *Diabetologia* 1996; 39: 298–305.

16 Alberti KGMM, Zimmet PZ. For the WHO Consultation Group: definition, diagnosis and classification of diabetes mellitus and its complications. Part 1: diagnosis and classification of diabetes mellitus. Provisional report of a WHO consultation. *Diabet Med* 1998; 15: 539–53.

17 De Vegt F, Dekker JM, Stehouwer CDA, Nijpels G, Bouter LM, Heine RJ. The 1997 American Diabetes Association criteria versus the 1985 World Health Organization criteria for the diagnosis of abnormal glucose tolerance. *Diabetes Care* 1998; 21: 1686–90.

18 DECODE Study Group. Will new diagnostic criteria for diabetes mellitus change phenotype of patients with diabetes? Reanalysis of European epidemiological data. *BMJ* 1998; 317: 371–5.

19 Shaw JE, de Courten M, Boyko EJ, Zimmet PZ. The impact on different populations of new diagnostic criteria for diabetes. *Diabetes Care* 1999; 22: 762–6.

20 Harris MI, Eastman RC, Cowie CC, Flegal KM, Eberhardt MS. Comparison of diabetes diagnostic categories in the US population according to 1997 American Diabetes Association and 1980–85 World Health Organization diagnostic criteria. *Diabetes Care* 1997; 20: 1859–62.

21 Unwin N, Alberti KGMM, Bhopal R, Harland J, Watson W, White M. Comparison of the current WHO and new ADA criteria for the diagnosis of diabetes mellitus in three ethnic groups in the UK. *Diabet Med* 1998; 15: 554–7.

22 Chang C-J, Wu J-S, Lu F-H, Lee H-L, Yang Y-C, Wen M-J. Fasting plasma glucose in screening for diabetes in the Taiwanese population. *Diabetes Care* 1998; 21: 1856–60.

23 Gimeno SGA, Ferreira SRG, Franco LJ, Iunes M, the Japanese–Brazilian Diabetes Study Group. Comparison of glucose tolerance categories according to World Health Organization and American Diabetes Association diagnostic criteria in a population-based study in Brazil. *Diabetes Care* 1998; 21: 1889–92.

24 Ko GTC, Chan JCN, Yeung VTF *et al.* Combined use of a fasting plasma glucose concentration and HbA$_{1c}$ or fructosamine predicts the likelihood of having diabetes in high-risk subjects. *Diabetes Care* 1998; 21: 1221–5.

25 Wiener K, Roberts NB. The relative merits of haemoglobin A$_{1c}$ and fasting plasma glucose as first-line diagnostic tests for diabetes mellitus in non-pregnant subjects. *Diabet Med* 1998; 15: 558–63.

26 Gomez-Perez FJ, Aguilar-Salinas CA, Lopez-Alvarenga JC, Perez-Jauregui J, Guillen-Pineda LE, Rull JA. Lack of agreement between the World Health Organization category of impaired glucose tolerance and the American Diabetes Association category of impaired fasting glucose. *Diabetes Care* 1998; 21: 1886–8.

27 Harris MI, Flegal KM, Cowie CC *et al.* Prevalence of diabetes, impaired fasting glucose, and impaired glucose tolerance in US adults. The Third National Health and Nutrition Examination Survey, 1988–94. *Diabetes Care* 1998; 21: 518–24.

28 Balkau B, Shipley M, Jarrett RJ *et al.* High blood glucose concentration is a risk factor for mortality in middle-aged nondiabetic men. *Diabetes Care* 1998; 21: 360–7.

29 Barrett-Connor E, Ferrara A. Isolated postchallenge hyperglycemia and the risk of fatal cardiovascular disease in older women and men. *Diabetes Care* 1998; 21: 1236–9.

30 Shaw JE, Hodge AM, de Courten M, Chitson P, Zimmet PZ. Isolated post-challenge hyperglycaemia confirmed as a risk factor for mortality. *Diabetologia* 1999; 42: 1050–4.

31 Barzilay JI, Spiekerman CF, Wahl PW *et al.* Cardiovascular disease in older adults with glucose disorders: comparison of American Diabetes Association criteria for diabetes mellitus with WHO criteria. *Lancet* 1999; 354: 622–5.

32 DECODE Study Group. Glucose tolerance and mortality: comparison of WHO and American Diabetes

Association diagnostic criteria. *Lancet* 1999; 354: 617–21.

33 Alberti KGMM. The clinical implications of impaired glucose tolerance. *Diabet Med* 1996; 13: 927–37.

34 Shaw JE, Zimmet PZ, de Courten M *et al.* Impaired fasting glucose or impaired glucose tolerance: what best predicts future diabetes? *Diabetes Care* 1999; 22: 399–402.

35 Larsson H, Berglund G, Lindgarde F, Ahren B. Comparison of ADA and WHO criteria for diagnosis of diabetes and glucose intolerance. *Diabetologia* 1998; 21: 1124–5.

36 Harris MI, Klein R, Welborn TA, Knuiman MW. Onset of NIDDM occurs at least 4–7 yr before clinical diagnosis. *Diabetes Care* 1992; 15: 815–19.

37 UK Prospective Diabetes Study Group. Intensive blood glucose control with sulphonylureas or insulin compared with conventional treatment and risk of complications in patients with type 2 diabetes (UKPDS 33). *Lancet* 1998; 352: 837–53.

38 UK Prospective Diabetes Study Group. Tight blood pressure control and risk of macrovascular and microvascular complications in type 2 diabetes (UKPDS 38). *BMJ* 1998; 317: 703–13.

39 The Heart Outcomes Prevention Evaluation Study Investigators. Effects of an angiotensin-converting enzyme inhibitor, ramipril, on cardiovascular events in high-risk patients. *N Engl J Med* 2000; 342: 145–53.

40 CDC Diabetes Cost-Effectiveness Study Group. The cost-effectiveness of screening for type 2 diabetes. *JAMA* 1998; 280: 1757–63.

41 Coutinho M, Gerstein HC, Wang Y, Yusuf S. The relationship between glucose and incident cardiovascular events. A metaregression analysis of published data from 20 studies of 95 783 individuals followed for 12.4 years. *Diabetes Care* 1999; 22: 233–40.

42 Herman WH, Smith PJ, Thompson TJ, Engelgau MM, Aubert RE. A new and simple questionnaire to identify people at increased risk for undiagnosed diabetes. *Diabetes Care* 1995; 18: 382–7.

43 Ruige JB, de Neeling JN, Kostense PJ, Bouter LM, Heine RJ. Performance of an NIDDM screening questionnaire based on symptoms and risk factors. *Diabetes Care* 1997; 20: 491–6.

44 Baan CA, Ruige JB, Stolk R *et al.* Performance of a predictive model to identify undiagnosed diabetes in a health care setting. *Diabetes Care* 1999; 22: 213–19.

45 Larsson G, Spjuth J, Ranstam J, Vikbladh I, Saxtrup O, Astedt B. Prognostic significance of birth of large infant for subsequent development of maternal non-insulin-dependent diabetes mellitus: a prospective study over 20–27 years. *Diabetes Care* 1986; 9: 359–64.

46 Welborn TA, Reid CM, Marriott G. Australian Diabetes Screening Study: impaired glucose tolerance and non-insulin-dependent diabetes mellitus. *Metabolism* 1997; 46 (Suppl. 1): 35–9.

47 Davies MJ, Williams DR, Metcalfe J. Community screening for non-insulin-dependent diabetes mellitus: self-testing for post-prandial glycosuria. *Q J Med* 1993; 86: 677–84.

48 Engelgau MM, Thompson TJ, Smith PJ *et al.* Screening for diabetes mellitus in adults. The utility of random capillary blood glucose measurements. *Diabetes Care* 1995; 18: 463–6.

49 Qiao Q, Keinanen-Kiukaanniemi S, Rajala U, Uusimaki A, Kivela SL. Random capillary whole blood glucose test as a screening test for diabetes mellitus in a middle-aged population. *Scand J Clin Lab Invest* 1995; 55: 3–8.

50 European Diabetes Policy Group. A desktop guide to type 2 diabetes mellitus. *Diabet Med* 1999; 16: 716–30.

51 Wahl PW, Savage PJ, Psaty BM, Orchard TJ, Robbins JA, Tracy RP. Diabetes in older adults. Comparison of 1997 American Diabetes Association classification of diabetes mellitus with 1985 WHO classification. *Lancet* 1998; 352: 1012–15.

52 Ko GTC, Chan JCN, Woo G, Cockram C. Use of the American Diabetes Association diagnostic criteria for diabetes in a Hong Kong Chinese population. *Diabetes Care* 1998; 21: 2094–7.

2: Does impaired glucose tolerance really exist, and if so what should be done about it?

John J. Nolan and Elaine Murphy

Introduction

Recent trends in the global prevalence of diabetes call for radical changes in public health strategy in relation to this disease. The prevalence of type 2 diabetes is currently escalating rapidly throughout the globe and in some regions doubling during intervals as short as 3–5 years [1]. This trend is most evident in areas undergoing rapid social and economic change with urbanization and industrialization. In the USA, it is now apparent that about 30% of new diabetes developing in children and adolescents has clinical features typical of type 2 diabetes. Prior to more dramatic recent changes in the demography of diabetes, there was already good epidemiological evidence that about half of all cases of frank type 2 diabetes were undiagnosed, unless specifically screened for [2]. Screening for diabetes needs to become an important public health priority but remains low on the political agenda in many countries. Currently, the American Diabetes Association (ADA) recommends screening based on the clinician's judgement in individual cases, particularly in high-risk individuals. For diabetes screening, the ADA favours fasting blood tests over the oral glucose tolerance test (OGTT) mainly because of convenience and cost [3]. This chapter will argue the merits of the OGTT and examine its potential as a tool to direct early clinical assessment and intervention in type 2 diabetes.

Background

Impaired glucose tolerance (IGT) was first defined in 1979, replacing a number of terms such as 'borderline diabetes', 'latent diabetes' and 'chemical diabetes' [4,5]. By definition, the diagnosis of IGT requires a standard OGTT during which plasma glucose is measured after an overnight fast and again

Table 2.1 Diagnostic criteria for diabetes mellitus, impaired glucose tolerance (IGT) and impaired fasting glucose (IFG).

Fasting plasma glucose (mmol/l)	
<6.1	Normal
>6.1 and <7.0	IFG
>7.0	Diabetes
2-hour plasma glucose (mmol/l)	
<7.8	Normal
>7.8 and <11.1	IGT
>11.1	Diabetes

2 hours after the ingestion of 75 g glucose [6]. An individual is classified as having IGT if the fasting plasma glucose concentration is less than that required for the diagnosis of diabetes and the 2-hour plasma glucose concentration is intermediate between the normal and the diabetic criteria. Recently, the diagnostic fasting plasma glucose threshold for diabetes has been lowered from 7.8 mmol/l to 7.0 mmol/l [7]. This has led to a new prediabetic fasting glucose classification, known as impaired fasting glucose (IFG). Table 2.1 summarizes the current diagnostic criteria and categories.

The issue of classification is one of the several difficulties with IGT, and is further complicated by the introduction of the new category of IFG. The main criticisms of IGT in the past have been its relative variability and instability, its clinical heterogeneity and uncertainty about its long-term implications for the development of diabetes and other diseases [8–11]. The OGTT itself has been in and out of favour, and has also been criticized for its variability. A recent argument in favour of the OGTT is the evidence from a large epidemiological survey that up to a third of undiagnosed subjects with diabetes had isolated postchallenge hyperglycaemia [12]. This study showed that OGTT screening of the subgroup with OGTT responses consistent with the new category of IFG would reduce the fraction with undiagnosed diabetes by half. The major goal of diabetes screening is not simply the quantitative classification of glycaemic responses but should be the prevention of microvascular and macrovascular complications of the disease. Earlier detection of those with frank hyperglycaemia offers the chance to limit at least the microvascular complications of retinopathy, neuropathy and nephropathy.

In contrast to those with frank diabetes, individuals with IGT are probably normoglycaemic most of the time, usually have normal levels of glycated haemoglobin and are protected from the microvascular complications of diabetes. However, it has been shown in various studies that subjects with IGT have an increased risk of macrovascular disease similar to those with frank type 2 diabetes [13,14]. It is interesting to note that Tominaga and colleagues have recently shown that IFG subjects do not have this cardiovascular risk, whereas IGT subjects from the same study have an approximately twofold increased cardiovascular mortality [15]. In a supporting Editorial, Baron makes the case that IGT itself should be regarded as a disease [16]. The accumulation of epidemiological evidence of this kind, along with advances in the understanding of the underlying pathophysiology of type 2 diabetes, is argument against the watertight categories of IFG, IGT and type 2 diabetes. This chapter will put the case for regarding IGT as the same disease as type 2 diabetes in many or even most cases. Different lines of research support this integrated understanding of diabetes, which is increasingly directed at the long-term cardiovascular consequences of the disease.

Pathophysiology of impaired glucose tolerance

IGT represents a state of abnormal glucose tolerance not yet sufficient for the diagnosis of diabetes. A simplistic view of IGT is that it represents a prediabetic condition. Type 2 diabetes is thought to be caused by both insulin resistance and reduced insulin secretion, thus IGT may be caused by either or both of these to a greater or lesser extent in any individual (Fig. 2.1). Prior to the development of IGT, a large cohort can be described as having compensated insulin resistance. This has been shown to be the case in several studies of normoglycaemic relatives of people with type 2 diabetes [17–20]. Progression

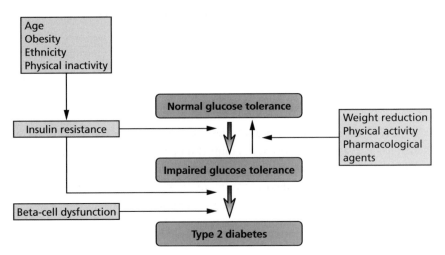

Fig. 2.1 Factors influencing the progression from normal glucose tolerance to IGT and to diabetes.

from normal glucose tolerance and compensated insulin resistance to IGT is a critical event in the evolution of diabetes and represents the onset of decompensated insulin resistance, where pancreatic insulin secretion begins to lag behind the challenge of a glucose load (Fig. 2.1). In relation to changes in insulin secretion, this relationship has been described as 'the Starling curve of the pancreas'.

The metabolic features of the IGT state have been studied by a number of groups, mostly in cross-sectional studies. Specific investigations have focused mainly on insulin secretion [21,22] or insulin action [23,24] in subjects with IGT. Taken together these studies show that subjects with IGT are more insulin resistant and hyperinsulinaemic than matched control subjects with normal glucose tolerance and that they have defects in the early insulin response to oral glucose. The exact aetiology and the relative contribution of these defects is no clearer in IGT than it is in type 2 diabetes, and presumably the causes are the same. Epidemiological evidence has accumulated to support a major role for environmental factors in the development of IGT, and its progression to diabetes [25–27]. Obesity [28], physical inactivity and ageing are all important and the background trend towards urbanization and industrialization in many countries appears to accelerate this process. The mechanisms of this process remain unclear. There is clearly a need for longitudinal studies in which the design would specifically address some of these unanswered questions.

Context and phenotype in impaired glucose tolerance

A major concern in relation to type 2 diabetes has been underdiagnosis and late diagnosis of the disease. Because diabetes is increasing in prevalence and because it is appearing in much younger subjects, earlier diagnosis is becoming more and more important. The OGTT glucose data alone constitute the minimal information available from the test and have a limited value outside a broader clinical context. Nonetheless, the glucose concentrations themselves, both fasting and 2-hour, are important predictors of the later development of diabetes, i.e. the higher the glucose, the more likely the eventual progression to frank diabetes. In an analysis of six prospective studies, including Caucasian, Hispanic, Mexican-American, African-American and Pima Indian subjects, the most important and consistent predictor of subsequent deterioration from IGT to diabetes was the level of fasting or postchallenge hyperglycaemia at baseline [29]. The addition of a simple history and physical examination provides more information which we propose would

I *History and family history*
Diabetes
Obesity
Hypertension
Dyslipidaemia
CHD/PVD

II *Clinical examination*
Obesity
Fat distribution
Signs of CHD/PVD

III *Repeat OGTT*
Fasting lipid profile
Fasting insulin/c-peptide

IV *Dietary consultation*

V *Consider*
Islet cell/GAD antibodies
Genetic markers
Models to estimate insulin resistance

CHD, coronary heart disease; GAD, glutamic acid decarboxylase; OGTT, oral glucose tolerance test; PVD, peripheral vascular disease.

improve the value of IGT as a classification. In particular, history and duration of hypertension, dyslipidaemia (particularly elevated triglycerides and low high-density lipoprotein (HDL) cholesterol) and obesity are important copredictors of diabetes, as is a positive family history for diabetes. Measurements of the degree of obesity in the patient and adipose tissue distribution are important markers of insulin resistance. Some individuals with IGT already have clinical evidence of atherosclerosis and end-organ damage, as is often the case in type 2 diabetes. Table 2.2 offers an approach to the phenotypic and metabolic characterization of patients with insulin resistance, IGT or diabetes.

Measurement of the insulin concentration in at least the fasting blood sample and ideally also in the 2-hour sample allows some simple estimation of the degree of insulin resistance of the subject [30]. We have recently developed a more detailed model for the calculation of insulin resistance, based on the glucose and insulin concentrations during a standard OGTT (fasting, 2-hour and/or 3-hour) [31] (Fig. 2.2). In this model the increase in glucose clearance from a remote single compartment after glucose ingestion

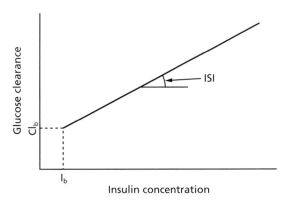

Fig. 2.2 The relationship between insulin concentration at steady state and glucose clearance. The insulin sensitivity index (ISI) can be approximated from the slope of the line and the glucose clearance value measured at basal insulin concentration (Cl_b and I_b).

is a linear function of the increment in insulin. The slope of the line is the (oral glucose) insulin sensitivity index (OGIS). Other mathematical models have used the OGTT as a basis for estimation of insulin sensitivity [32,33].

These various elements of clinical information add context to the OGTT and in particular to the IGT state. What is most at issue is the overall phenotype of the screened subject. Hypertension, dyslipidaemia and obesity are correlates of insulin resistance. Visceral fat distribution is more specific. Hyperinsulinaemia, both fasting and postchallenge, is consistent with insulin resistance, and of itself has been shown to be a powerful predictor of cardiovascular disease [34]. Antibody markers for autoimmune diabetes have a role in that they are of use in the detection of slow-onset or late-onset type 1 diabetes, sometimes referred to as LADA, which is often phenotypically different from type 2 diabetes [35]. As progress is made in the search for genetic causes of type 2 diabetes, there may be useful genetic markers in the future [36–38]. Table 2.2 summarizes an approach to setting the context and defining the phenotype in diabetes screening. This could constitute an approach to triage of screened individuals with IGT into a high-risk and a low-risk group.

A recently published Swedish study of more than 21 000 individuals has found a fourfold increased risk for IGT among obese subjects compared with normal-weight subjects [39]. Those subjects with IGT were also more likely to have first-degree relatives with diabetes, a higher mean body mass index (BMI), blood pressure and triglyceride level. However, this study also exposed the potential inadequacies of a population-based screening programme targetted towards obesity and a hereditary background of diabetes. Only 25% of subjects with IGT were obese (BMI > 30 kg/m²) and more than 70% reported no family history of diabetes. The concept of the 'metabolically obese', normal-weight individual who displays a cluster of dysmetabolic phenotypic characteristics despite maintaining a normal body weight may have important clinical implications for screening and prevention programmes [40]. In terms of cost–benefit, screening overweight 60 year olds might be effective but would only identify a small portion of the total IGT within this population. In other populations at higher risk of diabetes (Pima Indians, Nauruans and Hispanics) an inverse-U relationship exists between age and the progression from IGT to diabetes [29]. Diabetes develops at an earlier age in these genetically susceptible individuals, such that the progression rate declines with older age, rendering age-based screening programmes ineffective.

Consequences of impaired glucose tolerance

If an individual is found to have IGT, three important outcomes are possible:
1 Reversion to normal glucose tolerance.
2 Progression to the insulin resistance syndrome.
3 Progression to type 2 diabetes.

Because longitudinal studies that include glucose tolerance are lacking, we have a limited understanding of the natural history of these different pathways. However, a number of large epidemiological studies have given important clues. Overall, these studies show a consistent relationship between IGT and macrovascular disease, the most important health consequence of the insulin resistance syndrome. Progression from IGT specifically to type 2 diabetes is not necessary in order to cause cardiovascular disease. These large studies in general support a two-stage process during the evolution of abnormal glucose tolerance. The first phase of progression from normal glucose tolerance to IGT is driven by increasing insulin resistance, with its various causes. The second phase of progression from IGT to type 2 diabetes coincides with a fall in beta-cell insulin secretion (Fig. 2.1).

It has long been known that prediabetic abnormality in glucose tolerance could still be a risk factor for cardiovascular disease. For example, in the Whitehall study, a large cohort of non-diabetic male civil servants underwent a prospective study of cardiovascular outcomes in relation to various baseline risk factors including a 2-hour glucose tolerance measurement after a 50-g glucose load [41,42]. This study showed an independent risk value for glucose well below the current 7.8 mmol/l threshold for IGT. Similarly the Honolulu Heart Study [43] and the Rancho Bernardo Study [44] have followed large cohorts of non-diabetic subjects for cardiovascular outcomes and have shown a continuously increased risk of coronary heart disease

(CHD) with increasing glucose levels. In the latter study, age-adjusted mortality from ischaemic heart disease doubled in men as the fasting plasma glucose increased from 5 mmol/l to 7 mmol/l and tripled in women as the fasting plasma glucose increased from 6 mmol/l to 7.2 mmol/l. In the San Luis Valley study the prevalence of CHD was increased approximately twofold in non-Hispanic men and women with IGT compared to those with normal glucose tolerance [45]. Two-hour glucose levels predicted the development of CHD in men in the Paris Prospective study, but this effect was not significant after adjustment for triglyceride and fasting insulin [46]. A meta-analysis of the various cohort studies in non-diabetic populations has concluded that the increased risk of cardiovascular disease increased continuously with glucose levels above 4.2 mmol/l [47].

Intervention in impaired glucose tolerance

Several issues drive intervention studies in individuals with IGT. First, if progression to diabetes can be prevented, this will presumably diminish the likelihood of developing specific diabetes-related microvascular complications. Whether preventing the onset of diabetes will result in any significant reduction in macrovascular disease remains unclear. It is likely that restoration of normoglycaemia, together with improvements in obesity, dyslipidaemia, hypertension and overall insulin sensitivity, will be required rather than prevention of glycaemic deterioration alone.

Dietary and lifestyle modification, with or without pharmacological treatment, have been the basis for intervention studies to date [48–59]. Parameters examined include glycaemia, weight loss, anthropometric indices, lipids and blood pressure. While there is a general tendency for an improvement in obesity, not all long-term intervention studies have shown a consistent improvement in IGT. In particular, of two 10-year studies examining the effects of dietary advice and tolbutamide on individuals with IGT and 'borderline' diabetes, one, the Swedish study reported by Sartor *et al.*, showed a reduction in progression to diabetes in the tolbutamide-treated subjects compared with the control group, while the second, the Bedford study, found no difference between the two groups [56,57]. Of note, in the Swedish study less than 40% of patients actually completed the tolbutamide arm of the study. Some benefits have been seen over 1–2 years with the sulphonylureas, glibenclamide, glipizide and gliclazide, with regard to improvements in glucose tolerance, but weight gain can be a problem in these subjects [53–55].

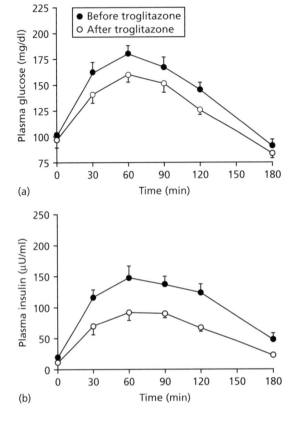

(a)

(b)

Fig. 2.3 OGTT glucose (a) and insulin (b) responses in obese subjects before and after 3 months' treatment with troglitazone.

Although early studies with phenformin showed no protective effect against the development of diabetes, the biguanide metformin appears to be more effective [58]. Metformin significantly reduced the conversion rate to diabetes from 16% in a placebo group to 3% in a group of Chinese subjects with IGT treated for 1 year ($P = 0.011$) [58]. Significant improvements were also noted in weight and insulin sensitivity (HOMA index, or homeostasis model of insulin resistance [30]). There were no differences in lipid parameters or blood pressure control. Conversion to normoglycaemia occurred in 85% of subjects treated with metformin compared with 51% of those receiving placebo. The thiazolidinedione, troglitazone, showed similar improvements in the glycaemic response to a glucose load with 80% of troglitazone-treated IGT subjects reverting to normal glucose tolerance compared with 48% of a placebo-treated group after 12 weeks [59]. In an earlier study, glucose tolerance was normalized in six of seven troglitazone-treated obese subjects with IGT and insulin resistance as determined by the euglycaemic–

hyperinsulinaemic clamp (Fig. 2.3) [60]. Treatment with troglitazone was associated with marked increases in insulin sensitivity as measured by a number of different methods despite strict maintenance of constant diet, physical exercise and weight during the 12-week treatment period [60]. It has more recently been clearly shown that troglitazone and metformin have complementary effects that improve abnormal glucose metabolism. While metformin primarily acts to reduce elevated hepatic glucose production, a defect mainly seen in fully established type 2 diabetes, troglitazone has a much greater effect on peripheral insulin resistance [61], a defect seen throughout the evolution of type 2 diabetes, and particularly in the phase of IGT. Troglitazone was introduced in 1997 in the US, and later for a brief period in Europe. It has now been withdrawn because of rare but unpredictable hepatotoxicity. Two further thiazolidinediones are now in use, rosiglitazone and pioglitazone, neither of which has been associated with hepatotoxicity. Several further insulin sensitizer drugs are in development, all directed at nuclear transcription target receptors. These agents must have important potential as diabetes prevention drugs of the future. Further testing of the prevention hypothesis with either lifestyle changes, metformin, acarbose or a combination is under way in the Early Diabetes Intervention Trial (EDIT) in the UK and in the US-based Diabetes Prevention Program [62].

Pharmacological intervention on a wide scale is expensive, may not provide any long-term benefits in terms of cardiovascular protection and may not be justified in IGT given that not all individuals with IGT will progress to diabetes. Lifestyle intervention studies, based on dietary advice with or without exercise advice or a structured exercise programme, suggest that improvements in glucose and lipid metabolism can be maintained for up to 6 years [48–51]. The degree of improvement in insulin resistance is proportional to any reduction in adiposity. The lifestyle programme, while it may be primarily targetted to the prevention of type 2 diabetes, is similar to that recommended for the prevention of cardiovascular disease. Cessation of cigarette smoking, a classic risk factor for atherosclerosis, should also be strongly encouraged. Once again, whether patients can sustain such lifestyle changes and whether such improvements are beneficial in the long term remains to be determined.

Conclusions

In conclusion, therefore, IGT can be regarded as a convenient and inexpensive biochemical marker of a severe metabolic dysfunction. IGT imparts an increased risk of cardiovascular disease similar to that of type 2 diabetes. IGT should not be regarded as a mild or 'borderline' condition. Clustering of IGT with central obesity, hypertension and dyslipidaemia represents a substantial management challenge, necessitating the control of multiple cardiovascular risk factors. More longitudinal studies are needed to prove that ameliorating IGT leads to a long-term reduction in the risk of cardiovascular disease. With the escalating incidence of IGT and type 2 diabetes it is likely that extensive public health education programmes will be required to target the large numbers of the population potentially at risk.

References

1 Zimmet PZ. Diabetes epidemiology as a tool to trigger diabetes research and care. *Diabetologia* 1999; 42: 499–518.

2 Harris MI *et al*. Prevalence of diabetes, impaired fasting glucose, and impaired glucose tolerance in US adults. The Third National Health and Nutrition Examination Survey, 1988–94. *Diabetes Care* 1998; 21: 518–24.

3 American Diabetes Association. Clinical practice recommendations, Screening for type 2 diabetes. *Diabetes Care* 2000; 23 (Suppl 1): S20–3.

4 National Diabetes Data Group. Classification and diagnosis of diabetes mellitus and other categories of glucose intolerance. *Diabetes* 1979; 28: 1039–57.

5 World Health Organization. *Diabetes Mellitus. Report of a WHO Study Group.* Technical Report Series no 727. Geneva: World Health Organization, 1985.

6 American Diabetes Association. Clinical practice recommendations. Report of the expert committee on the diagnosis and classification of diabetes mellitus. *Diabetes Care* 2000; 23 (Suppl 1): S4–19.

7 American Diabetes Association. Report of the expert committee on the diagnosis and classification of diabetes mellitus. *Diabetes Care* 1997; 20: 1183–97.

8 Stern MP, Morales PA, Valdez RA *et al*. Predicting diabetes: moving beyond impaired glucose tolerance. *Diabetes* 1993; 42: 706–14.

9 Keen H. Impaired glucose tolerance—not a diagnosis. *Diabetes Metab Rev* 1998; 14: S5–S12.

10 Alberti KGMM. The clinical implications of impaired glucose tolerance. *Diabet Med* 1996; 13: 927–37.

11 O'Rahilly S, Hattersley A, Vaag A, Gray H. Insulin resistance as the major cause of impaired glucose tolerance: a self-fulfilling prophecy? *Lancet* 1994; 344: 585–9.

12 The DECODE Study Group. Consequences of the new diagnostic criteria for diabetes in older men and women. The DECODE Study (Diabetes Epidemiology Collaborative Analysis of Diagnostic Criteria in Europe). *Diabetes Care* 1999; 22: 1667–71.

13 Haffner SM. Impaired glucose tolerance—is it relevant for cardiovascular disease? *Diabetologia* 1997; 40: S138–40.

14 Haffner SM. The importance of hyperglycaemia in the nonfasting state to the development of cardiovascular disease. *Endocrinol Rev* 1998; 19: 583–92.

15 Tominaga M, Eguchi H, Manaka H *et al*. Impaired glucose tolerance is a risk factor for cardiovascular disease but not impaired fasting glucose. *Diabetes Care* 1999; 22: 920–4.

16 Perry RC, Baron AD. Impaired glucose tolerance: why is it not a disease? [editorial] *Diabetes Care* 1999; 22: 883–5.

17 Meigs JB, D'Agostino RB, Wilson PWF *et al*. Risk variable clustering in the insulin

resistance syndrome: The Framingham Offspring Study. *Diabetes* 1997; 46: 1594–600.

18 Vaag A, Henriksen JE, Madsbad S, Holm N, Beck-Nielsen H. Insulin secretion, insulin action, and hepatic glucose production in identical twins discordant for non-insulin-dependent diabetes mellitus. *J Clin Invest* 1995; 95: 690–8.

19 Warram JH, Martin BC, Krolewski AS *et al.* Slow glucose removal rate and hyperinsulinemia precede the development of type II diabetes in the offspring of diabetic parents. *Ann Intern Med* 1990; 113: 909–15.

20 Beck-Nielsen H, Groop LC. Metabolic and genetic characterization of prediabetic states: sequence of events leading to non-insulin-dependent diabetes mellitus. *J Clin Invest* 1994; 94: 1714–21.

21 Byrne MM, Sturis J, Sobel RJ, Polonsky KS. Elevated plasma glucose 2-h postchallenge predicts defects in beta-cell function. *Am J Physiol* 1996; 270: E572–9.

22 Mitrakou A, Kelley D, Mokan M *et al.* Role of reduced suppression of glucose production and diminished early insulin release in impaired glucose tolerance. *N Engl J Med* 1992; 326: 22–9.

23 Lillioja S, Mott DM, Spraul M *et al.* Insulin resistance and insulin secretory dysfunction as precursors of non-insulin-dependent diabetes mellitus: prospective studies of Pima Indians. *N Engl J Med* 1992; 329: 1988–92.

24 Lillioja S, Mott DM, Howard BV *et al.* Impaired glucose tolerance as a disorder of insulin action. Longitudinal and cross-sectional studies in Pima Indians. *N Engl J Med* 1988; 318: 1217–25.

25 Weyer C, Bogardus C, Mott DM, Pratley RE. The natural history of insulin secretory dysfunction and insulin resistance in the pathogenesis of type 2 diabetes mellitus. *J Clin Invest* 1999; 104: 787–94.

26 Nijpels G. Determinants for the progression from impaired glucose tolerance to non-insulin-dependent diabetes mellitus. *Eur J Clin Invest* 1998; 28 (Suppl 2): 8–13.

27 Buchanan TA, Xiang A, Kjos S *et al.* Gestational diabetes: antepartum characteristics that predict postpartum glucose intolerance and type 2 diabetes in Latino women. *Diabetes* 1998; 47: 1302–10.

28 Ludvik B, Nolan JJ, Baloga J, Sacks D, Olefsky JM. Effect of obesity on insulin resistance in normal subjects and patients with NIDDM. *Diabetes* 1995; 44: 1121–5.

29 Edelstein S, Knowler WC, Bain RP *et al.* Predictors of progression from impaired glucose tolerance to NIDDM. An analysis of six prospective studies. *Diabetes* 1997; 46: 701–10.

30 Matthews DR, Hosker JP, Rudenski AS *et al.* Homeostasis model assessment: insulin resistance and beta-cell function from fasting plasma glucose and insulin concentrations in man. *Diabetologia* 1985; 28: 412–19.

31 Mari A, Pacini G, Ludvik B, Murphy E, Nolan JJ. A new method for assessing insulin sensitivity from the oral glucose tolerance test. *Diabetes* 1999; 48 (Suppl 1): 1251.

32 Matsuda M, DeFronzo RA. Insulin sensitivity indices obtained from oral glucose tolerance test: comparison with the euglycaemic insulin clamp. *Diabetes Care* 1999; 22: 1462–70.

33 Stumvoll M, Mitrakou A, Pimenta W *et al.* Use of the oral glucose tolerance test to assess insulin secretion and insulin sensitivity. *Diabetes* 1999; 48 (Suppl 1): 1312.

34 Despres JP, Lamarche B, Mauriege P *et al.* Hyperinsulinemia as an independent risk factor for ischemic heart disease. *N Engl J Med* 1996; 334: 952–7.

35 Zimmet P, Turner R, McCarty D, Rowley M, Mackay I. Crucial points at diagnosis. Type 2 diabetes or slow type 1 diabetes. *Diabetes Care* 1999; 22 (Suppl 2): B59–64.

36 Watanabe RM, Langefeld CD, Epstein M *et al.* Genome-wide linkage analysis of type 2 diabetes-related quantitative traits in the FUSION study. *Diabetes* 1999; 48 (Suppl 1): 46A.

37 Hanis CL, Boerwinkle E, Chakraborty R.

A genome wide search for human non-insulin dependent (type 2) diabetes genes reveals a major susceptibility locus on chromosome 2. *Nat Genet* 1996; 13: 161–6.

38 Mahtani MM, Widen E, Lehto M. Mapping of a gene for type 2 diabetes associated with an insulin secretion defect by a genome scan in Finnish families. *Nat Genet* 1996; 14: 90–4.

39 Lindahl B, Weinehall L, Asplund K, Hallmans G. Screening for impaired glucose tolerance: results from a population-based study in 21 057 individuals. *Diabetes Care* 1999; 22: 1988–92.

40 Dvorak R, DeNino WF, Ades PA, Poehlman E. Phenotypic characteristics associated with insulin resistance in metabolically obese normal-weight young women. *Diabetes* 1999; 48: 2210–14.

41 Fuller JH, Shipley MJ, Rose G, Jarret RJ, Keen H. Mortality from coronary heart disease and stroke in relation to degree of glycaemia: the Whitehall Study. *BMJ* 1983; 287: 867–70.

42 Fuller JH, Shipley MJ, Rose G, Jarret RJ, Keen H. Coronary-heart-disease risk and impaired glucose tolerance. The Whitehall Study. *Lancet* 1980; i: 1373–6.

43 Donahue RP, Abbott RD, Reed DM, Yano K. Post challenge glucose concentration and coronary heart disease in men of Japanese ancestry. Honolulu Heart Program. *Diabetes* 1987; 36: 565–76.

44 Scheidt-Nave C, Barrett-Connor E, Wingard DL, Cohn BA, Edelstein SL. Sex differences in fasting glycemia as a risk factor for ischaemic heart disease death. *Am J Epidemiol* 1991; 133: 565–76.

45 Rewers M, Shetterly SM, Baxter J, Marshall JA, Hamman RF. Prevalence of coronary heart disease in subjects with normal and impaired glucose tolerance and non-insulin dependent diabetes mellitus in a biethnic Colorado population. *Am J Epidemiol* 1992; 135: 1321–9.

46 Fontbonne A, Charles MA, Thibult N *et al.* Hyperinsulinaemia as a predictor of coronary heart disease mortality in a healthy population: the Paris Prospective Study, 15 year follow-up. *Diabetologia* 1991; 34: 356–61.

47 Gerstein HC. Glucose: a continuous risk factor for cardiovascular disease. *Diabet Med* 1997; 14: S25–S31.

48 Eriksson KF, Lindgarde F. Prevention of type 2 (non-insulin dependent) diabetes mellitus by diet and physical exercise. The six year Malmo feasibility study. *Diabetologia* 1991; 34: 891–8.

49 Ramaiya KL, Swai ABM, Alberti KGMM, McLarty D. Lifestyle changes decrease rates of glucose intolerance and cardiovascular (CVD) risk factors a six-year intervention study in a high risk Hindu Indian sub-community. *Diabetologia* 1992; 35 (Suppl 1): A60.

50 Bourn DM, Mann JI, McSkimming BJ, Waldron MA, Wischart JD. Impaired glucose tolerance and NIDDM. Does a lifestyle intervention program have an effect? *Diabetes Care* 1994; 17: 1311–19.

51 Eriksson J, Lindstrom J, Valle T *et al.* Prevention of type II diabetes in subjects with impaired glucose tolerance: the Diabetes Prevention Study (DPS) in Finland: study design and 1-year interim report on the feasibility of the lifestyle intervention programme. *Diabetologia* 1999; 42: 793–801.

52 Papoz L, Job D, Eschwege E *et al.* Effect of oral hypoglycaemic drugs on glucose tolerance and insulin secretion in borderline diabetic patients. *Diabetologia* 1978; 15: 373–80.

53 Ratzman KP, Witt S, Schulz B. The effect of long term glibenclamide treatment on glucose tolerance, insulin secretion and serum lipids in subjects with impaired glucose tolerance. *Diabet Metab* 1983; 9: 87–93.

54 Cederholm J. Short-term treatment of glucose intolerance in middle-aged subjects by diet, exercise and sulphonylurea. *Ups J Med Sci* 1985; 90: 229–42.

55 Karunakaran S, Hammersley MS, Morris RJ, Holman RR, for the Fasting Hyperglycaemia Study Group. Randomized controlled trial of sulphonylurea in 227 subjects with persistent fasting hyperglycaemia. *Diabetes* 1995; 44 (Suppl 1): 160A.

56 Sartor G, Schersten B, Carlstrom S, Melander A, Norden A, Persson G. Ten year follow-up of subjects with impaired glucose tolerance. Prevention of diabetes by tolbutamide and diet regulation. *Diabetes* 1980; 29: 41–9.

57 Keen H, Jarrett RJ, McCartney P. The ten year follow-up of the Bedford survey (1962–72): glucose tolerance and diabetes. *Diabetologia* 1982; 22: 73–8.

58 Li CL, Pan Y, Lu JM *et al*. Effect of metformin on patients with impaired glucose tolerance. *Diabet Med* 1999; 16: 477–81.

59 Antonucci T, Whitcomb R, McLain R, Lockwood D. Impaired glucose tolerance is normalized by treatment with the thiazolidinedione troglitazone. *Diabetes Care* 1997; 20: 188–93.

60 Nolan JJ, Ludvik B, Beerdsen P, Joyce M, Olefsky JM. Improvement in glucose tolerance and insulin resistance in obese subjects treated with troglitazone. *N Engl J Med* 1994; 331: 1188–93.

61 Inzucchi SE, Maggs DG, Spollett G *et al*. Efficacy and metabolic effects of metformin and troglitazone in type II diabetes mellitus. *N Engl J Med* 1998; 338: 867–72.

62 Diabetes Prevention Program Research Group. The diabetes prevention program (DPP). *Diabetes* 1997; 46 (Suppl 1): 138A.

3: Is gestational diabetes important, and worth screening for?

Lois Jovanovic and David J. Pettitt

Introduction

There is no controversy that overt diabetes during pregnancy is a major health risk for both the mother and the fetus, but there is still debate over the optimal approach for screening, diagnosis and management of milder elevations of maternal glucose levels. Many feel that aggressive, active management of maternal hyperglyaemia does not affect outcome. Thus, the treatment is all directed toward planning early delivery before the fetus dies. This chapter presents the argument that universal screening for elevations of maternal glucose and aggressive management of the maternal glucose levels can normalize the outcome of pregnancies complicated by gestational glucose intolerance or gestational diabetes.

Definitions of gestational diabetes: the screening controversies

Gestational diabetes mellitus (GDM) is a diagnosis to be applied only to women in whom glucose intolerance is first detected during pregnancy [1]. The definition applies regardless of whether insulin is used for treatment or whether the condition persists after the pregnancy. It does not exclude the possibility that unrecognized glucose intolerance may have antedated the pregnancy [2]. There is general agreement on the basic underlying concepts of this disorder, but here the accord ends: the glucose concentration at which the diagnosis is to be made, the number of tests and abnormal values needed for diagnosis and the need for screening procedures to detect unsuspected disease are all subjects for continuing discussion and disagreement.

Several groups have developed criteria for diagnosing GDM [1–9], none of which has enjoyed universal acceptance. Two definitions remain in wide

Table 3.1 WHO criteria for gestational impaired glucose tolerance and diabetes.

Plasma glucose	Gestational impaired glucose tolerance	Gestational diabetes mellitus
Fasting	<7.8 mmol/l	≥7.8 mmol/l
	<140 mg/dl	≥140 mg/dl
	and	*or*
2-hour	7.8–11.0 mmol/l	≥11.1 mmol/l
	140–199 mg/dl	≥200 mg/dl

use: those of the World Health Organization (WHO) [1,7,8] and the National Diabetes Data Group (NDDG) [3] with the American Diabetes Association (ADA) [9]. Unfortunately, advocates of each steadfastly refuse to accept the criteria of the other; while agreeing that the best definition has yet to be found neither has enjoyed universal acceptance.

The WHO criteria

The WHO definition of gestational diabetes dates from a technical report of a WHO Study Group on Diabetes in 1980 [7], which recommended that the diagnostic procedures and criteria for pregnant women should be the same as those proposed for all adults, and that the management of gestational impaired glucose tolerance (GIGT) be the same as for diabetes [8]. The procedure for diagnosis consists of a 75-g oral glucose tolerance test (OGTT) on the morning after an overnight fast. Diabetes is diagnosed if the fasting plasma glucose concentration is at least 7.8 mmol/l or the 2-hour glucose concentration is at least 11.1 mmol/l (Table 3.1). Impaired glucose tolerance (IGT) is diagnosed if the fasting glucose is <7.8 mmol/l and the 2-hour glucose is at least 7.8 mmol/l but less than 11.1 mmol/l. Until recently, these criteria were universally accepted for the diagnosis of diabetes and IGT in non-pregnant adults; the WHO criteria for the diagnosis of GDM therefore have the advantage of employing a standard test that yields directly comparable results.

However, as a definition of GDM and GIGT, these criteria are irrational. The glucose concentrations used to define diabetes correspond to the thresholds above which the diabetes-specific complications of retinopathy and nephropathy begin to occur, while the concentration used to define IGT identifies individuals at particularly high risk of developing diabetes. No data on complications of the pregnancy or on its outcome were considered in selecting the criteria for use in pregnant women. It was generally recognized that a diabetic glucose concentration of 11.1 mmol/l was too high for safety during pregnancy, so the GIGT was arbitrarily included in the definition.

The NDDG/ADA definition

The NDDG criteria, first published in 1979 [3], have no more to recommend them than do the WHO criteria. These criteria were based on a statistical approach developed by O'Sullivan and Mahan in the late 1950s [10], and subsequently modified. Diagnosis employs the 100-g OGTT, which was widely used in the USA at that time. GDM is diagnosed if the patient's glucose concentration exceeds the population mean by at least two standard deviations, at any two of four points—fasting, and 1, 2 and 3 hours after the oral load.

The original glucose concentrations reported by O'Sullivan and Mahan [10] were measured in whole blood using the Somogyi–Nelson method, whereas glucose is currently measured in serum or plasma using a glucose oxidase method. Therefore, the NDDG converted the original whole-blood concentrations into comparable plasma concentrations (Table 3.2). However, Carpenter and Coustan [11] pointed out that this conversion ignored other non-glucose reducing substances, which explains why specific glucose assays read about 5 mg/dl (0.28 mmol/l) lower than the Somogyi–Nelson method. Accordingly, they therefore proposed that 5 mg/dl should be subtracted from the original data (Table 3.2); this approach has recently been endorsed by the Fourth International Workshop Conference on Gestational Diabetes [2]. Sacks et al. [12] further refined the criteria by measuring 995

Table 3.2 NDDG criteria: glucose concentrations during a 100-g glucose tolerance test measured by various methods.

	Whole blood		Serum	
	O'Sullivan and Mahan [10]	NDDG [3]	Carpenter and Coustan [11]	Sacks [12]
Fasting	90 mg/dl 5.0 mmol/l	105 mg/dl 5.8 mmol/l	95 mg/dl 5.3 mmol/l	96 mg/dl 5.3 mmol/l
1-hour	165 mg/dl 9.2 mmol/l	190 mg/dl 10.6 mmol/l	180 mg/dl 10.0 mmol/l	172 mg/dl 9.5 mmol/l
2-hour	145 mg/dl 8.1 mmol/l	165 mg/dl 9.2 mmol/l	155 mg/dl 8.6 mmol/l	152 mg/dl 8.4 mmol/l
3-hour	125 mg/dl 6.9 mmol/l	145 mg/dl 8.1 mmol/l	140 mg/dl 7.8 mmol/l	131 mg/dl 7.3 mmol/l

duplicate samples both by the Somogyi–Nelson method and by the current glucose oxidase method, and developed an empirical formula by linear regression (Table 3.2). This procedure avoided the biases introduced by both the NDDG and the Carpenter and Coustan conversions and represents the truest conversion to date; however, it has been largely ignored, perhaps because the earlier numbers were rounded to the nearest 5 mg/dl for 'easy memorization' [10].

There are other problems inherent in the O'Sullivan and Mahan criteria. First, there is no biological rationale for defining a disease purely on a statistical distribution of laboratory values in the population, regardless of whether or not the disease is present; there is no reason to assume that exactly 2.5% of the population is affected. Instead, some correlation of glucose concentrations with an outcome of interest is needed. In this case, it was shown that the women with higher glucose concentrations during pregnancy were at higher risk of developing diabetes subsequently, but the impact on any aspect of the pregnancy or its outcome was not examined.

Second, if a statistical cut-off point is to be used, the population must be a non-diseased population rather than the 'unselected' population chosen for this analysis—which included some undoubtedly diabetic but previously undiagnosed subjects. Including subjects with abnormally high values both raises the mean and increases the spread of the glucose concentrations and therefore the standard deviation; the upper limit of 'normal' (mean plus two standard deviations) is therefore spuriously high. By excluding women who clearly had diabetes (albeit previously undiagnosed), O'Sullivan and Mahan estimated that diagnostic postload glucose concentrations would have been 5 mg/dl lower at each of their four time points [10].

Third, even if a non-diseased population were used and one accepted the validity of using a statistical cut-off point to define disease, there is no rationale for requiring a cut-off point to be met at two time points during the test. This completely invalidates any attempt to justify the statistical approach; O'Sullivan and Mahan abandoned their purely statistical approach because it was considered 'expedient' to do so [10].

The use and interpretation of the NDDG criteria are further complicated by the common practice in the USA of screening with a 50-g oral glucose load under uncontrolled conditions and only testing those women with a 1-hour postload concentration of at least 140 mg/dl (7.8 mmol/l). Carpenter and Coustan [11] have found a sufficient number of women with GDM with screening concentrations between 130 and 140 mg/dl, and have thus recommended the lower level (130 mg/dl, 7.2 mmol/l) to be used for screening.

Further changes were recently proposed at the Fourth International Workshop-Conference on Gestational Diabetes Mellitus. In addition to adopting the Carpenter and Coustan modification of the O'Sullivan criteria, it was recommended to omit all testing and screening on low-risk women and to consider using a 75-g glucose load [2]. The former recommendation has met with opposition [13,14], while the criteria proposed for the 75-g load require extremely high glucose concentrations at two of the three time points during the glucose tolerance test.

Evidence-based diagnostic criteria for GDM?

Several direct comparisons of outcomes using both sets of criteria have shown that the WHO criteria identify more adverse outcomes than those of the NDDG [15–17], but there is insufficient evidence to favour one set of criteria over the other.

It is easy to understand the reluctance of any practitioner to adopt either of these criteria, especially if he or she is comfortable with the other. In the USA, the American College of Obstetricians and Gynecologists endorses the NDDG criteria, making it difficult for specialists to use any others.

In the future, more rational criteria should become available. There is currently a multicentre international trial under way to correlate the results of the 75-g OGTT with pregnancy outcomes [18]. These data should help to define the best criteria for diagnosing GDM and the best protocol for identifying women at risk.

Does active management affect outcome?

Gestational diabetes is a common obstetric complication, with fetal macrosomia as the main problem, affecting up to 40% of the offspring of these pregnancies. Other neonatal complications attributed to gestational diabetes include respiratory distress syndrome, hypocalcaemia, hyperbilirubinaemia and hypoglycaemia. Macrosomia is associated with increased rates of secondary complications such as operative delivery, shoulder dystocia and birth trauma. The cause of fetal macrosomia in gestational diabetes remains controversial. The Pedersen hypothesis claims that macrosomia is due to fetal hyperinsulinaemia, a consequence of maternal hyperglycaemia [19]. Early studies by O'Sullivan and Mahan [10] supported this hypothesis, in that insulin therapy to normalize maternal blood glucose levels was found to reduce the frequency of macrosomia compared with routine prenatal care or treatment with diet therapy alone. Numerous studies [20–23] subsequently reported that vigorous efforts to optimize maternal glycaemic control decreased rates of macrosomia, caesarean section and neonatal complications. Other studies, however, have continued to report increased rates of macrosomia and perinatal morbidity despite tight maternal glycaemic control [21,24].

Conflicting reports on the efficacy of good glycaemic control in reducing perinatal morbidity have led to suggestions that factors other than hyperglycaemia are more important in causing macrosomia and related morbidities. However, our view—supported by the balance of evidence in the following discussion—is that sustaining normoglycaemia will prevent macrosomia. This approach demands aggressive management, starting with diet and moving on to insulin.

Dietary strategies to prevent macrosomia

The ADA has not produced specific dietary guidelines for gestational diabetic women, and for those who are obese, there is even less advice. In the ADA Clinical Practice Recommendations 1999 [25], the only advice is: 'Nutritional recommendations for women with pre-existing and gestational diabetes should be based on a nutritional assessment. Monitoring blood glucose levels, urine ketones, appetite and weight gain can be a guide to developing an appropriate individualized nutritional prescription and meal plan, and to making adjustments to the meal plan throughout pregnancy to ensure desired outcomes.' Clearly, specific dietary advice is lacking.

The optimal dietary prescription would provide the caloric and nutrient needs to sustain pregnancy, without causing postprandial hyperglycaemia. The search for a euglycaemic diet has been difficult: for example, the meal plan endorsed by the ADA (35 kcal/kg pregnant weight, composed of 50–60% carbohydrates) caused excessive weight gain and also caused severe postprandial hyperglycaemia which necessitated insulin therapy in 50% of patients [26] (Table 3.3). The logical step would be to restrict energy intake to below this level.

Hypocaloric diets have been advocated for use in pregnancy since the nineteenth century, for the prevention of eclampsia and pre-eclampsia as well as in diabetic patients [27]. Recommendations for energy needs were recently reviewed by the National Academy of Science (NAS) [28], but this report contains no specific guidelines for lean, healthy individuals with diabetes, nor for the obese, gestational diabetic woman. The caloric needs of obese,

Table 3.3 Comparison of ADA and euglycaemic diets.

Total daily calories if:	ADA diet	Euglycaemic diet
BMI = 80–120% IBW	35 kcal/kg IBW	30 kcal/kg IBW
BMI = 121–150% IBW	35 kcal/kg IBW	24 kcal/kg IBW
BMI ≥ 151% IBW	35 kcal/kg IBW	12 kcal/kg IBW
Calories as fat	<25% of total	≥40% of total
Calories as carbohydrate	>55% of total	<40% of total
Calories as protein	20% of total	20% of total
Dietary cholesterol	<25% of total	>40% of total
	<300 mg/day	<800 mg/day

BMI, body mass index; IBW, ideal body weight.

healthy women during pregnancy are addressed but are inconsistent with other data: the NAS recommends that no more than 7 kg needs to be gained during pregnancy by women who are >150% of ideal weight, whereas another study in morbidly obese women revealed that infant birth weight was optimal if maternal weight gain was <3 kg [28].

Caution is needed when attempting to limit energy intake in obese women with gestational diabetes, because diabetic women may be more vulnerable to protein malnutrition than non-diabetic women during pregnancy.

Magee *et al.* [29] compared a strict calorie-restricted 1200-kcal/day diet with a 2400-kcal/day diet as a treatment for obese subjects with GDM. After 6 weeks the two groups differed significantly in average glucose levels and fasting insulin levels, but fasting glucose levels and postglucose challenge levels were not significantly different. Ketonaemia and ketonuria developed in the calorie-restricted group after 1 week on the strict diet: the investigators concluded that an intake of 1200 kcal/day may adversely affect fetal well-being, and therefore did not recommend this. They then went on to study a moderately restricted diet of 1600 kcal/day [30]. After 1 week, this improved both fasting and mean 24-hour blood glucose by 20%, compared with 2400 kcal/day, and ketonaemia did not develop.

Role of ketones

Calorie restriction increases ketone production, which poses theoretical problems for the fetus, but the role of ketones in pregnancies complicated by diabetes remains controversial [31]. An initial evaluation of the offspring of mothers with ketonuria suggested these children might have lower IQ scores than expected [32]; however, this study has been questioned due to the methodology used and the concern that chorioamnionitis might have caused the intellectual impairment [30]. Rizzo *et al.* [33] studied 223 pregnant women and their offspring: 89 women with type 1 insulin-dependent diabetes, 99 with GDM and 35 with normal glucose tolerance. Intellectual function of the offspring (measured as scores on the Stanford–Binet tests) correlated inversely with the third-trimester β-hydroxybutyrate and free fatty acid plasma concentrations but not with the level of ketonuria. Thus, there may be a difference between starvation ketosis and the ketosis that develops with poorly-controlled diabetes [31]. Ketonuria develops in 10–20% of normal pregnancies after an overnight fast [34] and in the non-diabetic mother, and may in fact protect the fetus from starvation. Other studies [30] have shown improvements in glycaemic control with 1500–1800-kcal/day diets, without ketonuria.

Buchanan *et al.* [24] examined the glucose, insulin, free fatty acid and β-hydroxybutyrate responses to extended overnight fasts during the third trimester of pregnancy and compared these between two groups: obese women with normal glucose tolerance and age- and weight-matched women with gestational diabetes. After a 12-hour fast, plasma glucose, insulin and free fatty acids were higher in the gestational diabetic women, while β-hydroxybutyrate levels were similar in the two groups. When the fast was extended to 18 hours, glucose levels fell more rapidly in the group with gestational diabetes, but remained higher than in the obese normal women, while insulin levels declined equally in both groups. Free fatty acids increased by 44% above the 12-hour values in the obese women but did not rise further in those with gestational diabetes. Moreover, β-hydroxybutyrate levels remained virtually equal in the two groups. Therefore, brief periods of fasting are well tolerated by gestational diabetic women and mild carbohydrate restriction—perhaps coupled with longer spacing between meals—may be useful for the treatment of obesity in women with gestational diabetes.

The Diabetes in Early Pregnancy (DIEP) Study [20] revealed that low β-hydroxybutyrate levels during the first trimester are an independent predictor of macrosomia and may also influence spontaneous abortion and malformations [34–36]. β-Hydroxybutyrate levels in the diabetic group remained significantly higher than in the control group throughout the first trimester, although they fell as the trimester progressed. This study also showed that raised ketone levels are strongly correlated with poor glucose control in the diabetic group; by contrast, β-hydroxybutyrate levels in the controls negatively correlated with fasting glucose and thus probably reflect starvation. Interestingly, β-hydroxybutyrate levels in the first trimester seemed to predict macrosomia in the newborn, when birth weight was carefully controlled for gender and gestational week. This study also showed that the β-hydroxybutyrate levels were lower in women—whether diabetic or non-diabetic—who delivered a malformed infant or who had a spontaneous abortion.

Further systematic studies of β-hydroxybutyrate levels throughout normal and diabetic pregnancy and in gestational diabetic women are obviously warranted to determine their impact on and birth weight and outcome.

Diets designed to minimize postprandial hyperglycaemia

The risk of diabetic fetopathy that results from maternal hyperglycaemia should be reduced when the peak postprandial glycaemic response is blunted; it follows that reducing carbohydrate intake specifically might be beneficial.

To date, there have been no randomized controlled trials specifically focusing on the optimal diet for either the lean or the obese gestational diabetic woman. One diet which has been proven to provide the needs of pregnancy but does not cause excessive weight gain or hyperglycaemia consists of 30 kcal/kg (of current pregnant weight) for normal-weight women, 24 kcal/kg for overweight women and 12 kcal/kg for morbidly obese women [26,37]. Carbohydrates account for 40% of the total calories and are distributed as described in Table 3.4. Compared with the recommended ADA diet for non-pregnant people, this so-called euglycaemic diet has less carbohydrate and more fat; its rationale is a study which showed that the postprandial glucose peak is directly related to the carbohydrate content of the meal [38]. In this study, 14 obese subjects (>130% ideal body weight) with gestational diabetes,

Table 3.4 The euglycaemic diet for gestational diabetic women. Calorie distribution to maintain normoglycaemia; diet calculation for women of 80–120% of ideal body weight. Adapted from Jovanovic [23] with permission.

Time	Meal	Fraction (kcal/24 h)	% of daily carbohydrate allowed
8.00 AM	Breakfast	2/18	10
10.30 AM	Snack	1/18	5
12.00 noon	Lunch	5/18	30
3.00 PM	Snack	2/18	10
5.00 PM	Dinner	5/18	30
8.00 PM	Snack	2/18	5
11.00 PM	Snack	1/18	10

who did not require insulin, were enrolled at 32–36 weeks of gestation. They were prescribed a total energy intake of 24 kcal/kg/day, with 12.5% of the total caloric requirement at breakfast, 28% at both lunch and dinner, and the remainder were divided among three snacks. Patients checked their blood glucose four times daily and kept a diet diary. The 1-hour postprandial glucose levels showed a significant correlation with percentage carbohydrate in the meal. This relationship was most striking at dinner and more variable at breakfast and lunch. To maintain a 1-hour postprandial capillary whole-blood glucose level <7.8 mmol/l requires ≤45% carbohydrates at breakfast, ≤55% at lunch and 50% at dinner. For better control (postprandial value <6.7 mmol/l), respective values of 33%, 45% and 40% are required. Also, glycaemic responses to a mixed meal are closely related to its carbohydrate content, and high carbohydrate diets do not improve glycaemic control in this context.

Thus, the optimal diet for the gestational diabetic woman is based on maternal glucose as the variable upon which the success or failure of a dietary prescription is based. Prescription of the euglycaemic diet is a useful starting point, but drug and nutritional therapy needs to be tailored to the postprandial glucose results from the woman's diary of glucose measurements. A diet-controlled gestational diabetic woman needs to monitor her blood glucose four times a day (fasting and 1 hour after each meal).

Insulin treatment for the gestational diabetic woman

When dietary strategies fail to achieve the glucose goals for the gestational diabetic woman, insulin therapy is needed. The type of insulin chosen should be based on the pattern of hyperglycaemia, and this can only be determined by frequent glucose monitoring, perhaps six times a day (before and 1 hour after each meal) [39].

The frequency of monitoring and the criteria for starting insulin remain controversial. Our programme has succeeded in normalizing the birth weight of the infants in Santa Barbara County, with a cost saving of over $1000 per pregnancy screened for gestational diabetes [40]. The following discussion outlines our approach.

If the fasting glucose (whole-blood capillary) exceeds 5 mmol/l, then iso-phane should be given before bed, beginning with doses of 0.2 unit/kg. If the postprandial glucose exceeds 6.67 mmol/l, then premeal rapid-acting insulin should be prescribed, beginning with a dose of 1 unit per 10 g of carbohydrate in the meal.

	Fraction of total insulin dose		
Time	Isophane	Soluble
Pre-breakfast	5/18	2/9
Pre-lunch		1/6
Pre-dinner		1/6
Bedtime	1/6	

Table 3.5 Initial calculation of insulin therapy for four injections a day*.

*Total insulin = 0.7 units × present pregnant weight in kilograms for weeks 1–18; 0.8 units × present pregnant weight in kilograms for weeks 18–26; 0.9 units × present pregnant weight in kilograms for weeks 26–36; 1.0 units × present pregnant weight in kilograms for weeks 36–40.

If both the fasting and postprandial glucose levels are elevated, or if postprandial hypoglycaemia can only be blunted at the expense of starvation, ketosis occurs, and an intensified regimen is prescribed, as for the type 1 diabetic woman [41,42] (Table 3.5). Normal pancreatic insulin production—of which about 50% comprises mealtime boluses—can be mimicked approximately by four injections a day of combinations of isophane and soluble insulin; three injections per day may be acceptable if the patient is willing to time her lunch to coincide with midday insulin peak from the morning isophane (Table 3.5).

The total daily dose of insulin should be based on body weight and gestational week (Table 3.5). In the first trimester an average insulin requirement is 0.7 units/kg/day, rising to 0.8 units/kg/day in the second and 9–1.0 units/kg/day during the third. In a massively obese woman, initial insulin doses may need to be increased to 1.5–2.0 units/kg/day to overcome the combined insulin resistance of pregnancy and obesity [39]. Twin gestations cause an approximate doubling of the insulin requirement throughout pregnancy. Smooth titration of insulin dosage demands frequent blood glucose monitoring, with at least 6 measurements each day.

Insulin lispro, a rapidly absorbed analogue of human insulin, mimics more closely the profile of postprandial insulin release and results in lower postprandial glucose concentrations; moreover, inappropriate hyperinsulinaemia is reduced, which may be related to its capacity to upregulate insulin receptors [43]. We assessed the safety and efficacy of insulin lispro in the treatment of gestational diabetes [44]. Forty-two gestational diabetic women in their second trimester who had failed to achieve normoglycaemia with diet alone were randomized to treatment with isophane and either soluble human insulin or insulin lispro. After 6 weeks of therapy, the insulin lispro group had significantly lower postprandial glucose levels (by about 1.0 mmol/l) without an increase in hypoglycaemic events. No increases in lispro-specific or insulin-specific antibodies were demonstrated in the insulin lispro group—an important issue because insulin only crosses the placenta when it is complexed with immunoglobulin. The lack of antibody formation against lispro should therefore minimize transplacental transfer of insulin lispro to the neonate. Consistent with this a subset of mothers who received a continuous intravenous infusion of insulin lispro at parturition [44] had measured circulatory concentrations of the analogue, but none could be detected in cord blood. Overall, insulin lispro proved to be as safe as soluble human insulin in the treatment of gestational diabetes, and resulted in a significantly lower postprandial glycaemia. Studies of the safety and efficacy of insulin analogues for the treatment of pregnant women with established type 1 and type 2 diabetes are still in progress.

Costs and benefits of GDM management

It is still not clear whether it is cost effective to screen all pregnant women for gestational diabetes and then to treat the detected case; unfortunately, evidence is sparse and only partially supportive. The most recent and comprehensive study looking at the costs and benefits of managing gestational diabetes was conducted by Kitzmiller and colleagues [45] using data gathered prospectively from three distinct gestational diabetes management programmes in New England and in Northern and Southern California. There were three parts to Kitzmiller's assessment: (i) cost identification, (ii) cost–effectiveness analysis and (iii) cost–benefit analysis.

Cost identification

The costs identified comprise 'all health resources required to diagnose GDM, monitor blood glucose, maintain blood glucose within targetted ranges and survey the gravida and fetus to ensure good outcomes'. These resources included the length of time each patient spent with each type of provider, the duration of blood glucose monitoring and insulin treatment as well as the number of non-stress tests (NSTs), ultrasound scans and amniocenteses. An average reimbursement rate (calculated according to information provided by 46 health insurance companies in Northern California) was applied to all three programmes to eliminate the effect of geographical pricing differences.

In Northern Californian and New England, management costs were calculated according to the treatment required and ranged from US$817–1500 for patients treated by diet alone to $1838–2089 for those requiring insulin. The Southern California programme (which differed by including patients requiring insulin treatment before 30 weeks' gestation) found premeal blood glucose monitoring to be cheaper than the postprandial monitoring group (US$3596 vs US$3770).

Cost–effectiveness analysis

This compared the calculated input costs associated with GDM treatment, to the outcome costs per patient. Costs of pregnancy outcomes included all healthcare resources used for inpatient antepartum care, delivery and postdelivery care. Some outcomes were expressed in non-monetary terms: percentage of patients requiring insulin therapy, antepartum admissions, deliveries <37 weeks, fetal macrosomia at birth (>4000 g), caesarean sections and neonatal intensive care unit (NICU) admissions. Using the difference between treatment groups for specific outcomes (e.g. NICU admissions, fetal macrosomia) as the denominator and the difference in treatment costs between the two groups as the numerator, Kitzmiller was able to compare the cost effectiveness of the two treatment groups in each of the three programmes. For example, although input costs were slightly higher postprandial than for the premeal glucose monitoring group in Southern California (see above), outcome costs were considerably lower for the latter (US$7495 vs US$8013) because of markedly lower caesarean section rates (24.2% vs 39.4%) and NICU admission (106.1 days/100 deliveries vs 127.3 days/100 deliveries. This data suggests that it costs only US$35 to prevent a caesarean section— which costs US$880 more than a normal vaginal delivery—by asking women to test their blood sugars after meals. This figure underestimates savings in that it does not include any psychological or long-term benefits of having a normal vaginal delivery rather than a caesarean section. Similarly, the additional cost of postprandial monitoring was US$25 in order to avoid 1 day in the NICU, which costs from US$1800 to US$2000.

Caesarean section and NICU admission rates were higher in women receiving insulin rather than diet therapy, which may reflect the fact that patients requiring insulin may have more severe glucose intolerance than women requiring only diet therapy.

Cost–benefit analysis

A cost–benefit analysis—which attempts to convert all treatment inputs and outcomes into monetary terms—was used only on the randomized, insulin-requiring patient groups in the Southern California programme. Here, for each extra US$1 spent on postprandial monitoring, approximately US$3 is saved by avoiding adverse outcomes; again, this figure does not include any cost estimation of psychological stress or long-term outcomes such as performance in school, development of obesity or glucose intolerance.

More research needed

The data presented by Kitzmiller *et al.* [45] from the Southern California programme suggest that intensive management of GDM with postprandial glucose monitoring benefits the mother and the baby (as well as the health insurance company). In future analyses, it would be interesting to consider the treatment and outcome costs associated with varying levels of blood glucose control. In addition, it would also be interesting to include the costs of screening the general pregnant population, for example with the 1-hour 50-g OGTT and follow-up 100-g OGTT used to identify the 355 women who participated in these management programmes. Lemen and colleagues [46] performed such an analysis in an adolescent pregnant population and found that the screening cost per case diagnosed was US$2292. They concluded that this may be prohibitively expensive, but did not compare this with the cost of complicated outcomes, such as NICU admissions and caesarean sections, which may be even higher in unidentified and untreated women. Thus, until there is a definitive report showing a cost–benefit to universal screening programmes and treatment in response to the diagnosis of gestational diabetes, issues surrounding the optimal means to identify and treat gestational diabetes will remain controversial.

Conclusions

Pregnancy is a time when serial metabolic changes in the mother are carefully regulated, to provide optimum substrate for both the mother and the fetus. Subtle perturbations in maternal metabolism can have implications not only for the index pregnancy but also for future generations. The focus of management during the past century has generally been to deliver a live infant from a live mother, and this goal is generally achieved at most centres. The challenge for the twenty-first century is to develop management strategies that provide not only a normal outcome for the index pregnancy, but also establish a maternal/fetal environment that does not place the mother, infant or subsequent generations at risk of abnormal glucose and insulin homeostasis with the concomitant risks of obesity, hypertension and diabetes mellitus. Thus, there should be no controversy, so that the goals for clinicians are to strive for as 'normal' metabolism as possible before, during and after each pregnancy.

Pregnancy represents a window of opportunity for healthcare providers to change lifestyle patterns toward habits that will be healthier for the individual as well as society. The challenge to clinicians is to provide information based on scientific evidence so that these goals can be accomplished.

Acknowledgements

The authors wish to thank Ms Jenna Beart for her valuable contribution to the section on the cost effectiveness of screening. In addition, we with to thank Ms Jeannine Glockler for help in the preparation of this manuscript.

References

1 WHO Study Group. *Prevention of Diabetes Mellitus.* Technical Report Series no 844. Geneva: World Health Organization, 1994.

2 Metzger BE, Coustan DR. Summary and recommendations of the fourth international workshop-conference on gestational diabetes mellitus. *Diabetes Care* 1988; 21: B161–7.

3 National Diabetes Data Group. Classification and diagnosis of diabetes mellitus and other categories of glucose intolerance. *Diabetes* 1979; 28: 1039–57.

4 Martin FIR for the Ad Hoc Working Party. The diagnosis of gestational diabetes. *Med J Aust* 1991; 155: 112.

5 Canadian Task Force on the Periodic Health Examination. Periodic health examination, 1992 update: 1. Screening for gestational diabetes mellitus. *Can Med Assoc J* 1991; 147: 435–43.

6 American College of Obstetricians and Gynecologists. *Diabetes and Pregnancy.* ACOG Technical Bulletin no 200. Washington DC: American College of Obstetricians and Gynecologists, 1994.

7 WHO Expert Committee on Diabetes Mellitus. Second report. WHO Technical Report Series no. 646. Geneva: World Health Organization, 1980.

8 World Health Organization. *Prevention of Diabetes Mellitus: Report of a WHO Study Group.* WHO Technical Report Series no 844. Geneva: World Health Organization, 1994.

9 Freinkel N, Josimovich J. Conference planning committee: American Diabetes Association Workshop-Conference on Gestational Diabetes: summary and recommendations. *Diabetes Care* 1980; 3: 499–501.

10 O'Sullivan JB, Mahan CM. Criteria for the oral glucose tolerance test in pregnancy. *Diabetes* 1964; 13: 278–85.

11 Carpenter MW, Coustan DR. Criteria for screening tests for gestational diabetes. *Am J Obstet Gynecol* 1982; 144: 768–73.

12 Sacks DA, Abu-Fadil S, Greenspoon JS, Fotheringham N. Do the current

standards for glucose tolerance testing in pregnancy represent a valid conversion of O'Sullivan's original criteria? *Am J Obstet Gynecol* 1989; 161: 638–41.

13 Moses RG, Moses J, Davis WS. Gestational diabetes: do lean young caucasian women need to be tested? *Diabetes Care* 1998; 21: 1803–6.

14 Moses RG, Moses M, Russell KG, Shier GM. The 75-g glucose tolerance test in pregnancy: a reference range determined on a low risk population and related to selected pregnancy outcomes. *Diabetes Care* 1998; 21: 1807–11.

15 Amadin RA, Famuyiwa OO, Adelusi BO. Glycemic response to 75 gms and 100 gms glucose load during pregnancy in Nigerian women. *Diabetologia Croatica* 1989; 18: 159–61.

16 Pettitt DJ, Bennett PH, Hanson RL, Narayan KMV, Knowler WC. Comparison of World Health Organization and National Diabetes Data Group procedures to detect abnormalities of glucose tolerance during pregnancy. *Diabetes Care* 1994; 17: 1264–8.

17 Deerochanawong C, Putiyanun C, Wongsuryrat M, Serirat S, Junayon P. Comparison of National Diabetes Data Group and World Health Organization criteria for detecting gestational diabetes mellitus. *Diabetologia* 1996; 39: 1070–3.

18 Metzger B for the Hyperglycemia and Adverse Pregnancy Outcome (HAPO) Group, personal communication, 1999.

19 Pedersen J. *The Pregnant Diabetic and Her Newborn.* Copenhagen: Munksgaard, 1967.

20 Jovanovic-Peterson L, Peterson CM, Reed GF *et al.* Maternal postprandial glucose levels and infant birth weight: the diabetes in early pregnancy study. *Am J Obstet Gynecol* 1991; 164: 103–11.

21 DeVeciana M, Major CA, Morgan MA *et al.* Postprandial versus preprandial blood glucose monitoring in women with gestational diabetes mellitus requiring insulin therapy. *N Engl J Med* 1995; 333: 1237–41.

22 Combs CA, Gunderson E, Kitzmiller JL, Gavin LA, Main EK. Relationship of fetal macrosomia to maternal postprandial glucose control during pregnancy. *Diabetes Care* 1992; 15: 1251–7.

23 Jovanovic L (ed). *Medical Management of Pregnancy Complicated by Diabetes*, 3rd edn. Alexandria, VA: American Diabetes Association, 2000.

24 Buchanan TA, Metzger BE, Freinkel N. Accelerated starvation in late pregnancy: a comparison between obese women with and without gestational diabetes mellitus. *Am J Obstet Gynecol* 1990; 162: 1015–20.

25 American Diabetes Association. Position statement: nutrition recommendations and principles for people with diabetes mellitus. *Diabetes Care* 1999; 22 (Suppl. 1): 1–11.

26 Jovanovic-Peterson L, Peterson CM. Dietary manipulation as a primary treatment strategy for pregnancies complicated by diabetes. *J Am Col Nutr* 1990; 9: 320–5.

27 Dexter L, Weiss S. *Preclamptic and Eclamptic Toxemia of Pregnancy.* Boston: Little, Brown, 1941.

28 King J (Chair Subcommittee on Nutritional Status and Weight Gain During Pregnancy), Allen L, (Chair Subcommittee on Dietary Intake and Nutrient Supplements During Pregnancy). *Nutrition During Pregnancy.* Washington, DC: National Academy Press, 1990.

29 Magee MS, Knopp RH, Benedetti TJ. Metabolic effects of 1200-kcal diet in obese pregnant women with gestational diabetes. *Diabetes* 1990; 39: 234–40.

30 Knopp RH, Magee MS, Raisys V. Hypocaloric diets and ketogenesis in the management of obese gestational diabetic women. *J Am Coll Nutr* 1991; 10: 649–67.

31 Jovanovic-Peterson L, Peterson CM. Sweet success, but an acid after taste? [editorial]. *N Engl J Med* 1991; 325: 959–60.

32 Churchill JA, Berrendes HW, Nemore J. Neuropsychological deficits in children of diabetic mothers. A report from the collaborative study of cerebral palsy. *Am J Obstet Gynecol* 1969; 105: 257–68.

33 Rizzo T, Metzger BE, Burns WJ, Burns K. Correlations between antepartum maternal metabolism and intelligence of

offspring. *N Engl J Med* 1991; 325: 911–16.

34 Mills JL, Knopp RH, Simpson JL *et al.* Lack of relation between malformation rates in infants of diabetic mothers to glycemic control during organogenesis. *N Engl J Med* 1988; 318: 671–6.

35 Jovanovic L, Metzger B, Knopp RH *et al.* β-hydroxybutyrate levels in type 1 diabetic pregnancy compared with normal pregnancy. *Diabetes Care* 1998; 21: 1–5.

36 Mills JL, Simpson JL, Driscoll SG *et al.* Incidence of spontaneous abortion among normal women and insulin dependent diabetic women whose pregnancies were identified within 21 days of conception. *N Engl J Med* 1988; 319: 1617–23.

37 Jovanovic-Peterson L, Peterson CM. Nutritional management of the obese gestational diabetic woman. *J Am Coll Nutr* 1992; 11: 246–50.

38 Peterson CM, Jovanovic-Peterson L. Percentage of carbohydrate and glycemic response to breakfast, lunch and dinner in women with gestational diabetes. *Diabetes* 1991; 40 (Suppl 2): 172–4.

39 Mulford MI, Jovanovic-Peterson L, Peterson CM. Alternative therapies for the management of gestational diabetes. *Clin Perinatol* 1993; 20: 619–34.

40 Jovanovic-Peterson L, Bevier W, Peterson CM. The Santa Barbara County Health Care Services Program: birthweight change concomitant with screening for and treatment of glucose-intolerance of pregnancy: a potential cost–effective intervention. *Am J Perinatol* 1997; 14: 221–8.

41 Jovanovic L, Druzin M, Peterson CM. Effect of euglycemia on the outcome of pregnancy in insulin-dependent diabetic women as compared with normal control subjects. *Am J Med* 1981; 71: 921–7.

42 Jovanovic-Peterson L, Peterson CM. Rationale for prevention and treatment of glucose-mediated macrosomia: a protocol for gestational diabetes. *Endocrine Pract* 1996; 2: 118–29.

43 Jehle PM, Fussgaenger RD, Kunze U, Dolderer M, Warchol W, Koop I. The human insulin analog insulin lispro improves insulin binding on circulating monocytes of intensively treated insulin dependent diabetes mellitus patients. *J Clin Endocrinol Metab* 1996; 81: 2319–27.

44 Jovanovic L, Ilic S, Pettitt D *et al.* The metabolic and immunologic effects of insulin lispro. *Diabetes Care* 1999; 22: 1422–7.

45 Kitzmiller JL, Elixhauser A, Carr S *et al.* Assessment of costs and benefits of management of gestational diabetes mellitus. *Diabetes Care* 1998; 21 (Suppl 2): B123–30.

46 Lemen PM, Wigton TR, Miller-McCarthey AJ, Cruikshank DP. Screening for gestational diabetes mellitus in adolescent pregnancies. *Am J Obstet Gynecol* 1998; 178: 1251–6.

4: What should we do about microalbuminuria?

Stephen M. Thomas

The description of a radioimmunoassay in 1963 by Keen and Chlouverakis [1] allowed the measurement of previously undetectable levels of urinary albumin. This led in 1969 to the landmark report that a proportion of patients with type 2 diabetes in Bedford had elevated urinary albumin excretion, so-called microalbuminuria [2]. The importance of microalbuminuria was not fully appreciated, however, until 1982 when groups in London and Denmark independently described that microalbuminuria was predictive of the later development of overt diabetic kidney disease (DKD) and progressive renal failure [3,4]. Since this time, the literature and knowledge of this phase of the diabetic kidney lesion has exploded.

The prevalence of microalbuminuria in type 1 diabetes is quoted as between 4% and 20% [5,6] and in type 2 diabetes around 20–36% [7], and as such is a significant problem in any diabetes clinic. In addition, it is now clear that the development of microalbuminuria is associated with widespread systemic abnormalities and has consequences not only for renal but also for cardiovascular disease in both type 1 and type 2 diabetes.

Significance of microalbuminuria for renal disease

Traditionally, the onset of DKD has been thought of as the presence of clinically detectable dipstick-positive proteinuria, equivalent to a urinary protein excretion of >300 mg/day. There is strong evidence of an individual susceptibility to DKD in type 1 and increasingly in type 2 diabetes [8]. This susceptibility seems to be genetic [9], but as yet there is no way of identifying those who are at risk of DKD, other than an early rise in urinary albumin excretion rate (AER).

Early studies on microalbuminuria used differing cut-off points of urinary AER but persistent microalbuminuria is now defined as an AER

Table 4.1 Predictive value of albumin excretion rate (AER) for diabetic kidney disease (DKD) in type 1 diabetes.

Group	Patients (no.)	Discriminant AER (µg/min)	Follow-up (years)	Percentage of patients developing DKD
Viberti *et al.* [3]	63	30	14	88
Parving *et al.* [4]	25	28	6	75
Mogensen *et al.* [14]	43	15	10	86
Microalbuminuria Collaborative study [68]	70	10	4	17
Mathiesen *et al.* [13]	71	70	6	100

between 20 and 200 µg/min (30 and 300 mg/day) in at least two of three consecutive collections [10]. Microalbuminuria can occur within a year of type 1 diabetes, although persistent elevation of AER is more common after 5 years [11]. Once persistent microalbuminuria has developed, the AER increases by between 7% and 18.6% per year [12].

Over 80% of patients with microalbuminuria progress to DKD [3,4,10,13,14] (Table 4.1), and at levels of urinary AER > 100 µg/min this rises to ~100%. The development of DKD is, however, a continuum from normal albumin excretion and any 'man-made' cut-off will inevitably lead to a degree of misclassification.

It has been traditional to consider microalbuminuria as a predictor of later disease, to the extent that it is commonly known as 'incipient nephropathy'. However, there is now important evidence from biopsy studies that this phase does not merely predict DKD but is associated with significant glomerular disease at the time of microalbuminuria. In type 1 diabetes, Walker *et al.* found patients with microalbuminuria to have glomerular basement membrane thickening, expansion of the mesangial matrix volume fraction and matrix volume as compared to normoalbuminuric controls [15]. Fioretto *et al.* came to a similar conclusion in those with an AER >31 µg/min, who had lesions which ranged up to the advanced changes seen in overt proteinuria. Interestingly, and in contrast to the experience of Walker *et al.*, they found that glomerular structure in those with 'low-level' microalbuminuria <31 µg/min was not significantly different from controls [16]. In addition, patients with microalbuminuria also have evidence of renal arteriolar hyalinosis [17] and interstitial expansion, the latter associated with a more rapid fall in glomerular filtration rate [18].

In type 2 diabetes, the significance of microalbuminuria is more controversial, as the incidence of other non-diabetic renal diseases may be higher

[19,20]. Microalbuminuria in type 2 diabetes may be associated with renal lesions with less severity and a greater heterogeneity as compared to Caucasian patients with type 1 diabetes [21]. Nevertheless, in studies of type 2 diabetes in Europe, patients with microalbuminuria had greater glomerular volume, mesangial sclerosis and arteriolar hyalinosis than non-diabetic control subjects [22], findings confirmed in a study in Japan [23].

Most patients have a normal glomerular filtration rate (GFR) when they develop overt DKD; however, GFR may fall, albeit within the normal range, even in microalbuminuria.

Thus, it may well be time to abandon the term 'incipient nephropathy' and recognize that the development of microalbuminuria indicates significant renal disease. Because, at lower levels of AER, ~20% of patients do not progress to overt DKD, early microalbuminuria may represent a more treatable phase of disease which should be targetted for intervention.

Significance of microalbuminuria for cardiovascular disease

In addition to the risk for advanced renal disease in diabetes, it is clear that microalbuminuria is an important marker of cardiovascular morbidity and mortality. Several studies have demonstrated this in type 2 diabetes. In one 'combined analysis' of eight cohorts studied, the overall odds ratio associated with microalbuminuria for death due to cardiovascular disease was 2.4 (95% CI 1.8–3.1) [7]. Indeed, in type 2 diabetes microalbuminuria is more predictive of cardiovascular death than it is of end-stage renal failure [24]. It is further suggested that in type 2 diabetes this increase in risk operates at levels of AER only minimally above the normal range and that an AER > 10 µg/min should be targetted for intervention [25].

This relationship with cardiovascular disease is not only true in type 2 diabetes, where patients tend to be older and to have greater cardiovascular risk factors, but also in type 1 diabetes. In a 23-year follow-up Messent et al. found a relative risk of cardiovascular mortality of 2.94 (95% CI 1.18–7.34) associated with microalbuminuria [26]. In addition, in a cross-sectional study Earle et al. found that microalbuminuria was an independent risk factor for silent myocardial ischaemia, suggesting that significant coronary artery lesions may already be present during the phase of microalbuminuria [27].

The reasons for the relationship between microalbuminuria and cardiovascular disease are complex. Whether, in fact, microalbuminuria is an independent risk factor for cardiovascular disease or whether the relationship results from a clustering of conventional risk factors is unclear [28].

Associations and consequences of microalbuminuria

Undoubtedly, the metabolic and haemodynamic associations of microalbuminuria are important in the associated increased renal and cardiovascular risk and some of these alterations will be considered further.

Blood pressure

Considerable debate centres on the links between blood pressure and microalbuminuria, with controversy over whether a rise in blood pressure predates the rise in AER or occurs after the development of microalbuminuria. In the UK Microalbuminuria Collaborative study, a longitudinal study of 137 patients with type 1 diabetes and normoalbuminuria at baseline, mean arterial pressure was higher from baseline in those who developed microalbuminuria as compared to those who remained normoalbuminuric [29] (Fig. 4.1). By contrast, in cohorts reported from Danish studies, the rise in blood pressure occurred after the development of persistent microalbuminuria [30]. This discrepancy is unresolved and is important, not least in the understanding of the pathogenic mechanisms involved in the development of DKD.

In type 2 diabetes, a study in Japan found blood pressure to be an important predictor of future microalbuminuria [31]. In Pima Indians, the level of arterial pressure, even before the onset of diabetes itself, predicts the subsequent development of elevated urinary albumin excretion [32].

In the hypertension in diabetes study, intensive treatment of blood pressure (mean 144/82 mmHg) resulted in a significant 29% reduction in the risk of microalbuminuria after 6 years, as compared with less tight control (mean 154/87 mmHg) [33]. Interestingly, the effect on microalbuminuria after 9 years was no longer statistically significant.

Therefore in type 1 diabetes it remains uncertain whether rises in blood pressure predate microalbuminuria or vice versa. In type 2 diabetes, there seems to be less controversy, with higher arterial pressures being a risk factor for the future development of microalbuminuria and with increasingly lower blood pressure targets for treatment advisable in this population.

During the phase of microalbuminuria in both type 1 and type 2 diabetes there is no doubt that both systolic and diastolic blood pressure, whether office or 24-hour measurements, rise with the AER [34–37]. In type 1 diabetes, the sitting blood pressure rises in the phase of microalbuminuria by an

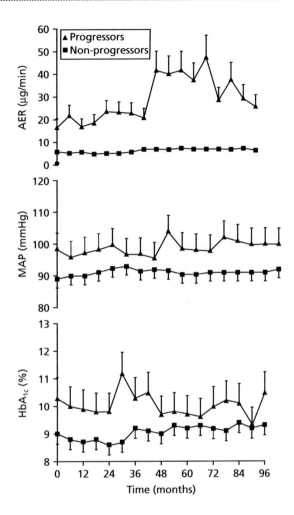

Fig. 4.1 Predictors of the development of microalbuminuria in type 1 diabetes [29].

average of 3–4 mmHg per year, compared to 1 mmHg per year in long-term normoalbuminuric and healthy controls [38].

The exact prevalence of hypertension in those with type 1 diabetes and microalbuminuria depends upon the changing definition of hypertension. In a Danish cohort study, the prevalence of hypertension, using World Health Organization (WHO) criteria (systolic blood pressure (SBP) ≥160 mmHg, diastolic blood pressure (DBP) ≥95 mmHg), was 15% in those with normal AER, 26% in those with microalbuminuria and 61% in those with macro-albuminuria [39]. When the criteria for hypertension from the 5th report of the Joint National Committee on Detection, Evaluation and Treatment of Hypertension (SBP ≥130 mmHg, DBP ≥80 mmHg) were used, the prevalence rose to 42%, 52% and 79% for normoalbuminuric, microalbuminuric and macroalbuminuric patients, respectively. This highlights the consequences for clinical practice of targetting ever lower blood pressures.

Lipid disturbances

Microalbuminuria is associated with a distinctly unfavourable lipid profile. In type 1 diabetes, this is in contrast to the generally beneficial profile seen in patients with good glycaemic control. Type 2 diabetes itself is, however, associated with deleterious changes in serum lipids, which are exaggerated in those with microalbuminuria. The concentrations of total cholesterol, very low density lipoprotein (VLDL) cholesterol, low-density lipoprotein (LDL) cholesterol, triglycerides and fibrinogen rise with increasing urinary AER in patients with type 1 diabetes [40]. In addition, there is an increase in LDL mass and atherogenic small dense LDL particles, which correlates with the plasma triglyceride concentrations. High-density lipoprotein (HDL) levels also tend to be reduced, with a disadvantageous alteration in their composition [41–43].

The importance of alterations in serum lipids was demonstrated by a recent longitudinal study of a hospital-based cohort of patients with type 2 diabetes in London. This study suggested that a significant portion of the excess risk associated with microalbuminuria was attributable to alterations in serum cholesterol (Table 4.2). This is of great importance and suggests serum lipids to be an important area of therapeutic intervention in those with microalbuminuria.

	CHD mortality	
	Risk ratio	95% CI
Age	2.0	(0.94–4.30)
Sex	3.8	(1.16–12.6)
Pre-existing CHD	2.7	(0.93–7.94)
HbA$_{1c}$	1.5	(1.01–2.32)
Serum cholesterol	2.5	(1.50–4.17)
Microalbuminuria (Y/N)	1.8	(0.56–6.04)

Table 4.2 Multivariate analysis of risk factors for coronary heart disease (CHD) mortality in type 2 diabetes. After Mattock et al. [28].

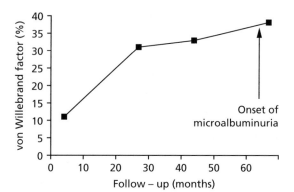

Fig. 4.2 Rise in von Willebrand factor precedes onset of microalbuminuria in type 1 diabetes. Adapted from Stehouwer *et al.* [50] with permission.

Endothelial dysfunction

There is good evidence of widespread endothelial dysfunction in diabetes even at the stage of microalbuminuria. Markers of endothelial dysfunction such as transcapillary albumin escape rate, circulating levels of Von Willebrand factor (vWf), plasminogen activator inhibitor 1 (PAI-1), thrombomodulin, homocysteine and fibrinogen are increased in microalbuminuria [44–49], although this may not purely reflect endothelial dysfunction.

A recent longitudinal study has shown that increases in vWf levels in patients with type 1 diabetes precede the development of microalbuminuria, occurring when the AER is in the normal range [50] (Fig. 4.2). Although these findings may reflect a continuum in the disease process, they may also suggest that detection of early endothelial dysfunction could be used to identify those at risk of developing DKD.

A new concept recently proposed is that of benign and malignant microalbuminuria, stratified according to the presence or absence of endothelial activation/dysfunction. The proponents suggest that classification of microalbuminuria according to whether or not there is endothelial damage identifies those with a greater risk. This 'malignant' microalbuminuria associated with endothelial activation may be more associated with diabetic microvascular complications [44] and with macrovascular damage. However this hypothesis needs to be tested and further explanation is necessary of the possible mechanisms involved. Within the glomerular capillary wall, the main barrier to protein loss lies not within the endothelium but more likely at the level of the podocyte, slit diaphragm and the basement membrane.

Thus, the additional clinical benefit of classifying by microalbuminuria and endothelial dysfunction is unproven, but these observations provide interesting new areas for investigation, and the interaction of endothelial damage and microalbuminuria merits further study.

Significance of microalbuminuria in pregnancy

An increase in urinary AER of between 40% and 200% occurs in otherwise normal pregnancies, mostly in the second and third trimester. The predictive value of microalbuminuria in pregnancy in diabetes is uncertain, although in some small studies it has been associated with preterm delivery in diabetic and non-diabetic pregnancies [51] and is suggested as a marker of subclinical pre-eclampsia by some but not all studies [52,53]. Several antenatal diabetes clinics are screening for microalbuminuria, but the precise significance of the observation needs to be determined in larger studies.

Microalbuminuria and ethnicity

Several studies now indicate that there is considerable ethnic variability in the risk of microalbuminuria in diabetes. In the UK, Asian Indians appear to be at increased risk of developing microalbuminuria but not other diabetic microvascular complications, as compared with Europid populations [54]. Interestingly, in Japanese populations, microalbuminuria does not seem to be associated with excess cardiovascular risk [55], although the reasons for this discrepancy are uncertain.

Management of microalbuminuria

Screening

Should we screen for microalbuminuria? It is true that there are few studies reporting the benefits of treatment of microalbuminuria with hard endpoints such as preservation of GFR, prevention of end-stage renal failure or reduction in mortality. The paucity of these studies is, in part, a reflection of the large patient number and long study duration necessary, factors that may preclude their performance indefinitely. In the interim, what should one say? There has been some debate in the literature as to the cost-effectiveness of screening for microalbuminuria. The high predictive power of microalbuminuria for overt DKD and vascular death and the clustering with risk factors for cardiovascular disease all seem to argue in favour of a screening programme backed up by appropriate intervention.

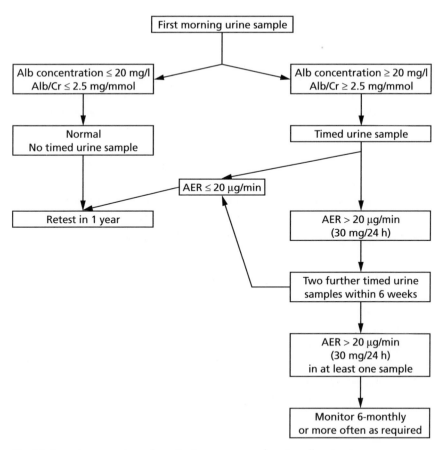

Fig. 4.3 Screening strategies and monitoring programme for microalbuminuria.

Screening can be performed in a number of ways. Sensitive stick tests are now available [56] and are convenient, as is an early morning albumin : creatinine ratio [57]. The 'gold standard' is still to measure AER in three timed urine samples; if therapeutic decisions are to be based upon the diagnosis of microalbuminuria, then ideally the diagnosis should be confirmed in this way. One suggested screening protocol is shown in Fig. 4.3.

Treatment

Blood pressure

Treatment of blood pressure is paramount and undisputed, the only controversy being what are appropriate target pressures and which agents should be used. In the UK Microalbuminuria Collaborative Study, the mean arterial pressure (MAP) remained at 90 mmHg or below throughout the period of follow-up in those who remained normoalbuminuric [29]. In keeping with this, a regression analysis by Mogensen suggested that in the microalbuminuric phase retardation of the rise of AER would require a MAP of ~92 mmHg (125/75) [58]. To date, however, these targets have not been validated in prospective intervention studies.

It is clear that the priority in antihypertensive treatment should be the attainment of good blood pressure control, although it is likely that our concept of what blood presure this implies may continue to change. A separate question is what agents should we primarily use to treat those with microalbuminuria.

Two large placebo-controlled studies investigated captopril treatment in normotensive patients with type 1 diabetes and microalbuminuria with a combined total of 235 patients studied [59]. Twenty-five of 114 placebo-treated patients (21.9%) and eight of 111 captopril-treated patients (7.2%) progressed to persistent clinical albuminuria over 24 months. There was a significant 69% (95% CI 31.7–86.1%) reduction in the risk of progression by captopril, which persisted after adjustment for differences in time-averaged mean arterial pressure. AER increased by an average of 14.2% per year in the placebo-treated group compared with a reduction of 9.6% (–18.6% to 0.4%) per year in the captopril-treated group.

The Italian Microalbuminuria study group compared the effect of lisinopril and nifedipine over 3 years in normotensive patients with type 1 diabetes and 'incipient nephropathy' [60]. Patients in both the lisinopril and the nifedipine group were less likely to progress to macroalbuminuria, with around a 60% risk reduction in both groups. Patients treated with lisinopril but not nifedipine were less likely to have a >50% increase in AER over baseline compared to placebo, and those treated with lisinopril had a significantly lower blood pressure during follow-up.

A meta-analysis of studies of type 1 diabetes with microalbuminuria or 'overt' proteinuria, treated for more than 4 weeks with antihypertensives, found that ACE I treatment reduced proteinuria more than treatment with beta-blockers, diuretics or calcium antagonists ('conventional therapy'), despite a similar average reduction in blood pressure. In a linear regression analysis, it was calculated that ACE I treatment would reduce proteinuria by 30% even if there was zero blood pressure change. Nifedipine treatment was associated with a rise in proteinuria, while conventional treatment in the analysis had no antiproteinuric effect without a blood-pressure-lowering effect [61].

Furthermore, a recent meta-analysis of clinical trials of ACE I in patients with type 1 diabetes and microalbuminuria found that ACE I therapy reduced progression to macroalbuminuria by 79%, with regression to normoalbuminuria occurring 2.64-fold more often on ACE I. In addition, the antiproteinuric effect of ACE I seemed to be greater in those with the highest AER, an 81% reduction at an AER of 200 μg/min compared with 26% at 20 μg/min [62].

Similarly, studies in type 2 diabetes have suggested the potential benefit of treatment with ACE inhibitors. Ravid *et al.* [63] studied 94 patients with type 2 diabetes with microalbuminuria randomly assigned to either enalapril or placebo. In those treated with enalapril, six of 49 patients progressed to overt DKD as compared with 19 of 45 placebo-treated patients.

In a study of Japanese patients with type 2 diabetes and microalbuminuria [64], 52 patients were divided into four groups. Twenty-six patients with a blood pressure ≥150/90 mmHg, who at the beginning of the study were on no treatment, were randomized to either enalapril or no treatment. A further 26 with blood pressure below this value on nifedipine were similarly randomized. After 4 years, both groups treated with enalapril had a significant fall in AER, whereas AER tended to increase in both the groups not on enalapril although no patients progressed to macroalbuminuria.

Interim results of the Appropriate Blood Pressure Control in Diabetes (ABCD) trial has highlighted a potential benefit of ACE inhibitors in myocardial protection in type 2 diabetes [65]. This trial aimed primarily at testing the effect on renal function of two contrasting levels of diastolic blood-pressure control and compared the effects of enalapril with a long-acting dihydropyridine, nisoldipine, with cardiovascular events considered as secondary endpoints. After 5 years, there was a significant difference in the number of fatal and non-fatal myocardial infarctions (25 in the nisoldipine group vs 5 in the enalapril group; risk ratio 9.5; 95% CI 2.3–21.4), and at the suggestion of the Data and Safety Monitoring Committee those with hypertension randomized to nisoldipine were reassigned to enalapril. Further confirmation may be necessary, but this is suggestive that ACE inhibitors may have cardioprotective as well as renoprotective effects.

Recently the MICRO-HOPE substudy of the Heart Outcomes Prevention Evaluation (HOPE) study [66] has published the benefits of treatment with an ACE inhibitor in patients with type 2 diabetes and microalbuminuria. The

HOPE study enrolled 3577 patients aged 55 years or older with a history of diabetes and at least one other cardiovascular risk factor (lipid abnormalities, hypertension, microalbuminuria or current smoking). Urinary AER was measured at baseline, 1 year and study end (4.5 years). Microalbuminuria was defined as an early morning albumin : creatinine ratio of 2 mg/mmol or higher in men and women. At baseline ~30% of patients had microalbuminuria, 553 of whom were randomly allocated to treatment with ramipril and 587 to placebo. The study was terminated by the data monitoring committee as ramipril lowered the risk of a primary combined end-point of myocardial infarction, stroke or cardiovascular disease (CVD) death by 25% and total mortality by 24%. Treatment with ramipril lowered the risk of overt nephropathy in all patients with diabetes. In addition, ramipril lowered the risk of the primary combined end-point in all patients with diabetes [66].

In most of the studies discussed above, ACE I treatment was associated with lower blood pressures than other treatments. This makes it difficult to determine whether there was any benefit to these agents independent of their effect on systemic blood pressure but it does imply at least that they are effective antihypertensives for these patients.

Recent advances in molecular genetics have raised the issue that individual responses to treatment with ACE I may be in part dependent upon the ACE genotype. A 287-bp (base pair) deletion in the ACE gene gives rise to a deletion (D) allele and an insertion (I) allele, with the suggestion of faster progression and may be less response to ACE inhibition in those homozygous for the D allele which is associated with higher plasma ACE levels [67]. In the future, therefore, it is conceivable that treatment may be tailored according to genotype.

In conclusion, the clear message is the importance of blood pressure control, which will often require more than one agent. Current data supports the use of ACE I as first-line therapy.

Glycaemic control

The Diabetes Control and Complications Trial (DCCT) research group in type 1 diabetes [68] and the UKPDS Prospective Diabetes Study (UKPDS) in type 2 diabetes [69] have shown that improved glycaemic control reduces the development of microalbuminuria. However, these studies and many smaller ones have included predominantly patients with normal AER at baseline.

There has been much debate over the years as to the importance of blood glucose control in the progression of microalbuminuria. Prospective small-scale studies in patients with microalbuminuria have failed to show any benefit in terms of progression of proteinuria or loss of GFR [70,71]. By contrast, a study in patients with type 1 diabetes and microalbuminuria demonstrated a benefit of improved glycaemic control for ~3 years on renal histology, with greater increases in basement membrane thickness, matrix/ mesangial volume and matrix star volume in patients on conventional rather than intensified insulin therapy [72].

In work in Minneapolis, the effect of solitary pancreas transplantation on renal histology in eight patients with type 1 diabetes was analysed at 5 and 10 years [73]. The thickness of the glomerular basement membrane did not change significantly from baseline to 5 years, but it had decreased by 10 years. The mesangial fractional volume and the mesangial–matrix fractional volume increased from baseline to 5 years; at 10 years these values were lower than at baseline or at 5 years. The mesangial-cell fractional volume also increased from baseline to 5 years and then decreased to the baseline value by 10 years.

The mean glomerular volume decreased from baseline to 5 years and did not change significantly thereafter. The change in the urinary albumin excretion rate from baseline to 10 years after transplantation was correlated with the change in mesangial fractional volume over that period.

Although this small study in no way supports the use of pancreas transplantation for the treatment of microalbuminuria, these reports would seem to question the existence of a metabolic 'point of no return'. It would therefore seem reasonable purely from a renal point of view to aim for as good glycaemic control as is practicable without significant hypoglycaemia.

Dietary treatment

The benefits of a reduction of protein intake has long been debated in the treatment of DKD. Reduction of dietary protein by ~50% has been shown to reduce the fractional clearance of albumin in patients with microalbuminuria and to lower GFR in patients with hyperfiltration, independently of changes in glucose control and blood pressure [74].

The St Vincent Declaration guidelines for type 1 diabetes recommend that it is probably reasonable to limit the protein intake in patients with micro-albuminuria to approximately 0.8–1 g/kg body weight per day and to consider a replacement of some animal protein with vegetable sources. Close monitoring is necessary when prescribing low-protein diets to minimize any ill-effects of such diets.

Smoking

There is evidence that smoking may be related to both the development and progression of microalbuminuria and DKD [75]. Although this evidence is not conclusive and the relationship weak, the strong association with cardiovascular disease means that smoking should be particularly discouraged in patients with microalbuminuria.

Summary

Microalbuminuria is associated with significant glomerular pathology and heightened cardiovascular risk. There are many associated systemic alterations which are amenable to treatment. Recent evidence supports the benefit of intervention at the phase of microalbuminuria in type 1 diabetes in particular. In type 2 diabetes treatment of those with microalbuminuria remains of great importance, it remains to be seen whether treatment of those with type 2 diabetes and a normal AER is as cost effective and beneficial as treatment of those with microalbuminuria.

References

1 Keen H, Chlouverakis C. An immunoassay method for urinary albumin at low concentration. *Lancet* 1963; ii: 913–14.

2 Keen H, Chlouverakis C, Fuller J, Jarrett RJ. The concomitants of raised blood sugar: studies in newly-detected hyperglycaemics. II. Urinary albumin excretion, blood pressure and their relation to blood sugar levels. *Guy's Hosp Rep* 1969; 118: 247–54.

3 Viberti GC, Hill RD, Jarrett RJ, Argyropoulos A, Mahmud U, Keen H. Microalbuminuria as a predictor of clinical nephropathy in insulin-dependent diabetes mellitus. *Lancet* 1982; i: 1430–2.

4 Parving HH, Oxenboll B, Svendsen PA, Christiansen JS, Andersen AR. Early detection of patients at risk of developing diabetic nephropathy. A longitudinal study of urinary albumin excretion. *Acta Endocrinol* 1982; 100: 550–5.

5 Microalbuminuria Collaborative Study Group United Kingdom. Microalbuminuria in type I diabetic patients. Prevalence and clinical characteristics. Microalbuminuria Collaborative Study Group. *Diabetes Care* 1992; 15: 495–501.

6 Parving HH, Hommel E, Mathiesen E *et al.* Prevalence of microalbuminuria, arterial hypertension, retinopathy and neuropathy in patients with insulin dependent diabetes. *BMJ Clin Res Edn* 1988; 296: 156–60.

7 Dineen SF, Gerstein HC. The association of microalbuminuria and mortality in non-insulin dependent diabetes mellitus. *Arch Intern Med* 1997; 157: 1413–18.

8 Krolewski AS, Fogarty DG, Warram JH. Hypertension and nephropathy in diabetes mellitus: what is inherited and what is acquired? *Diabetes Res Clin Prac* 1998; 39 (Suppl): S1–14.

9 Quinn M, Angelico MC, Warram JH, Krolewski AS. Familial factors determine the development of diabetic nephropathy

in patients with IDDM. *Diabetologia* 1996; 39: 940–5.

10 Mogensen CE, Keane WF, Bennett PH *et al*. Prevention of diabetic renal disease with special reference to microalbuminuria. *Lancet* 1995; 346: 1080–4.

11 Stephenson JM, Fuller JH. Microalbuminuria is not rare before 5 years of IDDM. EURODIAB IDDM Complications Study Group and the WHO Multinational Study of Vascular Disease in Diabetes Study Group. *J Diabetes and its Complications* 1994; 8: 166–73.

12 Barnes DJ, Viberti GC. Strategies for the prevention of diabetic kidney disease: early antihypertensive treatment or improved glycemic control? *J Diabetes and its Complications* 1994; 8: 189–92.

13 Mathiesen ER, Oxenboll B, Johansen K, Svendsen PA, Deckert T. Incipient nephropathy in type 1 (insulin-dependent) diabetes. *Diabetologia* 1984; 26: 406–10.

14 Mogensen CE, Christensen CK. Predicting diabetic nephropathy in insulin-dependent patients. *N Engl J Med* 1984; 311: 89–93.

15 Walker JD, Close CF, Jones SL *et al*. Glomerular structure in type-1 (insulin-dependent) diabetic patients with normo- and microalbuminuria. *Kidney Int* 1992; 41: 741–8.

16 Fioretto P, Mauer M. Glomerular changes in normo- and microalbuminuric patients with long-standing insulin-dependent diabetes mellitus. *Adv Nephrol* 1997; 26: 247–63.

17 Osterby R, Bangstad HJ, Nyberg G, Walker JD, Viberti GC. A quantitative ultrastructural study of juxtaglomerular arterioles in IDDM patients with micro- and normoalbuminuria. *Diabetologia* 1995; 38: 1320–7.

18 Rudberg S, Osterby R. Decreasing glomerular filtration rate—an indicator of more advanced diabetic glomerulopathy in the early course of microalbuminuria in IDDM adolescents? *Nephrology, Dialysis, Transplantation* 1997; 12: 1149–54.

19 Bangstad HJ, Osterby R, Dahl-Jorgensen K *et al*. Early glomerulopathy is present in young, type 1 (insulin-dependent) diabetic patients with microalbuminuria. *Diabetologia* 1993; 36: 523–9.

20 Bianchi S, Bigazzi R, Campese VM. Microalbuminuria in essential hypertension. *J Nephrol* 1997; 10: 216–19.

21 Fioretto P, Mauer M, Brocco E *et al*. Patterns of renal injury in NIDDM patients with microalbuminuria. *Diabetologia* 1996; 39: 1569–76.

22 Bertani T, Gambara V, Remuzzi G. Structural basis of diabetic nephropathy in microalbuminuric NIDDM patients: a light microscopy study. *Diabetologia* 1996; 39: 1625–8.

23 Kanauchi M, Ishihara K, Nishioka H, Nishiura K, Dohi K. Glomerular lesions in patients with non-insulin-dependent diabetes mellitus and microalbuminuria. *Intern Med* 1993; 32: 753–7.

24 Schmitz A, Vaeth M. Microalbuminuria: a major risk factor in non insulin dependent diabetes. A 10 year follow up study of 503 patients. *Diabet Med* 1988; 5: 126–34.

25 Macleod JM, Lutale J, Marshall SM. Albumin excretion and vascular deaths in NIDDM. *Diabetologia* 1995; 38: 610–16.

26 Messent JW, Elliott TG, Hill RD, Jarrett RJ, Keen H, Viberti GC. Prognostic significance of microalbuminuria in insulin-dependent diabetes mellitus: a twenty-three year follow-up study. *Kidney Int* 1992; 41: 836–9.

27 Earle KA, Mishra M, Morocutti A *et al*. Microalbuminuria as a marker of silent myocardial ischaemia in IDDM patients. *Diabetologia* 1996; 39: 854–6.

28 Mattock MB, Barnes DJ, Viberti G *et al*. Microalbuminuria and coronary heart disease in NIDDM: an incidence study. *Diabetes* 1998; 47: 1786–92.

29 Microalbuminuria Collaborative Study Group United Kingdom. Risk factors for development of microalbuminuria in insulin dependent diabetic patients: a cohort study. *BMJ* 1993; 306: 1235–9.

30 Mathiesen ER, Ronn B, Jensen T, Storm B, Deckert T. Relationship between blood pressure and urinary albumin excretion in development of microalbuminuria. *Diabetes* 1990; 39: 245–9.

31 Haneda M, Kikkawa R, Togawa M *et al.* High blood pressure is a risk factor for the development of microalbuminuria in Japanese subjects with non-insulin-dependent diabetes mellitus. *J Diabetes and its Complications* 1992; 6: 181–5.

32 Nelson RG, Pettitt DJ, Baird HR *et al.* Pre-diabetic blood pressure predicts urinary albumin excretion after the onset of type 2 (non-insulin-dependent) diabetes mellitus in Pima Indians. *Diabetologia* 1993; 36: 998–1001.

33 UKPDS Prospective Diabetes Study (UKPDS) Group. Tight blood pressure control and risk of macrovascular and microvascular complications in type 2 diabetes: UKPDS 38. UK Prospective Diabetes Study Group. *BMJ* 1998; 317: 703–13.

34 Sochett EB, Poon I, Balfe W, Daneman D. Ambulatory blood pressure monitoring in insulin-dependent diabetes mellitus adolescents with and without microalbuminuria. *J Diabetes and its Complications* 1998; 12: 18–23.

35 Garg SK, Chase HP, Icaza G, Rothman RL, Osberg I, Carmain JA. 24-hour ambulatory blood pressure and renal disease in young subjects with type I diabetes. *J Diabetes and its Complications* 1997; 11: 263–7.

36 Mitchell TH, Nolan B, Henry M, Cronin C, Baker H, Greely G. Microalbuminuria in patients with non-insulin-dependent diabetes mellitus relates to nocturnal systolic blood pressure. *Am J Med* 1997; 102: 531–5.

37 Equiluz-Bruck S, Schnack C, Kopp HP, Schernthaner G. Nondipping of nocturnal blood pressure is related to urinary albumin excretion rate in patients with type 2 diabetes mellitus. *Am J Hypertens* 1996; 9: 1139–43.

38 Mogensen CE. Systemic blood pressure and glomerular leakage with particular reference to diabetes and hypertension. *J Intern Med* 1994; 235: 297–316.

39 Tarnow L, Rossing P, Gall MA, Nielsen FS, Parving HH. Prevalence of arterial hypertension in diabetic patients before and after the JNC-V. *Diabetes Care* 1994; 17: 1247–51.

40 Jensen JS, Feldt-Rasmussen B, Borch-Johnsen K, Clausen P, Appleyard M, Jensen G. Microalbuminuria and its relation to cardiovascular disease and risk factors. A population-based study of 1254 hypertensive individuals. *J Human Hypertens* 1997; 11: 727–32.

41 Jones SL, Close CF, Mattock MB, Jarrett RJ, Keen H, Viberti GC. Plasma lipid and coagulation factor concentrations in insulin dependent diabetics with microalbuminuria. *BMJ* 1989; 298: 487–90.

42 Lahdenpera S, Groop PH, Tilly-Kiesi M *et al.* LDL subclasses in IDDM patients: relation to diabetic nephropathy. *Diabetologia* 1994; 37: 681–8.

43 Uusitupa MI, Niskanen LK, Siitonen O, Voutilainen E, Pyorala K. Ten-year cardiovascular mortality in relation to risk factors and abnormalities in lipoprotein composition in type 2 (non-insulin-dependent) diabetic and non-diabetic subjects. *Diabetologia* 1993; 36: 1175–84.

44 Fioretto P, Stehouwer CD, Mauer M *et al.* Heterogeneous nature of microalbuminuria in NIDDM: studies of endothelial function and renal structure. *Diabetologia* 1998; 41: 233–6.

45 Gruden G, Pagano G, Romagnoli R, Frezet D, Olivetti C, Cavallo-Perin P. Thrombomodulin levels in insulin-dependent diabetic patients with microalbuminuria. *Diabet Med* 1995; 12: 258–60.

46 Gruden G, Cavallo-Perin P, Bazzan M, Stella S, Vuolo A, Pagano G. PAI-1 and factor VII activity are higher in IDDM patients with microalbuminuria. *Diabetes* 1994; 43: 426–9.

47 Greaves M, Malia RG, Goodfellow K *et al.* Fibrinogen and von Willebrand factor in IDDM: relationships to lipid vascular risk factors, blood pressure, glycaemic control and urinary albumin excretion rate: the EURODIAB IDDM Complications Study. *Diabetologia* 1997; 40: 698–705.

48 Hofmann MA, Kohl B, Zumbach MS *et al.* Hyperhomocyst(e)inemia and endothelial dysfunction in IDDM. *Diabetes Care* 1997; 20: 1880–6.

49 Hofmann MA, Kohl B, Zumbach MS
et al. Hyperhomocyst(e)inemia and
endothelial dysfunction in IDDM.
Diabetes Care 1998; 21: 841–8.

50 Stehouwer CD, Fischer HR, van Kuijk
AW, Polak BC, Donker AJ. Endothelial
dysfunction precedes development of
microalbuminuria in IDDM. Diabetes
1995; 44: 561–4.

51 Perry IJ. Urinary microalbumin excretion
in early pregnancy and gestational age at
delivery. BMJ 1993; 307: 420–1.

52 Konstantin-Hansen KF, Hesseldahl H,
Pedersen SM. Microalbuminuria as a
predictor of pre-eclampsia. Acta Obstet
Gynecol Scand 1992; 71: 343–6.

53 Winocour PH, Taylor RJ. Early
alterations of renal function in insulin
dependent diabetic pregnancies and their
importance in predicting pre-eclamptic
toxaemia. Diabetes Res 1989; 10:
159–64.

54 Allawi J, Rao PV, Gilbert R et al.
Microalbuminuria in non-insulin-
dependent diabetes: its prevalence
in Indian compared with Europid
patients. BMJ Clin Res Edn 1988;
296: 462–4.

55 Araki S, Haneda M, Togawa M et al.
Microalbuminuria is not associated with
cardiovascular death in Japanese
NIDDM. Diabetes Res Clin Prac 1997;
35: 35–40.

56 Marshall SM, Shearing PA, Alberti KG.
Micral-test strips evaluated for screening
for albuminuria. Clin Chem 1992; 38:
588–91.

57 Marshall SM. Screening for
microalbuminuria: which measurement?
Diabet Med 1991; 8: 706–11.

58 Mogensen CE. High blood pressure as a
factor in the progression of diabetic
nephropathy. Acta Med Scand Suppl
1976; 602: 29–32.

59 The Microalbuminuria Captopril Study
Group. Captopril reduces the risk of
nephropathy in IDDM patients with
microalbuminuria. The Microalbuminuria Captopril Study Group.
Diabetologia 1996; 39: 587–93.

60 Crepaldi G, Carta Q, Deferrari G et al.
Effects of lisinopril and nifedipine on
the progression to overt albuminuria
in IDDM patients with incipient
nephropathy and normal blood pressure.
The Italian Microalbuminuria Study
Group in IDDM. Diabetes Care 1998;
21: 104–10.

61 Kasiske BL, Kalil RS, Ma JZ, Liao M,
Keane WF. Effect of antihypertensive
therapy on the kidney in patients with
diabetes: a meta-regression analysis.
Ann Intern Med 1993; 118: 129–38.

62 The Ace Inhibitors in Diabetic
Nephropathy Trialist Group E. When
should ACE inhibitors be used in IDDM?
A combined analysis of clinical trials.
Diabetologia 1998; 41 (Suppl 1):
(abstract) 4A.

63 Ravid M, Brosh D, Levi Z, Bar-Dayan Y,
Ravid D, Rachmani R. Use of enalapril to
attenuate decline in renal function in
normotensive, normoalbuminuric
patients with type 2 diabetes mellitus. A
randomized, controlled trial. Ann Intern
Med 1998; 128: 982–8.

64 Sano T, Hotta N, Kawanura T,
Matsumae H et al. Effects of long-term
enalapril treatment on persistent
microalbuminuria in normotensive type 2
diabetic patients: results of a 4-year,
prospective randomized study. Diabet
Med 1996; 13: 120–4.

65 Estacio RO, Jeffers BW, Hiatt WR,
Biggerstaff SL, Gifford N, Schrier RW.
The effect of nisoldipine as compared
with enalapril on cardiovascular
outcomes in patients with non-insulin-
dependent diabetes and hypertension.
N Engl J Med 1998; 338: 645–52.

66 Heart Outcomes Prevention Evaluation
(HOPE) Study Investigators. Effects of
Ramipril on cardiovascular and
microvascular outcomes in people with
diabetes mellitus: results of the HOPE
study and MICRO-HOPE substudy.
Lancet 2000; 355: 253–9.

67 Parving HH, Jacobsen P, Tarnow L et al.
Effect of deletion polymorphism of
angiotensin converting enzyme gene on
progression of diabetic nephropathy
during inhibition of angiotensin
converting enzyme: observational follow
up study. BMJ 1996; 313: 591–4.

68 The Diabetes Control and Complications Trial Research Group. The effect of intensive treatment of diabetes on the development and progression of long-term complications in insulin-dependent diabetes mellitus. *N Engl J Med* 1993; 329: 977–86.

69 UKPDS Prospective Diabetes Study (UKPDS) Group. Intensive blood-glucose control with sulphonylureas or insulin compared with conventional treatment and risk of complications in patients with type 2 diabetes (UKPDS 33). *Lancet* 1998; 352: 837–53.

70 Microalbuminuria Collaborative Study Group United Kingdom. Intensive therapy and progression to clinical albuminuria in patients with insulin dependent diabetes mellitus and microalbuminuria. *BMJ* 1995; 311: 973–7.

71 The Diabetes Control and Complications Trial Research Group. Effect of intensive diabetes treatment on the development and progression of long-term complications in adolescents with insulin-dependent diabetes mellitus. *J Pediatr* 1994; 125: 177–88.

72 Bangstad HJ, Osterby R, Dahl-Jorgensen K, Berg KJ, Hartmann A, Hanssen KF. Improvement of blood glucose control in IDDM patients retards the progression of morphological changes in early diabetic nephropathy. *Diabetologia* 1994; 37: 483–90.

73 Fioretto P, Steffes MW, Sutherland DE, Goetz FC, Mauer M. Reversal of lesions of diabetic nephropathy after pancreas transplantation. *N Engl J Med* 1998; 339: 69–75.

74 Cohen D, Dodds R, Viberti GC. Effect of protein restriction in insulin dependent diabetics at risk of nephropathy. *Br Med J Clin Res Edn* 1987; 294: 795–8.

75 Orth SR, Ritz E, Schrier RW. The renal risks of smoking. *Kidney Int* 1997; 51: 1669–77.

Management issues in type 2 diabetes

5: Is obesity realistically treatable in type 2 diabetes?

John Wilding

Introduction

Obesity is arguably the greatest challenge that remains in the management of diabetes, yet it is often conveniently dismissed as being untreatable, leading to almost total therapeutic nihilism, or at best a referral to the dietician. Yet obesity is the leading aetiological factor in the pathogenesis of type 2 diabetes, and underlies the current worldwide pandemic of this condition [1]. It is a major obstacle to the successful treatment of both type 1 and type 2 diabetes, with weight gain being second only to hypoglycaemia as a complication of treatment with insulin and sulphonylureas [2–4]. Many of the complications of diabetes and associated conditions, including dyslipidaemia, hypertension, ischaemic heart disease and stroke, could be considered as much complications of the associated obesity as they are of the diabetes itself. Even problems such as foot ulcers may be less likely to heal if the patient is obese. Of course, it is possible to argue that with modern antihypertensive, lipid-lowering and oral hypoglycaemic drugs, the adverse effects of obesity can be effectively neutralized, but this ignores the mechanical, psychosocial and quality of life effects of obesity that are often the major concern of obese patients [5]. Despite this scepticism, there is now a growing body of good evidence, much of it from randomized trials, that obesity is treatable in many patients with type 2 diabetes, and that effective management of this problem can improve important short-term outcome measures, such as HbA_{1c}, hypertension and dyslipidaemia. There is also evidence that effective obesity treatment may delay or even prevent diabetes in at-risk obese subjects, yet so far there has been little concerted effort to manage this growing health problem.

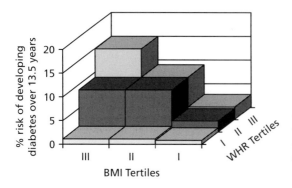

Fig. 5.1 The risk of developing diabetes is greatest in patients with a high waist circumference, indicating central obesity. Data from Ohlson *et al.* [8].

What is meant by obesity?

Although most epidemiological studies reporting the relationship between body weight and disease have used body mass index (BMI; weight in kg/height in m) [2]) as a measure of adiposity [6,7], it has recently become evident that this only tells part of the story. Measurements that take into account the amount of body fat, and particularly the distribution of body fat, are in fact much better than BMI at predicting who is likely to develop diabetes and the related metabolic abnormalities [8] (Fig. 5.1). Furthermore, in some populations (for example Asians living in the UK), substantially increased risk can occur at relatively low BMI, but with a relatively high waist : hip ratio, leading to the concept that such subjects are 'metabolically obese' [9]. Even this concept may not provide the entire picture, as recent research from animal models suggests that lipid deposits at other sites, notably within skeletal muscle, may contribute to insulin resistance and that lipid accumulation within the β-cells may impair their function, and ultimately lead to β-cell death [10].

Gluttony, sloth or just fat?

It is difficult to control for physical activity levels in epidemiological studies, and given the strong associations between obesity and physical inactivity, it is important to question the possible role of physical inactivity in the pathogenesis of type 2 diabetes, independent of body fat content. Even short periods of physical inactivity result in insulin resistance in non-diabetic subjects [11], and longer periods may contribute to lipid accumulation in muscle and dyslipidaemia, which may increase diabetes risk [12]. Hence, it is not entirely clear how much of the diabetes risk associated with obesity is in fact due to the low levels of physical activity seen in the obese population. Studies where rapid changes in nutrient availability occur, either using very low calorie diets, a protein-sparing modified fast or immediately following surgical treatment for obesity, suggest that flux of nutrients may be more important than was previously thought, as the metabolic improvement often precedes any decline in weight in these patients [13,14]. Furthermore, the content of the diet may also contribute to the associated metabolic risk, via a number of mechanisms, including hyperinsulinaemia with high levels of low glycaemic index carbohydrate, oxidative stress and the type of lipid in the diet [15], so that even for a given BMI or waist circumference, risk may vary according to the composition of the diet. Of course, each of these phenomena are interdependent, and it seems likely that these factors are all important in explaining the link between obesity, diabetes and the metabolic syndrome, but that some may predominate in certain individuals.

Does weight loss prevent diabetes?

There is now extensive evidence from animal studies, and a growing body of data from humans, that demonstrate that if obesity can be prevented or treated at an early stage, then diabetes is less likely to develop.

Animal studies

A number of studies in rats and mice with inherited syndromes of obesity, insulin resistance and diabetes have shown that if weight gain is prevented by energy restriction, or with anorectic drugs, then insulin sensitivity improves, and diabetes is less likely to develop [16]; the same is true in genetically normal animals made obese by feeding a highly palatable diet [17]. The most convincing animal data, perhaps of greater relevance to humans, is a long-term study in diabetes-prone Rhesus monkeys, which demonstrates that long-term energy restriction is effective at preventing the onset of diabetes [18].

Human studies

Epidemiological studies suggest that in subjects who intentionally lose weight, the chances of developing diabetes is reduced by up to 50% with a 5-kg weight loss [7]; diabetes-related death is also reduced by up to 40% [19]; this is also supported by a retrospective study in a Scottish diabetic clinic

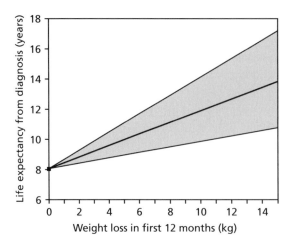

Fig. 5.2 Weight loss during the first 12 months from diagnosis of diabetes is predictive of life expectancy. Shaded areas indicate 95% confidence intervals. Adapted from Lean *et al.* [20] with permission.

population (Fig. 5.2). A number of intervention studies have looked at the effect of lifestyle intervention with diet and exercise at preventing or delaying the onset of type 2 diabetes, and several larger studies, with a treatment arm including lifestyle intervention, notably the Diabetes Prevention Program in the USA, are under way [21]. Studies in obese patients with impaired glucose tolerance in Sweden and China have demonstrated that even a modest weight loss of 2–4% is associated with improved insulin sensitivity and a reduced risk of progression to type 2 diabetes over a 6-year period [22,23]. This is supported by a recent analysis of data derived from studies of the antiobesity drug orlistat, which show improvements in glucose tolerance, and less risk of progression from normal to impaired glucose tolerance, or from impaired glucose tolerance to diabetes in treated patients who lost more weight [24]. Surgical studies, where profound weight loss has occurred, have produced some very impressive results. In a retrospective analysis of over 700 patients, treated for severe obesity with a gastric bypass procedure, Pories and colleagues have shown that of the 50% of these patients with impaired glucose tolerance (IGT) or type 2 diabetes, 80% remained normoglycaemic after up to 14 years follow-up [13]. The Swedish Obese Subjects study has now reported 2-year data on 845 surgically treated patients with severe obesity, compared with 845 matched controls managed by conventional means. Mean weight loss in the surgical group was 28 kg, vs 0.5 kg in the control group, and this was associated with a reduction in diabetes from 6.5% in the control group, to less than 0.5% in the intervention group (OR 0.02; 95% CI 0–0.16) (Fig. 5.3). These improvements were also associated with lower

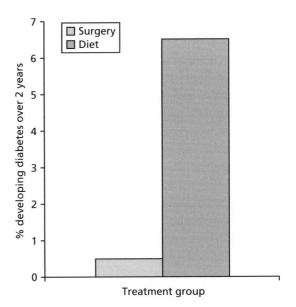

Fig. 5.3 Surgically induced weight loss is effective at preventing diabetes. Data from Sjostrom *et al.* [25].

blood pressure, and improved lipid profiles [25,26]. Taken together, these data imply that weight loss in obese patients is likely to reduce the incidence of type 2 diabetes, and that although the magnitude of the reduction is proportional to the degree of weight loss, beneficial effects are seen even with very modest weight loss in subjects at high risk by virtue of having glucose intolerance.

Can obesity be made safe?

Current management options for diabetes assume an approach that favours treating the metabolic and physical consequences of obesity, without necessarily addressing the underlying causes. Such approaches are certainly effective, and there is now a wealth of trial evidence to support the use of oral hypoglycaemic drugs and insulin to control hyperglycaemia (with a target HbA_{1c} below 7%), a range of antihypertensive drugs to reduce blood pressure to a target blood pressure below 140/85 mmHg, and use of lipid-lowering agents (principally statins) in most patients with a serum cholesterol above 5 mmol/l [27–29]. Thus, polypharmacy has become the norm in the diabetic clinic, and perhaps is allowing physicians, other healthcare professionals and patients to become complacent about treating the obesity that often underlies diabetes and associated metabolic disorders.

Thiazolidinediones—breaking the link between obesity and diabetes?

The newest class of drugs being used to treat diabetes, the thiazolidinediones, are agonists at the peroxisome proliferator activated receptor γ (PPAR-γ), and improve insulin resistance, and thus control of diabetes, principally by reducing the availability of non-esterified fatty acids (NEFA) as competition for glucose metabolism in skeletal muscle. Paradoxically, weight gain occurs with long-term treatment, but the amount of visceral fat is reduced, and the amount of sub-cutaneous fat increased [30]. In animal models the thiazolidinediones have been found to reduce triglyceride accumulation in islets [31], and reduce accumulation of fat in skeletal muscle [32]. Thus, this class of drugs appears to be able to dissociate some of the metabolic consequences of obesity from the obesity itself, and also remodel fat distribution in such a way that it is metabolically less harmful. Nevertheless, in animal models at least, prevention of thiazolidinedione-induced weight gain by energy restriction does result in greater improvements in metabolic control, indicating that such agents are not able to completely neutralize the adverse effects of obesity [17]. Newer agents in development include non-thiazolidinedione PPAR-γ agonists with antihypertensive properties [33], and agents which are also agonists at the PPAR-α receptor, the target for the fibrate group of drugs. Clearly, these agents have the potential to improve several aspects of the metabolic consequences of obesity simultaneously, but their effectiveness and future place in the range of therapies available for the obese diabetic patient remain to be clarified. Of course, while these drugs may offer some protection against the metabolic consequences of obesity, they will not improve other obesity-related problems such as breathlessness, joint pain or the risks associated with surgery.

Can the obese diabetic be treated with diet and lifestyle modification?

It is standard teaching that diet and exercise are the 'cornerstone' of management of type 2 diabetes, but what is the evidence that such interventions are effective at improving outcome measures such as glycaemic control, blood pressure and lipids, or perhaps more importantly, at influencing hard endpoints such as microvascular and macrovascular complications or mortality? This question is impossible to answer directly, as the study of lifestyle intervention versus no intervention at all has never, and probably will never, be carried out. Secondly, is it possible to improve outcomes by giving advice in a different way, or by using the techniques of behavioural psychology?

Dietary advice

There is a wealth of short-term studies demonstrating that weight loss with conventional 500–800-kcal deficit diets or with more rapid weight loss using, for example, a very low calorie diet [34] are effective at improving glycaemic control in patients with type 2 diabetes, but in general these interventions are difficult to sustain in the long term, and most patients regain the lost weight within 12 months [35].

The United Kingdom Prospective Diabetes Study (UKPDS) reported effects of dietary management alone, compared with sulphonylurea, metformin or insulin as primary treatment in obese patients with type 2 diabetes. Whilst it was clear that early intervention with pharmacological treatment results in superior results in terms of glycaemic control and outcome measures such as macrovascular complications, weight gain was a significant problem with all patients on pharmacological therapy, with the exception of the subgroup of obese patients treated with metformin, which was effectively weight neutral. Interestingly, this metformin-treated subgroup fared better overall, with a 32% reduction in diabetes-related endpoints (vs 12% for the main study) and a reduction in myocardial infarction (39% risk reduction) or death (36% risk reduction), which did not occur in the other intensively treated groups [36]. There are a number of potential explanations for this observation, but an effect secondary to the difference in weight between the groups is an interesting possibility.

Behaviour modification

A study by Wing *et al.* reports effects of a diet and behavioural programme on weight loss and glycaemic control over 2 years in patients with type 2 diabetes [37]. Mean weight loss in this study was 5.6%, and glycaemic control improved in proportion to the amount of weight lost. Patients losing 5% or more of body weight had improvements in HbA_{1c}, which fell by 1.6% in patients losing more than 10% of body weight. Although the intensive nature of this intervention, which included weekly group sessions, would make it an unrealistic option for the 100 million plus diabetic patients worldwide, the study is important in that it makes the point that behaviour change can result in meaningful weight loss in patients with type 2 diabetes, and that this weight loss does result in improved glycaemic control. Furthermore, many of the principles used in these studies are now incorporated into the advice given to many patients.

Drugs

The use of pharmacotherapy to help manage obese patients with diabetes has been controversial, and the withdrawal of the anorectic drugs fenfluramine and dexfenfluramine because of side-effects of primary pulmonary hypertension, cardiac valvular disease, and older amphetamine derivatives because of abuse potential, has understandably led to scepticism about the use of new agents. Nevertheless, two drugs, orlistat and sibutramine, have been found to be effective in patients with type 2 diabetes.

Orlistat

Orlistat is an intestinal lipase inhibitor that is not systemically absorbed; it results in failure to absorb about 30% of dietary fat [38], which would be expected to give a calorie deficit of about 200 kcal/day for an individual on a 2250-kcal diet of which 40% of calories come from fat (Fig. 5.4). In order to achieve a desired rate of weight loss of about 0.5 kg per week, a calorie deficit of 500 kcal/day is needed. The additional deficit must come from dietary restriction and increased physical activity; the side-effects of orlistat may help reinforce this, by helping patients to keep to a diet that is relatively low in fat. In trials of orlistat in non-diabetic subjects, the mean weight loss achieved is approximately 9.5 kg over 1 year (vs 5 kg for placebo); slight weight gain occurred during the second year of these studies, but this may be a consequence of the study design, as subjects were encouraged to follow a eucaloric diet for the second year of the study, with the aim of maintaining weight,

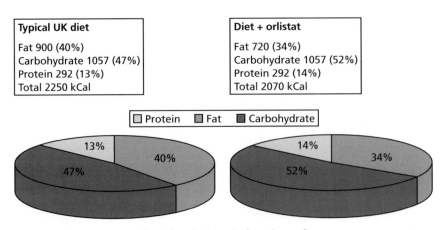

Typical UK diet
Fat 900 (40%)
Carbohydrate 1057 (47%)
Protein 292 (13%)
Total 2250 kCal

Diet + orlistat
Fat 720 (34%)
Carbohydrate 1057 (52%)
Protein 292 (14%)
Total 2070 kCal

□ Protein   ■ Fat   ■ Carbohydrate

13%   40%   47%

14%   34%   52%

Fig. 5.4 Orlistat treatment reduces the calorie intake from dietary fat.

rather than encouraging further weight loss [39,40]. A study designed to look at patients given revised dietary advice with the aim of producing continued weight loss is underway (the xenical diabetes obesity study, XENDOS) [41]. The reduced body weight seen in these studies was mostly fat, and the reductions in waist circumference seen indicate that a significant proportion of this was visceral fat. Modest reductions in blood pressure, lipids and insulin concentrations were seen in these normotensive subjects without hyperlipidaemia. Studies in subjects at greater cardiovascular risk are awaited.

One study using orlistat has looked specifically at the treatment of subjects with type 2 diabetes treated with sulphonylurea monotherapy, and has been reported in full [42]. This study randomized 391 subjects to receive either orlistat 120 mg tds or placebo for 1 year. Outcome measures included weight loss, reduction in waist circumference and improvement in HbA_{1c}. Other factors looked at included lipids, blood pressure and the dose of sulphonylurea needed to maintain diabetes control. Mean weight loss in the diabetic subjects treated with orlistat was 6.2% vs 4.3% with placebo. It should be noted that this is considerably less than is seen in non-diabetic subjects, and may reflect the difficulty that many patients with type 2 diabetes have in losing weight. Despite the relatively small difference in mean weight between the study groups, 49% of orlistat-treated patients achieved a weight loss of 5%, compared to 23% of placebo. This was associated with a mean improvement in HbA_{1c} of 0.4%. This may seem modest, but taken in the context of the epidemiological analysis of the UKPDS, and given the difficulty in maintaining glycaemic control in many patients with type 2 diabetes, this is certainly a significant improvement.

Sibutramine

Sibutramine is a selective serotonin and noradrenaline (norepinephrine) reuptake inhibitor that is now licensed in several countries for the treatment of obesity. When used in combination with a 500-kcal-deficit diet, it improves weight loss in non-diabetic subjects, with a mean weight loss of 5.5% at a dose of 10 mg and 7.2% at a dose of 15 mg, and has also been shown to promote weight maintenance when used in combination with a very low calorie diet [43]. A greater proportion of patients achieve a 5% or 10% weight loss with sibutramine than with placebo. Side-effects of sibutramine are related to its sympathomimetic action, and include a modest (4–6 beats per minute) rise in heart rate and a small increase in blood pressure in a minority of patients [44]. In diabetic patients treated with diet or oral agents, sibutramine is also effective at promoting weight loss, although, as with orlistat and other treatments for obesity in diabetic patients, less weight loss is seen in this patient group [45]. Weight loss is associated with improvements in HbA_{1c} that are proportional to the degree of weight loss; with significant improvements, specifically a reduction in HbA_{1c} of 0.4% seen in responders who lost >5% of body weight [46]. The results of larger studies in diet-, sulphonylurea- and metformin-treated patients are awaited.

A role for diabetes prevention?

Although patients enrolled in most of the studies of orlistat described above did not have diabetes, all patients had measurements of fasting glucose and insulin at baseline and at the end of the 1-year or 2-year treatment period, and underwent glucose tolerance testing at the start and end of the study. Patients not known to have diabetes, but who were found to have diabetes or impaired glucose tolerance not requiring treatment with oral hypoglycaemic drugs, were able to continue as subjects in these studies. This has allowed an analysis of all the available data, with the aim of determining if weight loss associated with orlistat treatment resulted in changes in insulin sensitivity, as assessed using the homeostasis model assessment (HOMA) method and also to see if patients' glucose tolerance category changed during the treatment period. Orlistat-treated patients had significantly greater improvements in their insulin resistance index after 1 year compared with placebo (–0.16 vs +0.18; $P = 0.003$). Greater improvements in insulin resistance index in the orlistat group were also observed after 2 years of treatment (–0.08 vs +0.39; $P < 0.001$). Furthermore, the improvement in insulin resistance was greatest in those patients who lost the most weight [47]. The area under the curve for glucose after the glucose challenge was less at 2 years in the orlistat-treated groups, and patients receiving active medication were less likely to deteriorate in glucose tolerance category from normal to impaired glucose tolerance or diabetes, or from impaired glucose tolerance to diabetes and those with impaired glucose tolerance or diabetes were more likely to improve [24] (Fig. 5.5). These data are consistent with studies of lifestyle intervention and with surgical studies indicating that significant weight loss can delay the onset, or perhaps prevent the development of type 2 diabetes in at-risk subjects.

Surgery

The prospect of using surgery to treat type 2 diabetes may seen drastic, but

Status at base line   **Status at 2 years**

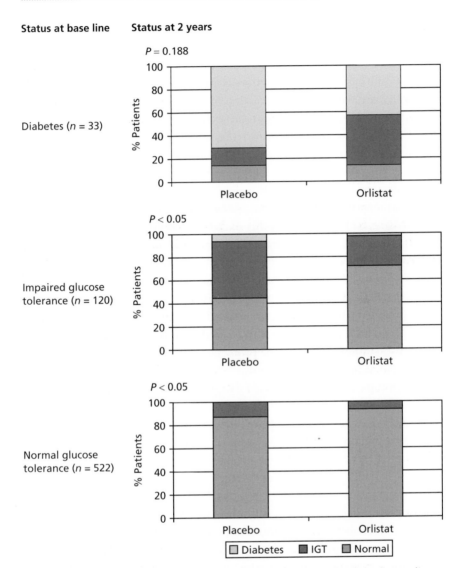

Diabetes (n = 33)

Impaired glucose
tolerance (n = 120)

Normal glucose
tolerance (n = 522)

Fig. 5.5 Data showing shift in glucose tolerance category over 12 months of placebo or orlistat treatment. Data from Heymsfield *et al.* [24].

some of the reported studies suggest that it may in fact be a very effective treatment for the condition, assuming that patients are selected appropriately. Surgical management is usually only advised for patients with severe obesity (BMI > 40 kg/m [2]), although some authorities are now suggesting that it may be used in patients with a BMI > 35 kg/m [2] if significant comorbidity is present. The procedures that are currently in use include the vertical banded gastroplasty (VBG), a variation of this (the Magenstrasse and Mill procedure) where the stomach is divided to reduced the risk of staple line failure, laporoscopic banding, and procedures which give a degree of malabsorption, such as gastric reduction with creation of a Roux-en-Y loop [48]. The latter procedure may result in dumping, and some vitamin malabsorption, but generally produces greater weight loss than the gastric reduction procedures. Surgical results are generally reported as percentage of excess weight lost, and results range from 50% for gastroplasty or banding to 60–70% for malabsorptive procedures. Such weight loss has been reported to result in improved metabolic control in patients with diabetes, reduced prevalence of new diabetes and reduction in other diabetes-associated comorbidity, such as hypertension and hyperlipidaemia. For example, in the retrospective series reported by Pories et al. treated with a gastric reduction procedure, combined with a Roux-en-Y loop, 121 of 146 patients (82.9%) with type 2 diabetes and 150 of 152 patients (98.7%) with impaired glucose tolerance maintained normal levels of plasma glucose, glycated haemoglobin, and insulin for up to 14 years [13]. The 2-year results from the Swedish Obese Subjects (SOS) study also support a significant protective effect of surgery, with an odds ratio for developing diabetes of 0.02 (95% CI 0–0.16) in the surgically treated group (see above and Fig. 5.3) [25]. However no study has specifically assessed the possible role of such procedures in treating type 2 diabetes in a prospective manner, but if the early results from the SOS study are confirmed long term, then this study will certainly be justified.

What of the future?

Obesity is clearly a major risk factor for type 2 diabetes, and a barrier to its effective treatment. The data now accumulating indicates that effective interventions for obesity are available that might delay or prevent the onset of this condition and that obesity management should become as much an accepted part of the therapeutic armoury for treating type 2 diabetes as oral hypoglycaemic drugs or insulin. Of course, such interventions will be expensive in terms of both time spent and drugs; the latter may be partly offset by a reduced requirement for oral hypoglycaemic drugs, antihypertensives and lipid-lowering agents. The current treatment strategies are not effective for everyone, and many patients are not ready to make the changes to their lifestyle that these require. However the development of drugs to treat obesity is still in its infancy, and our increasing understanding of the mechanisms controlling body weight is likely to lead to the development of new, perhaps more effective agents. Combination therapy for obesity is currently not considered to be safe, especially following the problems associated with phentermine–fenfluramine combinations in the USA; however, it is possible that combination therapy will re-emerge as newer agents with different modes of action are developed. The role of surgery is likely to be re-appraised once the results of the SOS study are available, but this is only likely to be a realistic option for a relatively small number of the most obese patients. Perhaps in the future we will stop thinking of ourselves as diabetologists, and instead concentrate on obesity as the greatest preventable and treatable cause of diabetes.

References

1 WHO Study Group. *Prevention of Diabetes Mellitus*. Geneva: WHO, 1997: 844.

2 United Kingdom Prospective Diabetes Study (UKPDS) 13: Relative efficacy of randomly allocated diet, sulphonylurea, insulin, or metformin in patients with newly diagnosed non-insulin dependent diabetes followed for three years. *BMJ* 1995; 310: 83–8.

3 Turner RC, Cull CA, Frighi V, Holman RR. Glycemic control with diet, sulfonylurea, metformin, or insulin in patients with type 2 diabetes mellitus—progressive requirement for multiple therapies (UKPDS 49). *JAMA* 1999; 281: 2005–12.

4 DCCT Research Group. The effect of intensive diabetes treatment on the development and progression of long-term complications in insulin-dependent diabetes mellitus: the Diabetes Control and Complications Trial. *N Engl J Med* 1993; 329: 977–86.

5 Narbro K, Agren G, Jonsson E *et al.* Sick leave and disability pension before and after treatment for obesity: a report from the Swedish Obese Subjects (SOS) study. *Int J Obesity* 1999; 23: 619–24.

6 Chan JM, Stampfer MJ, Ribb EB, Willett WC, Colditz GA. Obesity, fat distribution and weight gain as risk factors for clinical

diabetes in man. *Diabetes Care* 1994; 17: 961–9.

7 Colditz GA, Willett WC, Rotnitzky A, Manson JE. Weight-gain as a risk factor for clinical diabetes-mellitus in women. *Ann Intern Med* 1995; 122: 481–6.

8 Ohlson LO, Larsson B, Svardsudd K *et al.* The of influence body fat distribution on the incidence of diabetes mellitus. 13.5 years follow-up of the participants in the study of men born in 1913. *Diabetes* 1985; 34: 1055–8.

9 Ruderman N, Chisholm D, Pi-Sunyer X, Schneider S. The metabolically obese, normal-weight individual revisited. *Diabetes* 1998; 47: 699–713.

10 Buckingham RE, AlBarazanji KA, Toseland CDN *et al.* Peroxisome proliferator-activated receptor-gamma agonist, rosiglitazone, protects against nephropathy and pancreatic islet abnormalities in Zucker fatty rats. *Diabetes* 1998; 47: 1326–34.

11 Rosenthal M, Haskell WL, Solomon R, Widstrom A, Reaven GM. Demonstration of a relationship between physical training and insulin-stimulated glucose utilisation in normal humans. *Diabetes* 1983; 32: 408–11.

12 Eriksson J, Taimela S, Koivisto VA. Exercise and the metabolic syndrome. *Diabetologia* 1997; 40: 125–35.

13 Pories WJ, Swanson MS, MacDonald KG
   et al. Who would have thought it—an
   operation proves to be the most effective
   therapy for adult-onset diabetes-mellitus.
   Ann Surg 1995; 222: 339–52.

14 Wing RR, Blair EH, Bononi P, Marcus
   MD, Watanabe R, Bergman RN. Caloric
   restriction per se is a significant factor in
   improvements in glycemic control and
   insulin sensitivity during weight loss in
   obese NIDDM patients. Diabetes Care
   1994; 17: 30–6.

15 Storlien LH, Jenkins AB, Chisholm DJ,
   Pascoe WS, Khouri S, Kraegen EW.
   Influence of dietary fat composition on
   development of insulin resistance in rats:
   relationship to muscle triglyceride and
   ω-3 fatty acids in muscle phospholipid.
   Diabetes 1991; 40: 280–9.

16 Dubuc PU, Carlisle HJ. Food restriction
   normalizes somatic growth and diabetes
   in adrenalectomized ob/ob mice. Am J
   Physiol 1988; 255: R787–93.

17 Pickavance LC, Buckingham RE, Wilding
   JPH. Insulin-sensitising action of
   rosiglitazone is enhanced by food
   restriction. Diabetologia 1999; 42: S1
   (abstract).

18 Hansen BC, Bodkin NL. Primary
   prevention of diabetes mellitus by
   prevention of obesity in monkeys.
   Diabetes 1993; 42: 1809–14.

19 Williamson DF, Pamuk E, Thun M,
   Flanders D, Byers T, Heath C.
   Prospective study of intentional weight
   loss and mortality in never-smoking
   overweight US white women aged 40–64
   years. Am J Epidemiol 1995; 141:
   1128–41.

20 Lean MEJ, Powrie JK, Anderson AS,
   Garthwaite SPH. Obesity, weight loss and
   prognosis in type 2 diabetes. Diabet Med
   1990; 7: 228–41.

21 The Diabetes Prevention Program
   Research Group. The diabetes prevention
   program: design and methods for a
   clinical trial in the prevention of type 2
   diabetes. Diabetes Care 1999; 22:
   623–34.

22 Eriksson KF, Lindgarde F. Prevention
   of type-2 (non-insulin-dependent)
   diabetes-mellitus by diet and physical

23 Pan XR, Cao HB, Li GW et al. Effects of
   diet and exercise in preventing NIDDM in
   people with impaired glucose tolerance.
   Diabetes Care 1997; 20: 537–44.

24 Heymsfield SB, Segal KR, Hauptmann J
   et al. Effects of weight loss with orlistat
   on glucose tolerance and progression to
   impaired glucose tolerance and type 2
   diabetes in obese adults. Arch Intern Med
   2000, in press.

25 Sjostrom CD, Lissner L, Wedel H,
   Sjostrom L. Reduction in incidence of
   diabetes, hypertension and lipid
   disturbances after intentional weight loss
   induced by bariatric surgery: the SOS
   Intervention Study. Obesity Res 1999; 7:
   477–84.

26 Karason K, Wallentin L, Larsson B,
   Sjostrom L. Effects of obesity and weight
   loss on left ventricular mass and relative
   wall thickness: survey and intervention
   study. BMJ 1997; 315: 912–16.

27 United Kingdom Prospective Diabetes
   Study (UKPDS) 38: Tight blood pressure
   control and risk of macrovascular and
   macrovascular complications in type 2
   diabetes. BMJ 1998; 317: 703–13.

28 Anonymous. Effect of intensive blood
   glucose control with metformin on
   complications in overweight patients with
   type 2 diabetes (UKPDS 34). Lancet 1998;
   352: 854–65.

29 Ramsey LE, Williams B, Johnston JD,
   MacGregor GA, Poston L, Potter JF.
   British Hypertension Guidelines for
   hypertension management. BMJ 1999;
   319: 630–5.

30 Kelly IE, Han TS, Walsh K, Lean MEJ.
   Effects of a thiazolidinedione compound
   on body fat and fat distribution of
   patients with type 2 diabetes. Diabetes
   Care 1999; 22: 288–93.

31 Pickavance LC, Widdowson PS, Foster
   JR, Ishii S, Tanaka H, Williams G. The
   thiazolidinedione, MCC-555, prevents
   nitric oxide synthase induction in the
   pancreas of the Zucker Diabetic Fatty rat.
   Br J Pharmacol 1999; 128: 116–21.

32 Sreenan S, Keck S, Fuller T, Cockburn B,
   Burant CF. Effects of troglitazone on

substrate storage and utilization in insulin-resistant rats. *Am J Physiol Endocrinol Metab* 1999; 39: E1119–29.

33 Buchanan TA, Meehan WP, Jeng YY et al. Blood-pressure-lowering by pioglitazone—evidence for a direct vascular effect. *J Clin Invest* 1995; 96: 354–60.

34 Hanefield M, Weck M. Very low calorie diet therapy in obese non-insulin dependent diabetes patients. *Int J Obesity* 1989; 13: 33–7.

35 Wing RR, Blair E, Marcus M, Epstein LH, Harvey J. Year-long weight-loss treatment for obese patients with type-II diabetes—does including an intermittent very-low-calorie diet improve outcome. *Am J Med* 1994; 97: 354–62.

36 Turner RC, Holman RR, Stratton IM et al. Effect of intensive blood-glucose control with metformin on complications in overweight patients with type 2 diabetes (UKPDS 34). *Lancet* 1998; 352: 854–65.

37 Wing RR, Koeske R, Epstein LH, Nowalk MP, Gooding W, Becker D. Long-term effects of modest weight-loss in type-II diabetic patients. *Arch Intern Med* 1987; 147: 1749–53.

38 Zhi J, Melia AT, Guerciolini R et al. Retrospective population-based analysis of the dose–response (fecal fat excretion) relationship of orlistat in normal and obese volunteers. *Clin Pharmacol Ther* 1994; 56: 82–5.

39 Davidson MH, Hauptman J, DiGirolamo M et al. Weight control and risk factor reduction in obese subjects treated for 2 years with orlistat—a randomized controlled trial. *JAMA* 1999; 281: 235–42.

40 Sjostrom L, Rissanen A, Andersen T et al. Randomised placebo-controlled trial of orlistat for weight loss and prevention of weight regain in obese patients. *Lancet* 1998; 352: 167–72.

41 Torgerson J, Kappi M, Arlinger K, Bergmark G, Lantz H, Sjostrom L. The XENDOS study: logistics and outcome of recruitment. *Diabetes* 1998; 47: 1324.

42 Hollander PA, Elbein SC, Hirsch IB et al. Role of orlistat in the treatment of obese patients with type 2 diabetes—a 1-year randomized double-blind study. *Diabetes Care* 1998; 21: 1288–94.

43 Apfelbaum M, Vague P, Ziegler O, Hanotin C, Thomas F, Leutenegger E. Long-term maintenance of weight loss after a very-low-calorie diet: a randomized blinded trial of the efficacy and tolerability of sibutramine. *Am J Med* 1999; 106: 179–84.

44 Bray GA, Blackburn GL, Ferguson JM et al. Sibutramine produces dose-related weight loss. *Obesity Res* 1999; 7: 189–98.

45 Wing RR, Marcus MD, Epstein LH, Salata R. Type II diabetic subjects lose less weight than their overweight nondiabetic spouses. *Diabetes Care* 1987; 10: 563–6.

46 Finer N, Bloom SR, Frost GS, Banks LM, Griffiths J. Sibutramine is effective for weight loss and diabetic control in obesity with type 2 diabetes: a randomized, double-blind, placebo-controlled study. *Diabetes, Obesity and Metabolism* 2000; 2: 105–12.

47 Wilding JPH. Orlistat-induced weight loss improves insulin resistance in obese patients. *Diabetologia* 1999; 42 (Suppl 1): 807.

48 Mason EE. Past, present, and future of obesity surgery. *Obesity Surg* 1998; 8: 524–9.

6: What are the options for oral agent treatment of type 2 diabetes?

Michael Berger and Ingrid Mühlhauser

Therapeutic objectives

Before discussing the options for oral agent treatment of type 2 diabetes, it is mandatory to define the principal therapeutic objectives in terms of patient-orientated outcome goals [1]. First, patients' quality of life needs to be maintained as close to normal as possible by preventing acute complications and hyperglycaemia-related symptoms and by avoiding unnecessary iatrogenic interventions, such as unhelpful diagnostic procedures, a rigid dietary regimen and superfluous drugs and the risk of subsequent side-effects. Second, long-term complications must be prevented. In this context, the main medical problem of patients with type 2 diabetes is excessive cardiovascular morbidity and mortality. To a lesser extent, type 2 diabetic patients, especially when their disease develops at a younger age (e.g. below 60 years of age), are also at risk of microangiopathic complications.

This chapter discusses whether there is any positive evidence for treating type 2 diabetic patients with oral antidiabetic drugs to prevent their acute complications and symptoms and reduce their macrovascular or microvascular disease, comparing oral drugs with subcutaneous insulin treatment. Of the 90 167 publications on oral antidiabetic drugs identified in MEDLINE between 1966 and 1997, only two studies have ever attempted to investigate the effect of these drugs on vascular complications [2].

Sulphonylureas

The University Group Diabetes Program (UGDP) study failed to show any benefit of blood glucose lowering (by insulin) on macrovascular or microvascular disease in type 2 diabetes [3]; the use of tolbutamide, then the worldwide leading sulphonylurea drug, was associated with a significant increase in cardiovascular mortality [4]. However, with the exception of imposing a warning notice to be included in the product information on sulphonylurea drugs in the USA, there have been no interventions by the various national drug licensing authorities with regard to the continuous use of tolbutamide. Much of the criticism of the UGDP data on tolbutamide was related to their lack of pathophysiological plausibility [2]. During the past 15 years, however, it has been shown that sulphonylurea drugs close K^+_{ATP} channels in the myocardium and might interfere with ischaemic preconditioning, an internal autoprotective mechanism against myocardial necrosis that acts during hypoxia, such as during coronary artery disease [5,6]. Animal experimentation and some clinical investigations have demonstrated such potentially harmful side-effects for various sulphonylurea drugs. Thus, there is a growing body of indirect evidence that sulphonylureas may be hazardous in patients with coronary artery disease. In fact, the very substantial improvement in mortality rates in diabetic patients when they are switched to insulin therapy following an acute myocardial infarction, as shown in the Diabetes and Insulin-Glucose Infusion in Acute Myocardial Infarction (DIGAMI) study [7], might possibly be because the patients in the intervention group were completely taken off their sulphonylurea drugs [8,9]. However, the United Kingdom Prospective Diabetes Study (UKPDS), which had excluded patients with clinically relevant coronary artery disease, did not confirm any cardiotoxic effects of the two sulphonylureas investigated [10]; thus it may be concluded that there is no significant cardiotoxic effect of either glibenclamide or chlorpropamide in type 2 diabetic patients without clinically relevant coronary heart disease.

More important, though, was the conclusion of the UKPDS that intensive blood glucose control (achieving a medium HbA_{1c} level of 7.0% over 10 years, as opposed to a medium HbA_{1c} of 7.9% in the control group) was not associated with any measurable prevention of macroangiopathy (confirming the earlier findings of the UGDP [3]). HbA_{1c} reductions seen in the intervention groups were comparable for insulin, glibenclamide or chlorpropamide therapy. Like insulin treatment, glibenclamide did not reduce the risk of atherosclerotic complications, whereas chlorpropamide was clearly associated with an increase of blood pressure and the incidence of arterial hypertension [10]. When aiming to reduce the excessive cardiovascular morbidity and mortality in type 2 diabetes, therefore, it appears more effective to treat arterial hypertension, hypercholesterolaemia, to stop smoking and to take aspirin [1].

Turning to the microangiopathic complications, the UKPDS has impressively confirmed the hypothesis of the causal relationship between hyperglycaemia and microangiopathy for relatively young, early manifest type 2 diabetic patients. For the first time, it has become possible to calculate the size of the benefit achievable by intensive glycaemic control: the lowering of median HbA_{1c} levels from 7.9% to 7.0% during a period of 10 years has resulted in a statistically significant reduction of the absolute risk for any diabetes related end-point by 5.1% ($NNT_{10\ years}$ = 20; 95% CI 10–500) and for microangiopathic end-points by 2.8% ($NNT_{10\ years}$ = 36; CI not reported).

Although it is generally felt to be justified to extrapolate from these data to the even greater benefit that may be achievable when initially much higher HbA_{1c} levels are lowered by appropriate therapy, it is noteworthy that hard data, based upon randomized controlled trials, are only available for relatively young, early manifest type 2 diabetic patients in whom relatively good control (median HbA_{1c} 7.9%) was compared with very good control (median HbA_{1c} 7.0%) for a period of 10 years. There is no doubt that, for these patients, the use of glibenclamide is evidence-based, as it leads to a statistically significant reduction of microangiopathy. Following the principles of evidence-based medicine, it will now be up to patients to decide on their own HbA_{1c} target level depending on the risks they are prepared to take and the efforts they are prepared to make. To prepare patients for such a decision-making process will require innovative approaches in patient education and communication that do not seem to be currently available. In any case, such potential benefit of glibenclamide therapy must not be extrapolated to any other sulphonylurea drug. Thus, the end-point-related efficacy and safety of all other sulphonylurea drugs, such as glimepiride, gliclazide, etc., and also of the non-sulphonylurea insulin secretagogue repaglinide, must remain questionable until evidence to the contrary is accumulated.

Biguanides

Whereas the biguanide phenformin was associated with increased cardiovascular mortality in the UGDP study [11] and subsequently taken off the US market [2], metformin has remained part of the oral antidiabetic armamentarium in many European countries. Beginning in the late eighties, marketing activities promoted a worldwide 'renaissance of metformin'. Even though not a single patient-orientated outcome–benefit study had been documented, metformin was introduced on to the US market in 1995. For the first time, the UKPDS has provided some data to evaluate the efficacy and safety of metformin with regard to patient-orientated outcome objectives. Notwithstanding the fundamental criticism of the UKPDS [12] and its metformin section [13] in particular, the following data have been reported: in relatively young (mean age 53 years; newly manifest) type 2 diabetic patients with weight >120% ideal body weight (corresponding to a mean BMI of 31.8 ± 4.9 kg/m^2), the use of metformin monotherapy to achieve the goals of intensive glycaemic control (i.e. a mean HbA$_{1c}$ value of 7.4% during 10 years) was associated with a significant reduction of 'any diabetes related end-point', of diabetes-related and total mortality [14].

This finding has been criticized on methodological grounds, especially as the combination treatment of glibenclamide plus metformin (in normal weight and overweight patients) was associated with a statistically significant increase in total mortality. Whilst there are still questions about the validity of this part of the UKPDS data, any combination between glibenclamide and metformin in the treatment of type 2 diabetes must—at present—be discouraged, if the metformin data are accepted at all.

Other oral hypoglycaemic agents

In spite of the wealth of studies, product descriptions, publications and scientific and postgraduate fora, there is no information on whether any of the many other oral antidiabetic drugs are effective in preventing macroangiopathic or microangiopathic complications in type 2 diabetes. This is especially worrisome for some popular and relatively expensive drugs, such as acarbose and troglitazone—drugs for which there are additional doubts as to their safety and quality of life-related side-effects (e.g. flatulence with acarbose, potential liver damage with troglitazone).

Obesity

The negative effects of overweight in type 2 diabetes are often lamented—and of even more concern is any further increase in body weight during certain therapies, such as glibenclamide or insulin treatment, when compared with metformin. Previous epidemiological data [15,16] have repeatedly demonstrated that being overweight in type 2 diabetes is not necessarily associated with a negative prognosis—sometimes it seems as if the contrary is true. When comparing the control groups of 1138 almost normal-weight (BMI 27.8 ± 5.5 kg/m^2) and 411 overweight (BMI 31.8 ± 4.9 kg/m^2) type 2 diabetic patients, the UKPDS has shown that, after 10 years, there was no hazard of obesity with regard to any single or combined end-point analysed in the study [11,14].

Conclusions

Of the sulphonylurea drugs, only glibenclamide has been proven to be effective and safe for a subgroup of type 2 diabetic patients in the UKPDS study. By contrast, chlorpropamide was proven to be ineffective with regard to reducing microangiopathic late complications and it led to arterial hypertension—despite an identical improvement of glycaemia. Tolbutamide cannot be used because its alleged cardiotoxic effects have never been excluded. The efficacy and safety of sulphonylurea drugs need to be proven for every single drug—a group effect does not exist. There is a serious suspicion of a cardiotoxic effect of sulphonylureas in patients with coronary heart disease. Until relevant data have been accumulated from appropriate long-term studies, there is a case for sulphonylurea treatment being witheld from patients with coronary heart disease. Metformin appears to be effective in the monotherapy of obese people with type 2 diabetes, if the long list of contraindications is strictly observed and the patients' glycaemia can be well controlled on this regimen. Following the principles of evidence-based medicine, we suggest that any other oral antidiabetic drugs should not be used outside clinical trials.

References

1 Berger M, Mühlhauser I. Diabetes care and patient-oriented outcomes. *JAMA* 1999; 281: 1676–8.

2 Berger M, Richter B. Oral agents in the treatment of diabetes mellitus. In: Davidson JK, ed. *Diabetes Mellitus, A Problem Oriented Approach*, 3rd edn. New York: Thieme-Stratton, 2000: 415–36.

3 The University Group Diabetes Program. Effects of hypoglycemic agents on vascular complications in patients with adult-onset diabetes. VIII. *Diabetes* 1982; 31 (Suppl 5): 1–81.

4 The University Group Diabetes Program. A study on the effects of hypoglycemic agents on vascular complications in patients with adult-onset diabetes. I. *Diabetes* 1970; 19 (Suppl 2): 474–830.

5 Engler RL, Yellon DM. Sulfonylurea K⁺ATP blockade in type 2 diabetes and preconditioning in cardiovascular disease:

time for reconsideration. *Circulation* 1996; 94: 2297–301.

6 Leibowitz G, Cerasi E. Sulfonylurea treatment of NIDDM patients with cardiovascular disease: a mixed blessing? *Diabetologia* 1996; 39: 503–14.

7 Malmberg K, for the DIGAMI Study Group. Prospective randomized study of intensive insulin treatment on long-term survival after acute myocardial infarction in patients with diabetes mellitus. *BMJ* 1997; 314: 1512–15.

8 Mühlhauser I, Sawicki PT, Berger. M. Possible risk of sulphonylureas in the treatment of non-insulin-dependent diabetes mellitus and coronary artery disease [letter]. *Diabetologia* 1998; 41: 744.

9 Berger M, Mühlhauser I, Sawicki PT. Possible risk of sulphonylureas in the treatment of non-insulin-dependent diabetes mellitus and coronary artery

disease [letter]. *Diabetologia* 1997; 40: 1492–3.

10 UK Prospective Diabetes Group. Intensive blood glucose control with sulfonylureas or insulin compared with conventional treatment and risk of complications in patients with type 2 diabetes (UKPDS 33). *Lancet* 1998; 352: 837–53.

11 University Group Diabetes Program V. Evaluation of phenformin therapy. *Diabetes* 1975; 24 (Suppl 1): 65–184.

12 Ewart RM. The UKPDS: what was the question [letter]. *Lancet* 1999; 353: 1882.

13 Nathan DM. Some answers, more controversy from UKPDS. *Lancet* 1998; 352: 832–3.

14 UK Prospective Diabetes Group. Effect of intensive blood glucose control with metformin on complications in overweight patients with type 2 diabetes (UKPDS 34). *Lancet* 1998; 352: 854–65.

15 Klein R, Klein BE, Moss SE. Is obesity related to microvascular and macrovascular complications in diabetes? *Arch Intern Med* 1997; 157: 650–6.

16 Chaturvedi N, Fuller JH, the WHO Multinational Study Group. Mortality risk by body weight and weight change in people with NIDDM. *Diabetes Care* 1995; 18: 766–74.

7: Should obese type 2 diabetic patients be treated with insulin?

Matthew C. Riddle

As with other chapters in this book, this title poses an important but thorny question and a difficult management dilemma. Insulin is the only anti-hyperglycaemic agent powerful enough to normalize blood glucose control in many of the obese type 2 diabetic patients who predominate in the diabetic population; unfortunately, the use of insulin can cause particular problems in these very patients. Here, both sides of the argument will be discussed, in the context of studies that illuminate these issues. At the end, some tentative conclusions are offered, together with speculation on future approaches to this therapeutic challenge.

What is obesity? Obesity is commonly defined in relation to the weight range of the heaviest subset of a population, usually adjusted by height as the body mass index (BMI, kg/m^2). It can also be defined as body weight in excess of an 'ideal' value, determined by actuarial analysis, that confers longest survival in a given population. Other definitions are based on the proportion of body mass consisting of adipose tissue, or even the proportion accounted for by the visceral fat depot. None of these methods is easily generalized to populations that vary widely in age, ethnicity, nutritional patterns and vulnerability to illnesses.

Interestingly, the mean BMI of patients with type 2 diabetes seems to differ less between regions and countries than does the mean BMI in the general population. For instance, although people are more obese in the USA than in the UK [1], a cross-sectional survey found that patients with type 2 diabetes in the USA have an average BMI of around 30 kg/m^2, [2], close to the value of 29 kg/m^2 in recently diagnosed patients entering the United Kingdom Prospective Diabetes Study (UKPDS) [3]. For simplicity, this chapter will assume that a BMI > 30 kg/m^2 signifies clinically significant obesity.

There can be no doubt that obesity is becoming increasingly common [4]. The main reasons for the epidemic are falling physical activity, easy access to

94

fat-rich and calorie-dense foods and perhaps the decline of illnesses that previously limited life expectancy and the opportunity to gain weight [5]. Obesity leads to higher rates of illness and death in various ways, with type 2 diabetes featuring high on the list. Its incidence and prevalence are rising worldwide, and this is largely attributable to worsening adiposity. The rapidly increasing incidence of type 2 diabetes in young people is especially worrisome; in some parts of North America, one-third of patients diagnosed before the age of 20 have type 2 rather than type 1 diabetes [6].

Why does it matter whether obese patients use insulin?

Consensus on the need to treat hyperglycaemia in obese type 2 patients is now being reached, partly because the relationship between hyperglycaemia and tissue injury has grown clearer [7] and more importantly, because intervention trials show that early treatment of hyperglycaemia reduces complications independently of the type of diabetes or the adiposity of the patient. The adult type 1 patients in the Diabetes Control and Complications Trial (DCCT) [8], non-obese type 2 patients in the Kumamoto Study [9] and obese type 2 patients in the UKPDS [10] all showed remarkably similar benefits from intensified efforts to lower blood glucose. In each case, a reduction of haemoglobin A1c (HbA_{1c}) by 1% yielded 25–35% reductions in retinopathy and nephropathy, verifying that microvascular complications of diabetes are tightly linked to mean plasma glucose levels. These trials, supported by epidemiological evidence, show that keeping HbA_{1c} at or below 7% can slow the progression of microvascular complications. Vigorous treatment of hyperglycaemia above this level would therefore seem indicated for obese type 2 diabetic patients as for other groups, provided that the risks of treatment are acceptable.

The problem lies in exactly how to do this. All available treatments have limitations, some of them particularly problematical for obese patients. Weight control is difficult to achieve and maintain and, even when successful, does not prevent secondary failure of glycaemic control [11]. Sulphonylureas favour weight gain and become less effective over time as the capacity of the β-cell declines [12]. Although the UKPDS [10] showed no excess of vascular events with sulphonylureas (in fact, a trend towards fewer events), the recent findings that these drugs (especially tolbutamide and glibenclamide/glyburide) may adversely affect vascular adaption to ischaemia [13] have reawakened old fears about their safety [14,15]. Metformin cannot be used by some patients because of its side-effects, or contraindications such as renal insufficiency or congestive heart failure [16]. Moreover, the UKPDS showed that the development of secondary failure with metformin was no different from that with sulphonylureas, suggesting that continuing decline of β-cell function is inevitable once overt diabetes is present [17]. Further questions have arisen from a substudy within the UKPDS in which metformin, added to a sulphonylurea, was associated with more cardiovascular mortality than a sulphonylurea continued alone. Chance or an artefact of study design may have caused this, as the mortality rate dropped in the sulphonylurea-only subgroup after the unmasked randomization. However, an unexpectedly bad effect of the combination of these two drugs cannot be excluded entirely. Alpha-glucosidase inhibitors have limited glucose-lowering potency and cause flatulence [18]. Although concern about hepatic toxicity dominates current discussion of the thiazolidinediones [19], their tendency to cause weight gain and fluid retention may ultimately prove more important. Indeed, even with the best possible use of oral agents, hyperglycaemia often recurs. Insulin is ultimately needed by most patients if good glycaemic control is to be maintained, because it can always lower glucose if enough is given. However, many obese type 2 diabetic patients are not treated with insulin, for a variety of reasons; it could be said that the insulin resistance of obese patients is matched by the resistance of physicians to using insulin.

Obstacles to the use of insulin for obese patients

Some widely held views underly this reluctance.

Insulin is 'rarely effective'

Many people believe—and in medical practice the view is commonly expressed—that insulin is not very effective for obese patients. A notable example of this view appeared recently in the *Journal of the American Medical Association* in an article reporting experience from a regional health system in the USA between 1990–3 [20]. Over 700 patients with type 2 diabetes began using insulin but were still inadequately controlled 1 year later. Their degree of adiposity was not described, but a cross-sectional sample in the United States like this would be expected to have an average BMI of close to 30 kg/m^2. Their mean HbA$_{1c}$ fell from 9.3% at baseline only to 8.4% a year later. The authors concluded that 'insulin therapy was associated with increases in resource use and was rarely effective in achieving tight glycaemic control'. This view appears to have been accepted by many physicians and administrators who believe that insulin treatment is ineffective, strenuous, time consuming and costly, and that its introduction should be delayed until glycaemic control has become very poor. Whether insulin was used skilfully and to its full potential is, of course, debatable.

Injected insulin increases hyperinsulinaemia and cardiovascular events

A second concern relates to the pathophysiology of type 2 diabetes and its relationship to macrovascular disease. The last decade has brought much study, reviewing of literature and theorizing about the relationships between obesity, insulin resistance, hyperinsulinaemia, diabetes, hypertension, hyper-lipidaemia and cardiovascular events [21,22]. Most physicians are aware of the clinical entity comprising these elements, known variously as the Syndrome X or the insulin resistance, Reaven's or the cardiovascular dysmetabolic syndrome. Recognition of this syndrome has helped to establish a more comprehensive approach to the management of type 2 diabetes. Good evidence supports efforts to find and treat individual predictors of cardiovascular risk in obese patients, such as smoking, hypertension and hyperlipidaemia; indeed treating hypertension and dyslipidaemia in diabetic patients is proportionately just as helpful and in absolute terms more productive than in non-diabetic patients [23–27]. Study of insulin resistance has also led to new treatments and better understanding of older ones. The thiazolidinediones directly improve the insulin sensitivity of fat and muscle. Metformin's main therapeutic action has been traced to the liver [28], where it improves the response to insulin; its other effects—including limitation of calorie intake, weight loss and improvement of peripheral insulin sensitivity—appear more variable [16].

These benefits of attention to the insulin resistance syndrome are, unfortunately, accompanied by controversy about the possible dangers of insulin treatment. It has been argued that, as hyperinsulinaemia correlates with vascular events, it probably causes them. There is experimental support for this view, in that animal and laboratory studies suggest that high concentrations of insulin may harm vascular tissues [29]. Discussion of this point has recently become more complex, with better understanding of insulin-signalling pathways, and the identification of branches that protect against as well as ones that promote vascular disease [7]. In some large clinical surveys, multivariate analysis suggests that hyperinsulinaemia may be an independent cardiovascular risk factor even after adjustment for the effects of other risk factors [30], although others do not; for example, multivariate analysis of data from diabetic patients in the San Antonio Heart Study found that hyperglycaemia was an independent predictor of vascular events, whereas hyperinsulinaemia was not [31]. Another theoretical concern, that insulin administration may actually exacerbate insulin resistance, has been raised by the finding that experimental hyperinsulinaemia in humans may reduce the insulin sensitivity of tissues [32].

This debate has confused and worried clinicians, who might reasonably conclude that if the experts cannot agree on the risks and benefits of hyperinsulinaemia, then insulin should not be used aggressively for obese patients who already have high plasma insulin concentrations.

Insulin causes weight gain

Another part of the debate centres on weight. When patients begin taking insulin, they usually gain weight, especially when high dosages are needed. This weight gain is not due entirely to deposition of fat: significant fluid retention may occur, and lean tissue mass may also increase [33]. Restoration of lean tissue mass is especially likely (and indeed appropriate) when treatment follows prolonged periods of poor glycaemic control. For most patients, however, any weight gain is undesirable, while fluid retention may pose risks from dependent oedema in numb and poorly perfused feet and legs. It has also been suggested that weight gain—and especially central fat deposition— might also exacerbate insulin resistance and other metabolic abnormalities, and thus increase cardiovascular events [34].

Concern about weight gain after starting insulin treatment is compounded by limited understanding of its mechanisms. Retention of energy previously lost in the urine through glycosuria undoubtedly contributes. If a patient passes 100 g/day of glucose into the urine before treatment and none afterwards, then 400 calories are retained daily unless dietary intake declines or thermogenic loss increases. Also, patients may overeat to defend against or treat hypoglycaemia caused by insulin treatment. Yet another possibility is the direct stimulation of appetite by hyperinsulinaemia, but this theory has proved difficult to verify [35].

Short-term physiological studies

Much has been published on the use of insulin for type 2 diabetes [36,37]. The issues raised above have been brought into focus by some short-term studies of the physiological responses to insulin treatment.

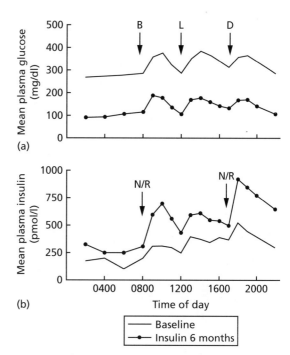

Fig. 7.1 Mean plasma glucose (a) and serum insulin (b) profiles for obese type 2 diabetic patients before and 6 months after starting intensive insulin treatment. The times of meals (B, breakfast; L, lunch; D, dinner) and insulin injections (N/R, NPH + Regular) are indicated by arrows. Adapted from Henry *et al.* [38] with permission.

The metabolic effects of 6 months' intensive insulin treatment of 14 obese patients no longer controlled by sulphonylureas were reported in an elegant study by Henry *et al.* [38]. Their subjects' mean age was 59 years, mean duration of diabetes was 7 years and mean BMI was 31 kg/m^2. Two to three weeks after sulphonylurea treatment was withdrawn, the patients began Isophane (NPH) and soluble (regular) insulin twice daily, seeking the best control possible. Fasting plasma glucose averaged 15.7 mmol/l at baseline and after 6 months declined nearly to normal; the mean HbA$_{1c}$ was 5.1% without hypoglycaemia. The average daily insulin dosage was 100 units. Both fasting and postprandial serum insulin concentrations increased, with mean concentrations 66% higher at 6 months (see Fig. 7.1).

The accompanying metabolic changes are of interest. The average weight increase was 8.7 kg, 80% of which occurred in the first 3 months. Estimated energy intake declined by 15%, from 2023 to 1711 calories/day. Fasting plasma triglyceride and total cholesterol concentrations fell markedly from 5.02 to 2.00 and 6.29 to 4.76 mmol/l, respectively, while low-density and high-density lipoproteins did not change. Overall, vigorous insulin treatment alone can almost normalize glucose levels in obese patients who retain some endogenous insulin, but at the cost of considerable weight gain.

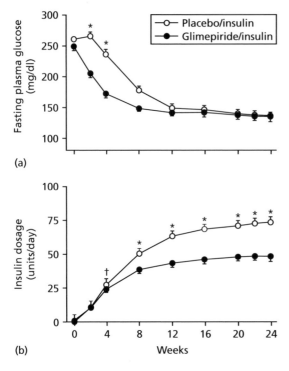

(a)

(b)

Fig. 7.2 Mean fasting plasma glucose (a) and daily insulin dosage (b) for obese type 2 diabetic patients beginning treatment with 70/30 insulin before dinner, with or without continued glimepiride. Insulin dosage was titrated to achieve a fasting plasma glucose concentration of 7.8 mmol/l. *$P < 0.001$, †$P < 0.05$ for significant between-group differences. Adapted from Riddle *et al.* [39] with permission.

Another study treated similar patients in a different fashion, perhaps more applicable to current clinical practice [39]. The 145 patients had a mean age of 58 years, mean duration of diabetes was 7 years and mean BMI was 33 kg/m². After an 8-week run-in on glimepiride treatment, they were randomized to insulin alone or insulin with continued glimepiride. Insulin was given as a single injection (of 70 : 30 isophane and soluble) before the main evening meal and the dosage titrated to achieve a fasting plasma glucose of 7.8 mmol/l. After 6 months, most subjects had reached this target level, although those continuing the sulphonylurea did so sooner; those receiving insulin alone showed initial worsening of glycaemic control, which was largely responsible for their drop-out rate of 15%. Mean daily insulin dosage was 78 units without and 49 units with continuing sulphonylurea. Glycaemic control improved in both groups, with HbA$_{1c}$ falling from 9.8% and 9.7% at baseline to 7.7% and 7.6%, respectively. Figure 7.2 shows the patterns of fasting plasma glucose and insulin dosage. Moderate glycaemic control was achieved, even in the very hyperglycaemic, very obese patients.

The metabolic consequences were similar to those described above [38], but less pronounced. Weight gain averaged 4.0 and 4.3 kg in the two groups;

Fig. 7.3 Three studies testing the effect of intensive insulin treatment on the sensitivity of peripheral tissues to insulin. In each study, glucose uptake was determined by the glucose-insulin clamp before and after insulin treatment. Data are expressed here as percentage of the glucose uptake found in matched non-diabetic control subjects from each study. Adapted from data from Scarlett *et al*. [40], Andrews *et al*. [41] and Garvey *et al*. [42].

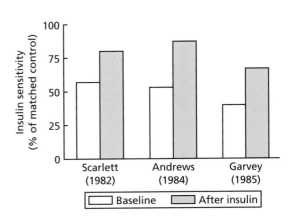

fasting serum insulin concentrations increased by 30% in both groups, while triglycerides declined by about 30% and blood pressure did not change.

Three small short-term studies examine the effects of insulin treatment on insulin sensitivity of tissues, measured using the glucose-insulin clamp [40–42]. In each, the duration of treatment was 2–4 weeks and the mean daily insulin dosage was high (110–198 units); comparable glycaemic control was achieved. In each study, insulin treatment improved insulin sensitivity, this improvement representing about half of the difference between the untreated patients and their matched non-diabetic controls (Fig. 7.3). These findings suggest that reversible glucose toxicity accounted for much of the insulin resistance, and that this could be eliminated by insulin treatment.

Finally, the effect of short-term treatment with insulin on lipoprotein metabolism was studied in seven type 2 diabetic patients who were not taking other glucose-lowering drugs [43]. The key finding was a reduction of very-low-density lipoprotein production accompanied by a 38% reduction of fasting triglyceride and a 17% reduction of low-density lipoprotein concentrations.

Long-term intervention studies

Two large, long-term studies that tracked clinical outcomes are particularly pertinent here: the UKPDS [10,17] and the Diabetes and Insulin-Glucose Infusion in Acute Myocardial Infarction (DIGAMI) Study [44].

The main part of the UKPDS included 3041 recently-diagnosed type 2 diabetic patients managed either with a conventional policy (i.e. lifestyle

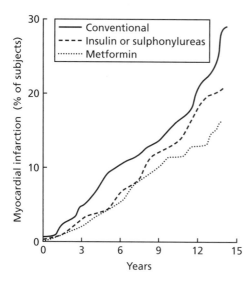

Fig. 7.4 Cumulative incidence of myocardial infarction in the substudy of obese subjects in the UKPDS, treated with 'conventional' dietary and lifestyle advice alone; or with insulin or sulphonylureas; or with metformin. Adapted from UKPDS 34 [17] with permission.

diet alone) or intensive treatment with either a sulphonylurea or insulin [10]. Their mean BMI after vigorous dietary treatment for at least 3 months was 27 kg/m². Over 10 years, the intensive treatment group had median Hb_{A1c} 0.9% lower than the conventional group and enjoyed a 25% reduction in microvascular end-points. All groups gained weight, but the intensive group gained more than the conventional with excess gains averaging 1.7 kg with glibenclamide, 2.6 kg with chlorpropamide and 4.0 kg with insulin. However, cardiovascular events were not increased by intensive treatment; indeed, the trend was towards fewer events with either sulphonylurea or insulin than with the conventional treatment policy.

Another part of the UKPDS protocol was devoted to 1704 more seriously obese patients (mean BMI, 31 kg/m²) [17]; 409 were randomized to treatment with insulin and the rest to a sulphonylurea, metformin or conventional policy. The effects of sulphonylurea and insulin treatment on weight were similar to those in the main part of the UKPDS. The excess weight gain over conventional policy was about 3 kg with glibenclamide, 4 kg with chlorpropamide and 5 kg with insulin. By contrast, metformin caused no weight gain relative to conventional policy. Strikingly, metformin reduced the rates of mortality and myocardial infarction compared with the conventionally treated group (see Fig. 7.4). It is possible that this apparent cardioprotective effect of metformin was, at least in part, attributable to its lack of tendency to cause weight gain. However, intensive treatment with either insulin or

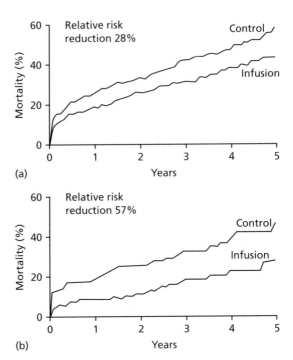

Fig. 7.5 Cumulative mortality rates in diabetic patients following myocardial infarction in the DIGAMI study. Intensive insulin treatment signficantly reduced mortality compared to conventional treatment in the whole group (a) and in a subset not previously using insulin and with a more favourable prognosis at admission (b). Adapted from Malmberg *et al.* [44] with permission.

sulphonylurea also showed a (statistically insignificant) trend toward fewer events, and there was no significant difference in cardiovascular outcomes between metformin and sulphonylurea or insulin.

   The DIGAMI study tested the immediate and longer term outcome of insulin treatment in diabetic patients who suffered myocardial infarction [43]. The 620 subjects' mean age was 68 years, median duration of diabetes was 8 years and mean BMI was 27. On admission, they were randomized to continued treatment at their physicians' discretion or to intensive treatment with intravenous insulin infusion for 48 h, followed by four injections of insulin daily for 5 years. As shown in Fig. 7.5, all-cause mortality was substantially lower in the intensively treated group; most of this effect appeared in the first few months but the between-group difference seemed to widen over time. When all subjects were considered, the relative risk reduction with intensive insulin treatment was 28% at 5 years. In a predefined subgroup of 272 patients who had not used insulin previously and were not seriously ill at entry, the risk reduction was 51%. A rationale for this benefit has been proposed, based mainly on the ability of injected insulin to suppress free fatty acid levels in plasma and thereby protect vulnerable myocardial tissue from the high oxygen demand provoked by metabolism of fatty acids [45]. These findings strongly challenge the view that insulin treatment increases cardio-vascular risk in type 2 diabetes. Indeed, they suggest that patients at highest risk should use insulin sooner rather than later.

Conclusions from clinical trials

These findings shed light on the common beliefs about the use of insulin. Although insulin is disappointingly ineffective in some clinical settings, rigorous studies show that it can be effective for obese patients when used skilfully. Concerns about adverse metabolic effects gain little support from short-term trials, although the weight gain caused by insulin treatment could be deleterious in the longer term. When hyperglycaemic, obese patients are treated with insulin, plasma insulin levels increase and glycaemic control improves; this is accompanied by at least short-term improvement in insulin sensitivity, no change in blood pressure and better lipid profiles. Triglyceride levels decline at least as much after treatment with insulin as with metformin or thiazolidinediones. Moreover, long-term medical outcomes are favourable. The UKPDS suggests that, at worst, insulin is neutral with respect to cardio-vascular events while the DIGAMI study argues that the highest-risk patients are protected by using insulin. However, all trials confirm weight gain with insulin treatment averaging 2–9 kg. The possibility that this gain has bad consequences needs further study.

The clinical challenge is therefore to optimize glycaemic control while minimizing weight gain. Aside from the best possible efforts to improve eating and exercise behaviours, the main tactics now available are basal insulin replacement and combining insulin with oral agents.

Basal insulin replacement

Several factors affect how much weight is gained when insulin treatment begins. If the patient loses weight before drug therapy, as before randomization in the UKPDS, weight may quickly increase through the combined effects of starting insulin and the inadvertent relaxation of efforts to improve lifestyle. If good effort begins or continues during insulin treatment, weight gain may be minimized. In addition, the greater the improvement of glycaemic control the more weight gain is likely. The way in which insulin treatment is started probably also plays a role. The data presented in Table 7.1 suggest that weight gain

Table 7.1 Weight gain associated with starting insulin in different ways. The studies shown differ in design; the mean BMI of the subjects, duration of the study, and the comparison group used are shown for each group.

	Baseline BMI (kg/m^2)	Duration of treatment (months)	Comparison against	Weight gain (kg)
Basal insulin				
Chow *et al.* [46]	24	6	Baseline	2.1
Landstedt-Hallin *et al.* [47]	26	4	Baseline	1.9
Yki-Järvinen *et al.* [48]	28	3	Oral agents	2.1
Cusi *et al.* [49]	30	4	Baseline	2.4
Riddle *et al.* [39]	33	6	Baseline	4.2
				Mean 2.5
Mealtime insulin				
Landstedt-Hallin *et al.* [47]	26	4	Baseline	3.4
Feinglos *et al.* [50]	31	4	Oral agents	3.2
				Mean 3.3
Basal + mealtime insulin				
Chow *et al.* [46]	24	6	Baseline	5.2
Yki-Järvinen *et al.* [48]				
2 injections	28	3	Oral agents	2.7
4 injections	28	3	Oral agents	2.9
Henry *et al.* [38]	31	6	Baseline	8.7
				Mean 5.7

may be less with the use of basal insulin (2.5 kg) [39–49] than with mealtime insulin (3.3 kg) [47,50] or basal plus mealtime insulin (5.7 kg) [38,46,48].

Combining insulin with metformin

Whether oral agents are continued or started together with insulin may also affect weight gain. Three recent trials, summarized in Table 7.2, show that combining metformin with insulin leads to less weight gain than the vigorous use of insulin alone [51–53]. In the most convincing of these [53], previous insulin treatment was intensified using three injections daily for a 2-month run-in period and resulted in Hb_{A1c} values averaging 7.6%. After randomization to metformin 1000 mg or placebo twice daily, intensive treatment was continued for 6 further months. The final Hb_{A1c} values were comparable in the two groups (7.0 vs 7.1%), but weight increased from baseline by 0.5 kg with insulin alone and decreased by 1.4 kg with metformin plus insulin.

Table 7.2 Three studies testing the effect of adding metformin (Met) while starting [51] or intensifying [52,53] insulin treatment are shown. In each case, customary doses of metformin given along with insulin markedly reduced the tendency to gain weight while glycaemic control improved.

	Yki-Järvinen et al. [51]		Aviles-Santa et al. [52]		Bergenstal et al. [53]	
	Ins	Ins + Met	Ins	Ins + Met	Ins	Ins + Met
Number of subjects	24	19	22	21	22	20
Duration of study (months)	12	12	6	6	4	4
Insulin dosage (units/day)						
Baseline	0	0	97	96	135	124
End	53	36	120	92	136	99
Hb_{A1c} (%)						
Baseline	10.1	9.7	9.1	9.0	7.2	7.7
End	7.9	7.2	7.6	6.5	7.0	7.1
Weight gain (kg)	4.6	0.9	3.2	0.5	0.5	–1.4
Weight benefit with metformin (kg)		–3.5	–	–2.7	–	–1.9

Future prospects

New therapeutic agents are being developed for type 2 diabetes, and some of these may aid the treatment of obese patients who are given insulin.

Thiazolidinediones

Three thiazolidinediones (troglitazone, rosiglitazone and pioglitazone) have been available in various countries. Only pioglitazone is currently officially approved for use when combined with insulin. Oedema and weight gain may occur and seem likely to be class effects of thiazolidinediones, although many patients with improved insulin sensitivity have no trouble with these side-effects. Figure 7.6 shows how metformin and troglitazone affect glucose and insulin levels when each is used in combination with continuous sub-cutaneous insulin infusion [54]. Both agents reduced insulin requirements and 24-h plasma insulin concentrations—metformin by about 30% and

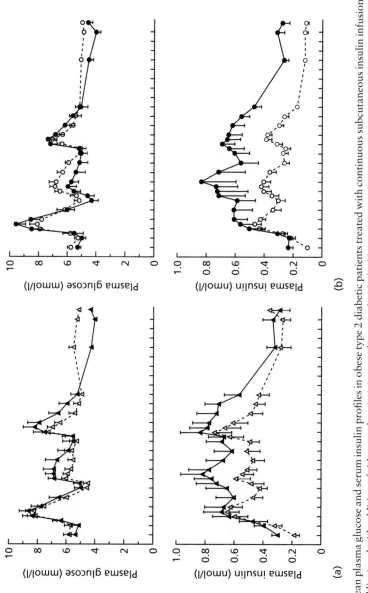

Fig. 7.6 Mean plasma glucose and serum insulin profiles in obese type 2 diabetic patients treated with continuous subcutaneous insulin infusion alone (CSII) (solid line) and with addition of either metformin (a) or troglitazone (b) (dashed line). Mean daily insulin requirements were 110 units without and 76 units with metformin 850 mg twice daily, and 102 units without and 48 units with troglitazone 400–600 mg daily. Adapted from Yu *et al.* [54] with permission.

troglitazone by about 50%—while there was no overall change in plasma glucose levels.

What does this effect of thiazolidinediones mean for obese patients taking insulin? Greater insulin sensitivity should allow lower doses of injected insulin and improved efficacy of any remaining endogenous insulin, which together might reduce glycaemic variability, decrease the risk of hypoglycaemia and limit weight gain. These benefits, if realized, could make treatment more acceptable to patients as well as providing better long-term glycaemic control. Also, there are hopes for other important benefits from thiazolidinediones: lower plasma insulin concentrations and/or direct tissue effects of thiazolidinediones may protect against vascular events [55], although experimental support for this hypothesis is currently limited to short-term physiological studies rather than outcome trials.

Insulin analogues

Insulin analogues [56] may also help. Insulin glargine, a long-acting analogue, may be available by late 2000. Studies in lean normal and type 1 diabetic subjects show that it has a highly reproducible and nearly peakless action profile that usually extends beyond 24 h. This analogue could theoretically be taken once daily at any time and deliver more predictable basal insulin levels, but whether it can decrease hypoglycaemic risk and weight gain when compared with available insulins must be tested.

The role of very rapidly-acting preparations of insulin (e.g. insulin lispro, insulin aspart, and the experimental inhaled insulin) for obese patients is not clear at present; these agents need further testing in this population.

Gut peptides

Ultimately, the holy grail for the treatment of obese patients with diabetes is an antihyperglycaemic agent that also physiologically controls excessive eating. Metformin approaches this ideal, but has a narrow balance between its therapeutic and unwanted effects; in particular, its satiety action and its tendency to cause nausea or to alter enjoyment of food seem to be closely related. Certain gut peptides may include regulation of appetite or satiety among their normal roles, and these might be exploited therapeutically. The β-cell peptide amylin and the intestinal glucagon-like peptide-1 (GLP-1) currently lead the pack. Both are secreted in response to eating, slow gastric emptying, reduce glucagon secretion and suppress food intake [57,58]. Pramlintide, a stable and less rapidly cleared analogue of amylin, is currently under development for improving glycaemic control, but must be given by injection [59]. Such gut peptides or their analogues might enhance the anti-hyperglycaemic effects of injected insulin while helping to control weight.

Conclusions

Should obese type 2 diabetic patients be treated with insulin? The evidence says yes, if the patient seems likely to benefit from a reduced risk of microvascular complications. Weight gain is the main difficulty, but this can be limited by providing basal insulin at first, especially in combination with metformin. The cascade of new therapeutic agents continues, and it is to be hoped that some may be usefully combined with insulin to improve glycaemic control while limiting weight gain.

References

1 Vanitallie TB. Prevalence of obesity. *Endocrinol Metab Clin NA* 1996; 25: 887–905.

2 Cowie CC, Harris MI. Physical and metabolic characteristics of persons with diabetes. In: The National Diabetes Data Group. *Diabetes in America*, 2nd edn. Bethesda, MD: National Institutes of Health, 1995: 117–64.

3 UK Prospective Study Group. UK Prospective Diabetes Study 27. Plasma lipids and lipoproteins at diagnosis of NIDDM by age and sex. *Diabetes Care* 1997; 20: 1683–7.

4 Mokdad AH, Serdula MK, Dietz WH, Bowman BA, Marks JS, Koplan JP. The spread of the obesity epidemic in the United States. 1991–98. *JAMA* 1999; 282: 1519–22.

5 Drewnowski A, Popkin BM. The nutrition transition: new trends in the Global Diet. *Nutr Rev* 1997; 55 (2): 31–43.

6 Rosenbloom AL, Joe JR, Young RS, Winter WE. Emerging epidemic of type 2 diabetes in youth. *Diabetes Care* 1999; 22: 345–54.

7 King GL, Brownlee M. The cellular and molecular mechanisms of diabetic complications. *Endocrinol Metab Clin NA* 1996; 25: 255–71.

8 DCCT Research Group. The effect of intensive treatment of diabetes on the development and progression of long-term complications of insulin-dependent diabetes mellitus. *N Engl J Med* 1993; 329: 1289–98.

9 Ohkubo Y, Kishikawa H, Araki E *et al.* Intensive insulin therapy prevents the progression of diabetic microvascular complications in Japanese patients with non-insulin-dependent diabetes mellitus. A randomized prospective 6-year study. *Diabetes Res Clin Prac* 1995; 28: 103–17.

10 UK Prospective Diabetes Study (UKPDS) Group. Intensive blood-glucose control with sulphonylureas or insulin compared with conventional treatment and risk of complications in patients with type 2 diabetes (UKPDS 33). *Lancet* 1998; 352: 837–53.

11 Hadden DR, Blair ALT, Wilson EA *et al.* Natural history of diabetes presenting age 40–69 years: a prospective study of the influence of intensive dietary therapy. *Q J Med* 1986; 59: 579–98.

12 Matthews DR, Cull CA, Stratton IM, Holman RR, Turner RC, the UK,

Prospective Diabetes Study Group. UKPDS 26: sulphonylurea failure in non-insulin-dependent diabetic patients over six years. *Diabet Med* 1998; 15: 297–303.

13 Klepzig H, Kober G, Matter C *et al*. Sulfonylureas and ischemic preconditioning. A double-blind, placebo-controlled evaluation of glimepiride and glibenclamide. *Eur Heart J* 1999; 20: 439–46.

14 Garratt KN, Brady PA, Hassinger NL, Grill DE, Terzic A, Holmes DR Jr. Sulfonylurea drugs increase early mortality in patients with diabetes mellitus after direct angioplasty for acute myocardial infarction. *J Am Coll Cardiol* 1999; 33: 119–24.

15 Goldner MG, Knatterud GL, Prout TE. Effects of hypoglycemic agents on vascular complications in patients with adult-onset diabetes: III. Clinical implications of UGDP results. *JAMA* 1971; 218: 1400–10.

16 Bailey CJ, Turner RC. Drug therapy: metformin. *N Engl J Med* 1996; 334: 574–9.

17 UK Prospective Diabetes Study (UKPDS) Group. Effect of intensive blood-glucose control with metformin on complications in overweight patients with type 2 diabetes (UKPDS 34). *Lancet* 1998; 352: 854–65.

18 Lebovitz HE. Alpha-glucosidase inhibitors. *Endocrinol Metab Clin NA* 1997; 26: 539–51.

19 Watkins PB, Whitcomb RW. Hepatic dysfunction associated with troglitazone. *N Engl J Med* 1998; 338: 916–17.

20 Hayward RA, Manning WG, Kaplan SH, Wagner EH, Greenfield S. Starting insulin therapy in patients with type 2 diabetes: effectiveness, complications, and resource utilization. *JAMA* 1997; 278: 1663–9.

21 Reaven GM. Role of insulin resistance in human disease. *Diabetes* 1988; 37: 1595–607.

22 Haffner SM. The insulin resistance syndrome revisited. *Diabetes Care* 1996; 19: 275–7.

23 UK Prospective Diabetes Study Group. Tight blood pressure control and risk of macrovascular and microvascular complications in type 2 diabetes. UKPDS 38. *BMJ* 1998; 317: 703–12.

24 Curb JD, Pressel SL, Cutler JA *et al*. Effect of diuretic-based antihypertensive treatment on cardiovascular disease risk in older diabetic patients with isolated systolic hypertension. *JAMA* 1996; 276: 1886–92.

25 Pyorala K, Pedersen TR, Kjekshus J *et al*. Cholesterol lowering with simvastatin improves prognosis of diabetic patients with coronary heart disease. *Diabetes Care* 1997; 20: 614–20.

26 Goldberg RB, Mellies MJ, Sacks FM *et al*. Cardiovascular events and their reduction with pravastatin in diabetic and glucose-intolerant myocardial infarction survivors with average cholesterol levels. *Circulation* 1998; 98: 2513–19.

27 Rubins HB, Robins SJ, Collins D *et al*. Gemfibrozil for the secondary prevention of coronary heart disease in men with low levels of high-density liproprotein cholesterol. *N Engl J Med* 1999; 341: 410–18.

28 Cusi K, Defronzo RA. Metformin: a review of its metabolic effects. *Diabetes Rev* 1998; 6: 89–131.

29 Stout RW. Insulin and atheroma, a 20-year perspective. *Diabetes Care* 1990; 13: 611–54.

30 Despres JP, Lamarche B, Mauriege P *et al*. Hyperinsulinemia as an independent risk factor for ishemic heart disease. *N Engl J Med* 1996; 334: 952–7.

31 Wei M, Gaskill SP, Haffner SM *et al*. Effects of diabetes and level of glycemia on all-cause and cardiovascular mortality. The San Antonio Heart Study. *Diabetes Care* 1998; 21: 1167–72.

32 Rizza RA, Mandarino LJ, Genest J, Baker BA, Gerich JE. Production of insulin resistance by hyperinsulinaemia in man. *Diabetologia* 1985; 28: 70–5.

33 Groop L, Widen E, Franssila-Kallunki A *et al*. Different effects of insulin and oral antidiabetic agents on glucose and energy metabolism in type 2 (non-insulin-dependent) diabetes mellitus. *Diabetologia* 1989; 32: 599–605.

34 Yki-Järvinen H, Ryysy L, Kauppila M *et al*. Effect of obesity on the response to insulin therapy in noninsulin-dependent

diabetes mellitus. *J Clin Endocrinol Metab* 1997; 82: 4037–43.

35 Rodin J, Wack J, Ferrannini E, Defronzo RA. Effect of insulin and glucose on feeding behavior. *Metabolism* 1985; 34: 826–31.

36 Edelman SV, Henry RR. Insulin therapy for normalizing glycosylated hemoglobin in type II diabetes. *Diabetes Rev* 1995; 3: 308–34.

37 Boyne MS, Saudek CD. Effect of insulin therapy on macrovascular risk factors in type 2 diabetes. *Diabetes Care* 1999; 22 (Suppl 3): C45–563.

38 Henry RR, Gumbiner B, Ditzler T, Wallace P, Lyon R, Glauber HS. Intensive conventional insulin therapy for type 2 diabetes: metabolic effects during a 6-month outpatient trial. *Diabetes Care* 1993; 16: 21–31.

39 Riddle MC, Schneider J, the Glimepiride Combination Group. Beginning insulin treatment of obese patients with evening 70/30 insulin plus glimepiride alone versus insulin alone. *Diabetes Care* 1998; 21: 1052–7.

40 Scarlett JA, Gray RS, Griffin J, Olefsky JM, Kolterman OG. Insulin treatment reverses the insulin resistance of type II diabetes mellitus. *Diabetes Care* 1982; 5: 353–63.

41 Andrews WJ, Vasques B, Nagulesparan M *et al.* Insulin therapy in obese, non-insulin-dependent diabetes induces improvements in insulin action and secretion that are maintained for two weeks after insulin withdrawal. *Diabetes* 1984; 33: 634–42.

42 Garvey WT, Olefsky JM, Griffin J, Hamman RF, Kolterman OG. The effect of insulin treatment on insulin secretion and action in type II diabetes mellitus. *Diabetes* 1985; 34: 222–34.

43 Taskinen MR, Packard CJ, Shepherd J. Effect of insulin therapy on metabolic fate of apolipoprotein B-containing lipoproteins in NIDDM. *Diabetes* 1990; 39: 1017–27.

44 Malmberg K, the DIGAMI Study Group. Prospective randomized study of intensive insulin treatment on long term survival after acute myocardial infarction in patients with diabetes mellitus. *BMJ* 1997; 314: 1512–15.

45 Apstein CS. Glucose-insulin-potassium for acute myocardial infarction. Remarkable results from a new prospective, randomized trial. *Circulation* 1998; 98: 2223–6.

46 Chow C-C, Tsang LWW, Sorensen JP, Cockram CS. Comparison of insulin with or without continuation of oral hypoglycemic agents in the treatment of secondary failure in NIDDM patients. *Diabetes Care* 1995; 18: 307–14.

47 Landstedt-Hallin L, Adamson U, Arner P, Bolinder J, Lins P-E. Comparison of bedtime NPH or preprandial regular insulin combined with glibenclamide in secondary sulfonylurea failure. *Diabetes Care* 1995; 18: 1183–6.

48 Yki-Järvinen H, Kaupilla M, Kujansuu Lahti J *et al.* Comparison of insulin regimens in patients with non-insulin-dependent diabetes mellitus. *N Engl J Med* 1992; 327: 1426–33.

49 Cusi K, Cunningham GR, Comstock JP. Safety and efficacy of normalizing fasting glucose with bedtime NPH insulin alone in NIDDM. *Diabetes Care* 1995; 18: 843–51.

50 Feinglos MN, Thacker CH, English J, Bethel MA, Lane JD. Modification of postprandial hyperglycemia with insulin lispro improves glucose control in patients with type 2 diabetes. *Diabetes Care* 1997; 20: 1539–42.

51 Yki-Järvinen H, Ryysy L, Nikkila K *et al.* Comparison of bedtime insulin regimens in patients with type 2 diabetes mellitus. *Ann Intern Med* 1999; 130: 389–96.

52 Aviles-Santa L, Sinding J, Raskin P. Effects of metformin in patients with poorly controlled insulin-treated type 2 diabetes mellitus. *Ann Intern Med* 1999; 131: 182–8.

53 Bergenstal R, Johnson M, Whipple D *et al.* Advantages of adding metformin to multiple dose insulin therapy in type 2 diabetes. *Diabetes* 1999; 47 (Suppl. 1): A47.

54 Yu JG, Kruszynska YT, Mulford MI, Olefsky JM. A comparison of troglitazone

and metformin on insulin requirements in euglycemic intensively insulin-treated type 2 diabetic patients. *Diabetes* 1999; 48: 2414–21.

55 Saleh YM, Mudaliar SR, Henry RR. Metabolic and vascular effects of the thiazolidine troglitazone. *Diabetes Rev* 1999; 7: 55–76.

56 Bolli GB, Dimarchi Park GD *et al.* Insulin analogs and their potential in the management of diabetes mellitus. *Diabetologia* 1999; 42: 1151–67.

57 Young AA. Amylin's physiology and its role in diabetes. *Curr Opin Endocrinol Diab* 1997; 4: 282–90.

58 Nauck MA. Glucagonlike peptide 1. *Curr Opin Endocrinol Diab* 1997; 4: 291–300.

59 Thompson RG, Pearson L, Schoenfeld SL, Kolterman OG, the Pramlintide in Type 2 Diabetes Group. Pramlintide, a synthetic analog of human amylin, improves the metabolic profile of patients with type 2 diabetes using insulin. *Diabetes Care* 1998; 21: 987–93.

8: Is the management of diabetic foot ulceration evidence based?

E. Ann Knowles and Andrew J. M. Boulton

Over the last decade the diabetic foot has emerged from a 'Cinderella' role when practitioners who were treating foot problems worked in isolation and were often ignorant of up-to-date practices. Care was previously based on the anecdotal experience of small numbers of healthcarers. Subsequently in many hospitals, resources have been rearranged and centres of excellence with their multidisciplinary foot care teams of doctors, nurses, podiatrists and orthotists have been established. As well as the staff in the foot clinic, other members of the team include the orthopaedic and vascular surgeons, and most importantly, the patient. Patients are key people in the team as their cooperation is essential when treating any foot problem.

One of the first multidisciplinary teams was established at Kings College Hospital in London [1]. This clinic showed that major amputations could be reduced with a multidisciplinary team approach. In our own clinic in Manchester, UK, a 42% reduction in amputations over a 3-year period was achieved [2]. It is important that team members are up to date with current practices and use procedures and treatments that are evidence based. This is difficult, as there are few evidence-based studies on the diabetic foot.

Why treat diabetic foot ulcers?

Foot ulcers that do not heal can be expensive to treat, with prolonged hospital stays and, for some patients, amputation. The Consensus Development Conference on diabetic foot wounds of the American Diabetes Association that met in Boston in 1999 recommended that foot ulcers should be treated to improve quality of life, control infection, maintain health status, prevent amputation and reduce costs [3]. Diabetic foot problems remain a major cause of lower limb amputation, particularly in those with lower limb ischaemia. This is expensive for the health services, and additionally the patient may no longer be able to work, and may need to depend on relatives and friends for support. We have still not all achieved the main aim of the St Vincent Declaration, which was to reduce the incidence of diabetic gangrene by 50% [4].

Causation

Diabetic foot ulcers are expensive, potentially limb threatening and, in many cases, potentially preventable. It is estimated that 15% of all people with diabetes will have a foot ulcer at some time during their life [5]. Patients with established neuropathy have an annual incidence of foot ulceration of 7.2% [6], and although the majority of patients are now treated as outpatients, 20% of all diabetes-related hospital admissions are for foot problems [7]. The costs are enormous.

In terms of causation, foot ulcers are 45–60% neuropathic, 25–45% neuro-ischaemic and 10% ischaemic [8], confirming that neuropathy is a major factor in foot ulceration. Neuropathy increases with poor glycaemic control, age and duration of diabetes [7], and is common (up to 50%) in older patients with type 2 diabetes [9].

Neuropathy

Somatic (sensorimotor) and autonomic nerves can be affected by neuropathy. A sensory deficit in the lower limbs causes loss of the protective pain sensation; patients will not feel the rub from a tight shoe, or any injury to the foot, and will continue to walk on an ulcerated foot and damage it further. Patients with autonomic neuropathy have reduced sweating and dry skin in the lower limbs and callus can build up under areas of high pressure. Cracks, fissures and breaks in the skin can occur, which make the foot susceptible to infection. The blood supply to the foot is also affected by sympathetic dysfunction, which invariably accompanies sensorimotor neuropathy; the arteriovenous shunts in the foot open and the increased blood flow results in bounding pulses and a warm foot.

Motor neuropathy can result in an alteration in foot shape and wasting of the intrinsic muscles of the foot (the plantar flexors and extensors) [8]. The typical high-risk cavus foot in diabetes with its high arch, prominent metatarsal heads and claw toes is in danger of ulceration (Fig. 8.1); but high foot pressures alone do not cause ulcers [10]. Patients with motor and sensory loss can develop an ulcer on the dorsum of the toes if their shoes do not have

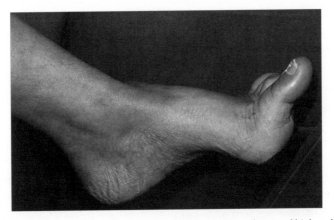

Fig. 8.1 High-risk foot with prominent metatarsal heads, clawing of toes and high arch.

Table 8.1 Factors that contribute to foot ulceration.	Neuropathy
	Peripheral vascular disease
	Foot deformity
	Callus
	Ill-fitting shoes
	Poor vision
	Elderly
	Nephropathy
	Poor glycaemic control

sufficient depth. Intrinsic factors in the causation of foot ulcers include peripheral neuropathy, peripheral vascular disease, nephropathy, limited joint mobility and foot deformity. The extrinsic factors include trauma, abnormal stresses, ill-fitting shoes and smoking. The diabetic foot does not ulcerate spontaneously; a combination of factors causes ulceration [9] (Table 8.1). There is a 50% annual risk of reulceration in any patient with a previous foot ulcer [9]. Screening is needed, but which tests should be used?

Vibration perception tests (vibration reception threshold: VPT) for neuropathy can be performed using a neurothesiometer (A.R. Horwell Ltd, London, UK), but is this the best test? Vibration perception increases with age [11] and it is known that any patient with a VPT > 25 has neuropathy [12]. Impaired vibration threshold is strongly associated with foot ulceration [9]. The height of a patient may also affect the vibration perception in the feet and ankles [13]. A rechargeable battery powers the neurothesiometer which is simple to use, but it is an expensive instrument that general practices and hospital clinics may not be able to afford. Some centres use a biosthesiometer

(Biomedical Instrument Co. Inc, Newbury, OH, USA) but this may not always be accurate if not correctly calibrated [14] and older machines could be electrically unsafe [15]. There is a small number of patients with small-fibre neuropathy and impaired pain and temperature sensation who are still able to feel the vibration of the neurothesiometer: a cold tuning fork may be needed to establish a diagnosis of neuropathy [16].

A tuning fork will also test vibration perception threshold and is cheaper to buy, but unlike the neurothesiometer is not specific. A middle C (128 Hz) tuning fork over the great toe will predict patients with severely reduced sensation who are at risk of ulceration and is a cheaper alternative to the neurothesiometer. A tendon hammer can be used to test ankle reflexes which, if absent, also predict foot ulcer risk.

Monofilaments [17] are increasingly being used as a test for neuropathy and in some centres are given to patients to test their feet at home, which may encourage them to examine their feet more often. The recommended sites to use are the great toe, heel and five metatarsal heads. The reproducibility of the monofilament is good [17]; any patient who cannot feel the 10-g mono-filament on the plantar surface of the foot has a high risk of ulceration [17].

The Semmes–Weinstein monofilament has a long nylon fibre that is embedded in a plastic handle and is used to test pressure sensation. Differ-ent grades of monofilament are available (1, 10, 75 g) but the grade most commonly used to identify patients at risk of foot ulceration is 10 g (5.07). The monofilament buckles at a force of 10 g and should be used on areas of the feet that are free of callus. The monofilaments are now available from several companies but the buckling force may be different in the various monofilaments [17].

Neurotips (Owen Mumford, Oxford, UK) are disposable, made of plastic with a sharp metal end and a blunt end, and are used to test sensation. In the past needles and hatpins have been used for pinprick sensation; these are not advisable as the skin can be punctured, causing infection.

The simplified neuropathy deficit score [18] is an excellent predictor for the 'at-risk' foot. It involves a scoring system based upon simple clinical assessment of three sensory modalities on the hallux, and presence or absence of the ankle reflexes.

The ischaemic foot

Peripheral vascular disease is more common in diabetic patients [19], and is an important contributory factor in foot ulceration and amputation [9]. The foot is often cool with absent foot pulses. Intermittent claudication is the first sign of peripheral vascular disease that can progress to rest pain as circulation deteriorates. Neuropathy may mask the symptoms of claudication and rest pain, and it is therefore important to distinguish between neuropathy and vascular disease. There is a relationship between patients who present with a black toe and vascular disease in other parts of the body: they are more at risk of myocardial infarction and amputation and this risk is increased in smokers [20]. Patients should be encouraged to stop smoking, and hypertension and dyslipidaemia should be controlled.

Palpation of the foot pulses helps to determine the vascular status of the feet, but the presence of a foot pulse does not exclude significant peripheral vascular disease [9]. Doppler blood pressures allow the calculation of the ankle-brachial pressure index (ABPI), although the accuracy of this test must be questioned due to the false high readings caused by calcification or stiffness of the arteries. Doppler blood pressure will detect large vessel disease, but may not detect small vessel disease. An ABPI of <0.9 usually indicates angiogram-positive disease [9]. Listening to the waveforms is also useful; the loss of the normal triphasic waveform suggests vascular disease [8].

Ischaemic ulcers may fail to improve or be slow to heal, and angiography is recommended in all patients if there is no improvement after 2 weeks [19]. Angiography is also recommended in any patient prior to the consideration of amputation. Poor glycaemic control can also impair wound healing, whereas near normoglycaemic control from diagnosis can help prevent the development of neuropathy [8].

Wound classification

Although several wound classifications have been developed, no system has been universally accepted. Many practitioners classify diabetic foot ulcers using the Wagner classification [21] (Table 8.2), which is a simple system but only determines the depth, neuropathic/ischaemic and infected state of the

Table 8.2 The Wagner classification.

Grade 0	No ulcer
Grade 1	Superficial ulcer
Grade 2	Deep ulcer
Grade 3	Osteomyelitis
Grade 4	Gangrene of forefoot
Grade 5	Gangrene of whole foot

Table 8.3 The University of Texas classification system for diabetic foot wounds.

	0	1	2	3
A	Pre- or postulcerative lesion completely healed	Superficial wound	Wound penetrating to tendon or capsule	Wound penetrating to bone or joint
B	Infection	Infection	Infection	Infection
C	Ischaemia	Ischaemia	Ischaemia	Ischaemia
D	Infection and ischaemia	Infection and ischaemia	Infection and ischaemia	Infection and ischaemia

ulcer. Harkless *et al.* have introduced a modified wound classification system (The University of Texas Diabetic Foot Classification) that includes a diabetic foot risk categorization [22] as well as a classification system for diabetic foot wounds [23] (Table 8.3), and provides more details about ischaemia and infection. The Wagner classification [21] does not give all the information that is needed and it may be advisable to change to a different system that provides more details about the condition of the foot ulcer. Further research is needed to find a system that is a simple guide to treatment and will predict outcomes. However, a preliminary study [24] suggests that the University of Texas wound classification system, which grades ulcers according to depth, and stages them according to ischaemia and infection, is superior to the Wagner classification.

Foot examination

Classifying foot ulcers is part of the initial foot examination for all new ulcers. Both feet are examined for any corns, calluses, ulcers, signs of ischaemia, infection or injury, and foot deformity; and gait is observed. Details of medical history, medication, and previous foot ulcers are recorded. Wound location, area, depth, appearance and odour should be included in the clinical assessment and recorded in the notes.

All people with diabetes should have their feet examined as part of their annual review. This should be done more often in patients with at-risk feet, but whose responsibility is it to examine the feet? Patients who are asked to remove their shoes and socks before seeing the doctor do not necessarily have their feet examined [25]. It is important that we all take the trouble to look at our patients' feet on a regular basis. If we do not bother to look at their feet when they come to clinic, we cannot expect them to examine their feet at home.

Many patients, particularly the elderly and patients with type 2 diabetes, do not attend a hospital diabetes clinic, and are cared for in the community by their GP, practice nurse and chiropodist. Hospital and community health-carers all need education about diabetic footcare, so that they can recognize foot problems, educate their patients and know who to contact if a problem occurs.

Debridement

It is, of course, essential that all foot ulcers are debrided and this is usually done by a podiatrist who removes callus and devitalized tissue. Callus build up can increase the incidence of foot ulceration and regular callus debridement is therefore essential. Callus increases vertical shear and is predictive of ulceration [10], acting as a foreign body and increasing foot pressures. Haemorrhage under callus requires urgent treatment, as there may be an ulcer forming beneath it. When the ulcer has been debrided it is cleansed, measured and an appropriate dressing applied; any sinuses present should be probed. The simple act of adequate debridement has been shown to have a positive influence on wound healing [26].

Dressings

Choice of dressing is important but can be influenced by the nurse, podiatrist or consultant; or even by the visit of a representative of a wound care company! Dressings can help to prevent further trauma, minimize the risk of infection and optimize the wound environment [27], but most dressings are not specifically designed for use on diabetic foot ulcers. A systematic review of wound dressings for diabetic foot ulcers that was funded by the UK NHS Health Technology Assessment Programme was undertaken [27]. After searching 18 electronic databases, 11 studies on dressings and diabetic foot ulcers were found that met their criteria. Many of the studies were small and some used dry gauze dressings as the comparator; further studies are needed. Evidence-based practice should be used if possible when selecting a dressing, and this will be influenced by the condition of the wound.

The use of hydrocolloid dressings on diabetic foot ulcers is controversial; there are some practitioners who insist they should not be used [28]. Anecdotal reports of inappropriately used hydrocolloid dressings causing infections and deterioration in diabetic foot wounds suggest that care must be taken when using hydrocolloid dressings [28]. However, if used correctly and changed at least two to three times a week, so that the wound can be inspected, they can be efficacious in the treatment of superficial neuropathic ulcers with medium to low amounts of exudate. Hydrocolloid dressings do not absorb excessive amounts of exudate, and thus maceration of the ulcer and surrounding skin can occur. Patients with vascular ulcers can experience 'drawing' pains in the wound if hydrocolloid dressings are used; a more suitable wound covering is a foam dressing such as Lyofoam.

Alginate dressings are made from seaweed and are available from several manufacturers. These dressings should not be used to pack sinuses or small ulcers as they can plug the wound, causing a build up of exudate [29]. Other dressings include hydrogels for sloughy ulcers and foam dressings. Iodine-based dressings can help to heal ulcers that are infected with methicillin-resistant *Staphylococcus aureus* (MRSA).

Care must be taken when selecting a dressing; practitioners should carefully assess the wound and have knowledge of available wound care products. The frequency of the dressing change will be influenced by the presence of exudate or infection, the condition of the wound and the stage of wound healing (sloughy, necrotic, granulating), and daily dressings may be needed. Frequent dressing changes can increase the cost of wound care and gauze can stick and traumatize the wound when removed. When ulcers have healed the new tissue is fragile and care must be taken to ensure that reulceration does not occur.

New dressings

Wound care companies have become increasingly involved with dressings for diabetic foot ulcers and several new but very expensive products are now available. Although expensive, these dressings can be cost effective if the healing time is less or if amputation or hospital admissions are avoided. Diabetic foot ulcers are chronic wounds that may not heal with conventional treatment; recurrent injury and infection can occur. The wound may not progress beyond the inflammatory/proliferative process of healing. The use of these new dressings may benefit some patients, provided that pressure relief, wound debridement and infection control are addressed.

Evidence from several controlled trials with recombinant human platelet-derived growth factor (Becaplermin) [30] used in resistant, non-infected neuropathic ulcers not responding to conventional treatment have shown reduced healing times and an increased incidence of complete healing.

Cultured human dermis (Dermagraft) [31] is a skin replacement therapy made from neonatal dermal fibroblasts that are cultured *in vitro* onto a bioabsorbic mesh. This living metabolically active tissue has to be handled very carefully and needs to be kept at −80°C and thawed prior to application on the wound. This product has received some criticism because of post hoc change of analysis and exclusion of certain patients. Further studies are in progress.

Larvae therapy

Debridement using a scalpel is the usual method of removing callus and some slough, but care needs to be taken with vascular ulcers. A hydrogel or enzymatic agent will debride sloughy ulcers but a more efficient method used by some centres is maggots (Fig. 8.2). The larvae are supplied by Brigend Hospital in Wales (UK) and are delivered by courier [32]. They are derived from the green bottle fly (*Lucilia sericata*) and their antimicrobial secretions can combat some clinical infections including streptococcus A, staphylococcus A and some resistant strains of bacteria such as MRSA [32]. The larvae also remove necrotic tissue and stimulate fibroblast activity *in vitro* [32]. Anecdotal evidence shows that larvae therapy is effective on some diabetic foot ulcers [33], but more published randomized-controlled studies are needed.

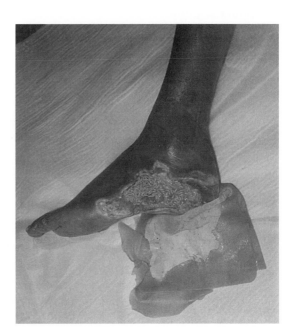

Fig. 8.2 Larvae therapy for foot ulcer. The hydrocolloid dressing was used to protect the surrounding skin.

Antibiotics and infection

Infection in the diabetic foot commonly occurs and delays wound healing. Infections in the diabetic foot are polymicrobial and need broad-spectrum antibiotics, which are effective against commonly known pathogens. There are few evidence-based studies to help in the choice of antibiotics; those few controlled studies were recently reviewed by Caputo [34]. Clinically infected ulcers are generally treated with broad-spectrum antibiotics such as co-amoxiclav or clindamycin (which penetrates well to bone); overuse of anti-biotics can lead to resistant organisms; and the use of antibiotics can increase the cost of care [3]. In a recent retrospective study [35] it was found that MRSA was more common in patients who had been previously treated with antibiotics, and their wounds took longer to heal than patients who did not have MRSA. Some practitioners routinely treat all foot ulcers with antibiotics. Uncomplicated, not clinically infected neuropathic foot ulcers should heal, provided there is adequate wound care and pressure relief, without the need for antibiotics [36]. Frequent follow-up is required and signs of infection such as erythema, warmth and tenderness must be looked for at each visit.

Consultation with the microbiologist when choosing antibiotics may be needed. Antibiotics such as clindamycin and co-amoxiclav can occasionally cause *Clostridium difficile* diarrhoea [8]; patients should be warned about this prior to treatment.

Osteomyelitis

Any non-healing ulcer must be probed and the foot X-rayed to help exclude osteomyelitis. Visible bone usually indicates osteomyelitis [37], and surgical intervention to resect infected bone may be needed to encourage healing [3]. Osteomyelitis is difficult to treat conservatively; a long course of treatment with antibiotics is needed [3].

Pressure relief

Pressure relief is essential when treating foot ulcers and must be addressed. Bed rest will heal ulcers, but care in hospital is expensive and it is difficult to keep an otherwise well patient in bed. Other methods of pressure relief include moulded insoles, footwear, felt padding, hosiery and casts.

In the UK the Scotchcast boot [38] is often used, whereas in the USA the 'gold standard' is the total contact cast [39]. Both casts require the expertise

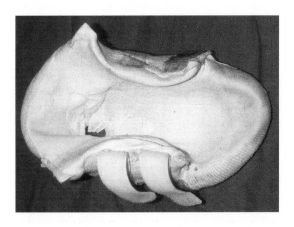

Fig. 8.3 Scotchcast boot (well worn) with window for heel ulcer.

of personnel who are trained to apply them. The Scotchcast boot (Fig. 8.3) is a well-padded, fibreglass cast, which extends from just beyond the toes to above the ankle. It has a windowed area under the ulcer site and although usually made as a removable cast, it can also be non-removable. Casts should be worn at all times when walking, including visits to the toilet at night. If there is an ulcer on the heel the cast can be made with a heel cap and this cast can be worn in bed as well. Compliance can be a problem with a removable cast that may not be worn all the time.

The total contact cast [39] is a minimally padded plaster of Paris cast, which can be covered with a layer of fibreglass. It extends from below the knee to the toes, which are enclosed in the cast. The total contact cast is contraindicated if ischaemia or wound infection is present. One advantage of the total contact cast is that it is non-removable, but there is the danger of rubs if the cast is not correctly applied. With the total contact cast 30% of pressure is taken by the leg on the cast wall [40].

Milroy Paul who, in the 1930s, was using casts to treat the foot ulcers of patients with leprosy [41] has influenced our work with casts for diabetic foot ulcers. However, 70 years later on and many centres are still not using any form of casting despite their effectiveness, and many do not run a diabetic foot clinic. There are few published studies suggesting that casts are effective, but anecdotal reports [38–42] and personal experience certainly suggest that they are. A trial to compare the Scotchcast boot and the total contact cast may decide which is most effective. Other centres use different but equally effective casts, such as the Hope boot [43], the Neofract boot [44] and a modified cast which podiatrists in Newcastle have devised [45].

Some companies are making off-the-shelf products to relieve pressure. Aircast (Aircast Ltd Partnership, London, UK) make a removable cast with inflatable air pockets. In a study of 25 patients, Foster *et al.* [46] healed 76% of their ulcers using an Aircast with few associated problems. Manufactured casts are useful for clinics that do not have practitioners who are skilled in making casts. Manufactured casts may be cheaper than the total costs of the materials for casts that require regular renewal.

Pressure sores

Patients with sensory loss are susceptible to pressures sores (Fig. 8.4) which often occur on the heel and can be limb and life threatening. Vigilance is needed, and part of any care plan must include the inspection of both heels on a daily basis and provision of adequate pressure relief for any immobile patient. The use of a pressure risk assessment such as the Waterlow score [47] will help to determine who is at risk and should be repeated if the pressure risk changes. Pressure-relieving devices such as leg troughs that lift the heel off the bed are useful in the prevention of pressure sores. Patients who are immobile can quickly develop pressure sores from resting their heels on a bed or stool.

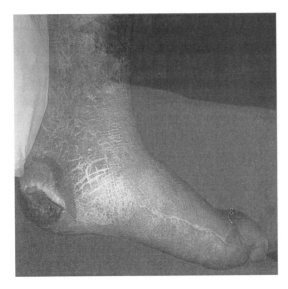

Fig. 8.4 Pressure sore on heel following amputation of leg that led to amputation of other leg.

Silicone

The atrophy of the fat pads under the metatarsal heads makes the foot vulnerable to ulceration. In the USA a podiatrist has successfully injected small amounts of liquid silicone for 25 years under high pressure points and vulnerable areas of the foot [48]. In the first randomized-controlled trial of injected silicone in the neuropathic foot, its efficacy was confirmed; it was shown to reduce plantar pressures measured by the optical pedobaragraph, and weight-bearing ultrasound studies show an increase in subcutaneous tissue depth under the metatarsal heads [49].

Approval has been sought for its use in this and other countries, but the controversy over the use of silicone breast implants may influence some practitioners; further trials and experience are needed of injected silicone in the high-risk diabetic foot.

Footwear

One of the commonest causes of foot ulceration is ill-fitting shoes; shoes must be assessed and if needed prescribed footwear provided.

The orthotist is an essential part of the team and should have knowledge of diabetic foot problems and know which shoes to provide. Companies now have a good selection of colours and styles of shoes and patients should be allowed to choose their prescribed footwear. The shoe must have sufficient depth to accommodate the foot and any pressure-relieving insoles. Patients are encouraged to break their shoes in gradually and eventually wear them at all times when walking.

We know that some of our patients do not wear their prescribed footwear [50] or may only put them on when they come to the clinic. The shoes we supply are expensive and budgets are limited; patients who do not wear their prescribed footwear are more likely to reulcerate [51].

Education

Education is also important, but although patients may have excellent knowledge of appropriate footcare, they do not always put that knowledge into practice and can be non-compliant [52]. It is difficult to convince patients with sensory loss and no symptoms that their feet are at risk of ulceration. Some patients who cannot reach or feel their feet may need to ask a relative or friend to do the examination for them.

Why do patients not comply? Patients must understand how their foot ulcer occurred. Their feet are not always their main priority; if neuropathic patients continue to walk on an ulcerated foot, infection may be 'pumped' through the foot and, despite this, early medical advice may not be sought. Some patients have distorted beliefs about neuropathy, which they link with poor circulation and amputation [52]; prescribed footwear or casts may not be worn, as no discomfort is felt from their ulceration. A change in behaviour is needed and we must persuade patients to try to modify their lifestyle to allow their foot ulcers to heal. Educational footcare literature should be in large print for visually impaired patients, and leaflets should be easy to understand, be relevant to that particular patient's problem and cover essential aspects of foot care [53]. Non-compliant patients who do not or will not follow advice remain a problem; if all else fails an emergency contact number should be given to them in case a foot problem occurs.

How should we organize foot ulcer care?

It has been shown that a multidisciplinary team of doctors, chiropodists, nurses and an orthotist is effective in reducing amputations (Table 8.4) [1,2]. Good liaison between other disciplines in both primary and secondary care is essential, and should also include the vascular and orthopaedic surgeons. There should be consistent advice from all team members [53] to avoid confusion, and leaflets and printed literature should be easy to understand, relevant to that patient, and more detailed for those at risk. Educational material must be reviewed. All healthcarers who care for people with diabetes should know how diabetes affects the feet, how to recognize and to whom to refer a foot problem to. Patients should be given an emergency contact number in case a problem does occur.

Multidisciplinary
Available for emergencies
Up-to-date knowledge
Preventative treatment
Education
Audit
Register of foot ulcers and amputations
Evidence-based practice
Prescribed footwear and orthoses

Table 8.4 Essentials of a footcare team.

There should be provision for early/urgent referral for all patients with new ulcers or foot problems who may need to be seen between clinics. Criteria for referral will help to ensure that the referral is relevant for the clinic. All new foot ulcer patients should have their feet screened and their ulcer assessed. Moulded insoles and extra-depth/bespoke shoes should be supplied to patients if their own footwear is unsuitable; shoes and insoles must be regularly reviewed and renewed or repaired, to maintain adequate pressure relief. It is cost effective to treat outpatients early to prevent amputations and hospital admissions. Patients whose ulcers have healed should continue to be seen by the podiatrist for preventative treatment. If the foot clinic is too busy they should be seen by an experienced podiatrist or a high-risk foot clinic could be established.

All people with diabetes should have their feet screened at annual review and more often if their feet are 'at risk'. Prevention really is better than cure; shoes and socks must always be removed and both feet examined. Team members must be up to date with wound care products and other aspects of diabetic foot care so that they can provide the best treatment. Liaison with community staff regarding treatment and dressings will help to maintain continuity of care and avoid confusion for the patient. Education is important and should include the patient and any relative or carer.

Audit and registration of foot ulcers and amputations will provide evidence of practice and could secure increased funding for future clinics as patient numbers increase.

Diabetic neuroarthropathy (Charcot foot)

The Charcot foot presents a challenge for many practitioners, with the occurrence of gross deformities that can lead to ulceration over bony prominences (Fig. 8.5). There is little evidence-based practice as to how to treat the Charcot foot [54], and various centres use different methods of treatment. There is general agreement, however, that significant immobilization is needed, and some centres favour total contact casting [55]. Intravenous pamidronate has also recently been shown to be helpful, in a randomized, placebo-controlled trial [56].

Conclusions

In the last decade, much progress has been made in diabetic foot research,

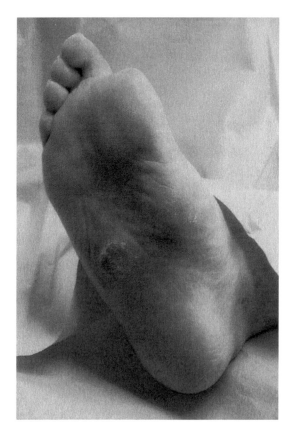

Fig. 8.5 Charcot foot—note callus build up under bony prominences.

and evidence-based practice should increase in the next decade. Randomized-controlled studies must have sufficient patients for statistical power and to overcome patient variability [3]. Evidence-based practice could lead to better services and falling costs but extra budgets may be needed to initiate this. Relying on tradition and intuition is no longer good enough; the educational needs of our staff must be assessed to enable them to introduce evidence-based practice, which could influence patient care and future trials.

References

1 Edmonds ME, Blundell MP, Morris ME, Thomas ME, Cotton LT, Watkins PJ. Improved survival of the diabetic foot: the role of a specialised clinic. *QJ Med* 1986; 60: 763–71.

2 Thomson FJ, Veves A, Ashe H *et al.* A team approach to diabetic foot care: the Manchester experience. *The Foot* 1991; 1: 75–82.

3 American Diabetes Association.

Consensus Development Conference on Diabetic Foot Wound Care. *Diabetes Care* 1999; 22: 1354–60.

4 Diabetes Care and Research in Europe. The St Vincent Declaration. *Diabet Med* 1990; 7: 360.

5 Palumbo PJ, Melton IJ. Peripheral vascular disease and diabetes. In: Harris MI, Hamman RF, eds. *Diabetes in America*. NIH Publications no 85–1468. Washington: US Government Printing Office, 1985: 1–21.

6 Abbott CA, Vileikyte LR, Williamson SH, Carrington A, Boulton AJM. Multi-centre study of the incidence and predictive risk factors for diabetic foot ulceration. *Diabetes Care* 1998; 21: 1071–5.

7 Williams DRR. The size of the problem: epidemiological and economic aspects of foot problems in diabetes. In: Boulton AJM, Connor H, Cavanagh PR, eds. *The Foot in Diabetes*, 2nd edn. New York: Wiley, 1994: 15–24.

8 Shaw JE, Boulton AJM. The diabetic foot. In: Davies AH, Beard JD, Wyatt MG, eds. *Essential Vascular Surgery*, 2nd edn. Philadelphia: WB Saunders, 2001: in press.

9 Shaw JE, Zimmett PZ, Boulton AJM. The epidemiology of diabetic neuropathy. *Diabetes Rev* 1999; 7: 245–52.

10 Veves A, Murray HJ, Young MJ, Boulton AJM. The risk of foot ulceration in diabetic patients with high foot pressures: a prospective study. *Diabetologia* 1992; 35: 660–3.

11 Coppini DV, Young PJ, Wong C, Macleod AF, Sonksen PH. Outcome on diabetic foot complications in relation to clinical examination and quantitative sensory testing. A case-controlled study. Age adjusted vibration perception test is better than sensitivity in clinical tests. *Diabet Med* 1998; 15: 765–71.

12 Klenerman L, McCabe C, Cogley D, Lang P, White M. Screening for patients at risk of diabetic foot ulceration in a general diabetic outpatient clinic. *Diabet Med* 1996; 13: 561–3.

13 Wiles PG, Pearce SM, Rice PJS, Mitchell JMMO. Vibration perception threshold.

Influence of age, height, sex and smoking, and calculation of accurate centile values. *Diabet Med* 1991; 8: 157–61.

14 Masson EA, Boulton AJM. Calibration problems with the biosthesiometer. *Diabet Med* 1990; 7: 261–2.

15 Watts GF, Shaw KM, Long G. A warning on the use of the biosthesiometer [letter]. *Diabet Med* 1986; 3: 91.

16 Edmonds ME, Foster AVM. *Managing the Diabetic Foot*. Oxford: Blackwell Science, 2000.

17 McGill M, Molyneaux L, Yue DK. Use of Semmes–Weinstein 5.07/10 gram monofilament: the long and short of it. *Diabet Med* 1998; 15: 615–17.

18 Young MJ, Boulton AJM, Williams DRR, Mcleod AF, Sonksen PH. A multicentre study of the prevalence of diabetic neuropathy. *Diabetologia* 1993; 36: 150–4.

19 Tooke JE. European consensus document on central limb ischaemia: implications for diabetes. *Diabet Med* 1990; 7: 544–6.

20 Shaw TN, Logan A, Lomax GA, Eccles K, Jones GR. Diabetic black toe is a marker for fatal myocardial infarction. *Pract Diabetes* 1998; 15: 43–4.

21 Wagner FW. Algorithms of diabetic foot care. In: Levin ME O'Neal FW, eds. *The Diabetic Foot*. St Louis: CV Mosby, 1983: 290.

22 Armstrong DG, Lavery LA, Harkless LB. Treatment-based classification system for assessment and care of diabetic feet. *Ostomy Wound Manag* 1996; 42: 50–8.

23 Armstrong DG, Lavery DG, Harkless LB. Validation of a diabetic wound classification system: the contribution of depth, infection, and vascular disease to the risk of amputation. *Diabetes Care* 1998; 21: 855–9.

24 Oyibo S, Jude E, Tarawneh I, Armstrong DG, Harkless LB, Boulton AJM. A comparison of two diabetic foot classification systems. *Diabet Med* 2000; 17 (Suppl 1): 54.

25 Cohen SJ. Potential barriers to diabetes care. *Diabetes Care* 1983; 6: 499–500.

26 Steed DL, Donohoe D, Webster MW, Lindsley L. Effect of extensive

debridement and treatment on the healing of diabetic foot ulcers. *J Am Coll Surg* 1996; 183: 61–4.

27 Callum N, Majid O'Meara S, Sheldon T. Use of dressings: is there an evidence base? In: Boulton AJM, Connor H, Cavanagh PR, eds. *The Foot in Diabetes*, 3rd edn. Chichester: John Wiley, 2000: 153–68.

28 Foster AVM, Spencer S, Edmonds ME. Deterioration of diabetic foot lesions under hydrocolloid dressings. *Pract Diabetes Int* 1997; 14: 62–4.

29 Lawrence IG, Lear JT, Burden AC. Alginate dressings and the diabetic foot ulcer. *Pract Diabetes Int* 1997; 14: 61–2.

30 Wieman TJ, Smiell JM, Yachin SU. Efficacy and safety of a topical gel formulation of recombinant human platelet-derived growth factor-BB (Becaplermin) patients with chronic neuropathic foot ulcers. *Diabetes Care* 1998; 21: 822–7.

31 Gentzkow G, Iawaski S, Hershon K *et al.* Use of dermagraft, a cultured human dermis to treat diabetic foot *Ulcers Diabetes Care* 1996; 21: 1230–10.

32 Thomas S, McAndrews AM, Hay N, Bourgiose S. The antimicrobial activity of maggot secretions: results of a preliminary study. *J Tissue Viability* 1999; 9: 127–32.

33 Rayman A, Stansfield G, Woollard T, Mackie A, Rayman G. Use of larvae in the treatment of the diabetic necrotic foot. *Diabetic Foot* 1998; 1: 7–13.

34 Caputo GM. The rational use of antimicrobial agents in diabetic foot infections. In: Boulton AJM, Connor H, Cavanagh PR, eds. *The Foot in Diabetes*, 3rd edn. Chichester: John Wiley, 2000: 143–52.

35 Tentolouris N, Jude EB, Smirnoff I, Knowles EA, Boulton AJM. Methicillin-resistant *Staphylococcus aureus*: an increasing problem in a diabetic foot clinic. *Diabet Med* 1999; 1: 767–71.

36 Chanteleau E, Tanudjaja T, Altenhofer F, Ersanli Z, Lacigova S, Metzger C. Antibiotic treatment for uncomplicated neuropathic foot ulcers in diabetes: a controlled trial. *Diabet Med* 1996; 13: 159.

37 Grayson ML, Gibbons GW, Balogh K, Levin E, Karchmer AW. Probing to bone in infected pedal ulcers: a clinical sign of underlying osteomyelitis in diabetic patients. *JAMA* 1997; 273: 721–3.

38 Burden AC, Jones GR, Jones R, Blandford RL. Use of a 'Scotchcast' boot in treating diabetic foot ulcers. *BMJ* 1983; 286: 1555–7.

39 Mueller MJ, Diamond JE, Sinacor DR *et al.* Total contact casting in treatment of diabetic plantar ulcers. Controlled clinical trial. *Diabetes Care* 1989; 12: 384–8.

40 Shaw JE, Hsi WL, Ulbrecht JS, Norkitis A, Becker MB, Cavanagh PR. The mechanism of plantar unloading in total contact casts: implications for design and clinical use. *Foot Ankle Int* 1997; 18: 809–17.

41 Coleman WC, Brand PW, Birke JA *et al.* The total contact cast: a therapy for plantar ulceration on insensitive feet. *J Am Podiatr Med Assoc* 1984; 74: 548–52.

42 Jones R, Beshay SA, Curryer GJ, Burden AC. Modification of the Leicester (Scotchcast) boot. *Pract Diabetes* 1989; 6: 118–20.

43 Williams A. The Hope removable walking cast: a method of treatment for diabetic/neuropathic ulceration. *Pract Diabetes Int* 1994; 11: 20–3.

44 Page S, Crooke G, Peacock I. 'Neofract' boots for diabetic neuropathic foot ulcers. *Pract Diabetes Int* 1995; 12: 135–7.

45 Whyte I. The Newcastle Optima slipper: a new method of casting. *Diabetic Foot* 1998; 1: 95–102.

46 Foster A, McColgan M, Edmonds M. Aircast—a new treatment for diabetic foot ulceration. *Diabet Med* 1998; 15: S22.

47 Waterlow J. Pressure sores: a risk assessment card. *Nursing Times*; 1985; 81: 45–55.

48 Balkin SW, Kaplan L. Injectable silicone and the diabetic foot: a 25-year report. *Foot*, 1991; 2: 83–8.

49 Van Schie CHM, Whalley A, Vileikyte L, Wignall T, Hollis S, Boulton AJM. The use of injected liquid silicone in the diabetic foot: a randomised-

controlled trial. *Diabetes Care* 2000;
23: 634–8.

50 Knowles EA, Boulton AJM. Do patients
with diabetes wear their prescribed
footwear? *Diabet Med* 1996; 13: 1064–8.

51 Chantleleau E, Haage P. An audit of
cushioned footwear: relation to patient
compliance. *Diabet Med* 1994; 11:
114–16.

52 Vileikyte L. Psychological aspects of
diabetic peripheral neuropathy. *Diabetes
Rev* 1999; 7: 387–94.

53 Connor H. Footcare advice: what do
we tell our patients and what should

we tell them? *Pract Diabetes Int* 1997;
14: 75–7.

54 Shaw JE, Boulton AJM. The Charcot foot.
Foot 1995; 5: 65–70.

55 McGill M, Molyneux L, Bolton T, Ioannou
K, Uren R, Yue DK. Response of Charcot's
arthropathy to contact casting: assessment
by quantitative techniques. *Diabetologia*
2000; 43: 481–4.

56 Jude EB, Selby PL, Donohue M *et al.*
Pamidronate in diabetic Charcot
neuropathy: a randomized placebo
controlled trial. *Diabet Med* 2000; 17
(Suppl 1): 54.

Management issues in type 1 diabetes

9: Is even moderate control of diabetes feasible in adolescents?

Stephen A. Greene

The aim of this chapter is to confirm that the answer is yes!

This may seem overoptimistic to those advising on the care of type 1 diabetes in adolescents, who are well aware that adolescence is a particular time of overall poor glycaemic control. Acute problems of poor glycaemic control include ketoacidosis and hypoglycaemia, and the potential development of chronic microvascular complications is also brought into stark focus in this age group.

These issues raise the challenge of why some teenagers and some health services caring for young people with diabetes achieve better results than others. Are there inherent physiological problems with adolescents with diabetes, or do they fail to comply with therapy? Can clinical services be changed to improve glycaemic control? Would these moves be at the expense of destroying the spirit of adolescent development and change?

Are adolescents poorly controlled?

Several surveys of large cohorts show conclusively an inexorable deterioration in glycaemic control in adolescence, compared with younger children. These include recent studies that overcame the problem of comparison of glycosylated haemoglobin (HbA_{1c}) from different centres by the use of a central laboratory assay: the Diabetes Control and Complications Trial (DCCT) Research Group [1], the Danish Study Group [2], the French Study Group [3] and the Scottish Study Group for the Care of the Young Diabetic (SSGCYD) [4]. Our data in Scotland from the DIABAUD2 project (the National audit project of the Scottish Study Group for the Care of the Young Diabetic) showed that 11–15-year-old patients had an average HbA_{1c} of 9.6% (girls) and 9.4% (boys); this was substantially higher than in children aged 4–10 years, namely 8.7% (girls) and 8.7% (boys) (Fig. 9.1). In both young children

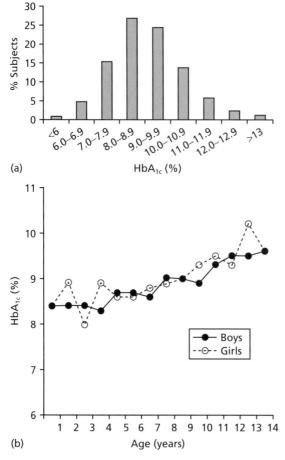

Fig. 9.1 Distribution of HbA_{1c} in 1670 children and teenagers throughout Scotland. $n = 1670$ patients <15 years' age. Data from DIABAUD 2 Project by the Scottish Study Group for the Care of the Young Diabetic [4].

and teenagers, there is a right-skewed distribution of HbA_{1c}, with some children and teenagers having extremely poor metabolic control; in Scotland, fewer than 25% maintain their HbA_{1c} at <8%.

Is this picture universal? The distribution of HbA_{1c} among different centres appears similar, although certain clinical teams appear to obtain better overall outcome for their patients. In DIABAUD2, we demonstrated significant influences on glycaemic control of various factors, which included age, gender, body mass index, social circumstances and family history. However, these associations accounted for less than 20% of the variation in glycaemic control. Marked geographical inequalities in glycaemic con-

Fig. 9.2 DIABAUD 2 Project [4]: centre differences (mean and 95% confidence intervals, expressed as the mean of the deviations from predicted HbA$_{1c}$) adjusted for factors known to influence glycaemic control (age, gender, body mass index, season, social circumstances and family history). Mean HbA$_{1c}$ in Scotland is 8.9%. If there were no centre effect, all values would lie on the zero line.

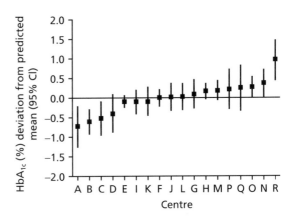

trol were demonstrated—after adjustment for factors associated with poor glycaemic control—with significant and major differences between clinical centres in median HbA$_{1c}$ of 8.2–9.6% (Fig. 9.2). A survey of the resources in each clinical centre revealed differences in the distribution of medical staff, variations in the performance of clinical tasks, discrepancies in offering 24-hour contact and home care, and differences in methodologies for investigations. However, these did not appear to influence individual or average clinical glycaemic control.

The Hvidore Study Group on Childhood Diabetes examined blood glucose control in an international cross-sectional study of 2873 children and adolescents in 22 centres from 18 countries [5]. The mean HbA$_{1c}$ for the entire cohort was 8.6%. This was equivalent to 8.3% in the DCCT Study and compared well with the intensively-treated group of teenagers in that study who had a mean HbA$_{1c}$ of 8.1%. Overall, however, the goal of near normal glycaemia was achieved in only a few. Intriguingly, major differences existed between centres, with a range in mean HbA$_{1c}$ from 7.3% to 10.1%. No obvious factors determining glycaemic control emerged from this limited assessment of the patients' clinical management and the resources available to each centre. Surprisingly, no significant impact on glycaemic control was found with different insulin regimens; indeed, one of the centres has reported 'good' overall control (clinic mean HbA$_{1c}$ 7.6%) using standard twice-daily regimens [6]. Control deteriorated again significantly throughout adolescence, despite an increase in insulin dose and number of daily insulin injections (2, 3, 4 or more).

Why are adolescents poorly controlled?

Physiological and psychological studies

Is the deterioration in glycaemic control seen in the adolescent with type 1 diabetes somehow preordained? Is the poor glycaemic control inherent in the changing physiology of adolescence, or is it related to behavioural changes in the management of the diabetes? Should we accept lower standards of glycaemic control in this age group, or should we alter our strategies in an attempt to achieve good glycaemic control?

Physiological changes in glucose metabolism during adolescence

Non-diabetic subjects show increasing insulin resistance, reflected in changes in fasting insulin levels, while moving from childhood into puberty [7]. There are also major changes in fasting insulin-like growth factor 1 binding protein and growth hormone concentrations in association with the puberty growth spurt [8]. Recently marked abnormalities suggestive of insulin resistance in normal teenagers in their insulin and glucose response to a standard meal have been shown [9]—which must reinforce current concern over the emergence of type 2 diabetes among the young, and which is following the 'epidemic' of obesity [10,11]. These general changes in the population seem likely to affect at least some patients with type 1 diabetes; an increase in body fat, reflecting both the insulin resistance and hormonal changes of puberty, may also lead to impairment of glucose metabolism.

These physiological changes in glucose metabolism appear to be heightened in adolescents with type 1 diabetes. Increased insulin dosages are often needed to maintain a similar level of glycaemia in patients moving from childhood to adolescence. Insulin-like growth factor levels decrease significantly during puberty and there are major increases in IGF binding-protein and growth hormone concentrations [8]. Body composition changes—notably fat accumulation—can be quite marked in teenagers with diabetes, particularly in girls [12].

Behavioural, social and cultural changes in adolescence

Adolescence is a critical time for young people with or without diabetes. Diabetic individuals need to take responsibility for the management of their own diabetes [13–15], and experience the relationship between their own actions, blood glucose levels and physical symptoms, which all influence beliefs about diabetes and its management. These are formative years in the development of such beliefs, which, once fully integrated and accepted by the young person, may prove difficult to change. Therefore, they are in the unenviable position of facing the same developmental tasks and demands as all young people, but with the additional burden of learning to manage their diabetes. The main challenge is to improve diabetes control through this transitional phase, without depriving young people of the appropriate age-related experiences [16]

The complex array of diabetes and general developmental issues has generated a wealth of literature on the psychological aspects of paediatric chronic illness, and diabetes in particular. Research has focused primarily on the relationship between adolescents and their families, with support and cohesion within the families being consistently associated with better metabolic control and self-care [17]. Furthermore, having to take early responsibility for diabetes care—especially without parental involvement—is predictive of lower concordance, poor control and diabetic ketoacidosis [18]. However, there is a paucity of research on the role of the adolescent's peer group in relation to concordance, at a time when peer influence becomes important. It has been recommended that 'greater attention be paid to the social context' in which the adolescent lives [19–23]. The few studies that have been conducted indicate that peers are an important source of emotional support, and that this support is essential for optimal self-care and emotional well-being [22–25].

Our group investigated macro- and microcultural influences on the health strategies and beliefs of young people and professional health carers in adolescents with diabetes. In a cross-cultural study in Scotland and Italy, anthropological methodology was used that highlighted significant social and cultural influences on concordance with diabetes regimens [26–27]. In practical terms, the following observations were made in the Scottish diabetes service.

• Patients with good control were more likely to be rewarded with fewer clinic visits, which could intensify their sense of isolation.

• Responsibility was encouraged at an early age, separating the young diabetic from family and peer support.

• Parents and peers were excluded at an age irrespective of development, i.e. categorization was by age, not individual ability and preference.

• Exclusion of the parents obscured non-concordance, suggesting 'normal progress towards adulthood and independence'.
• Breakdown of reciprocal social networks that provided community support for the young diabetic patient. This contrasted with considerable reciprocity between the health carers (e.g. conferences, team meetings, social support network).

Healthcare professionals comply with British social pressures to concentrate on the individuality of their patients, irrespective of their social situations, to make them accountable for their own illness. There is a mismatch between the health goals of the young person with diabetes and the healthcare professionals supporting them. This is compounded by the 'medicalization of adolescence'—the expectation that adolescence is a medical entity—and leads automatically to disruption of health. Health carers expect poor concordance in young people and there is a notion of low success and that 'good concordance is viewed as abnormal in this age'. This leads in turn to the expectation that diabetes management strategies are damned in this group from the outset.

Unmanageable diabetes in the teenager

The natural history of type 1 diabetes prior to the discovery of insulin in 1921–22 was failed treatment, leading to death, classically in older children and the older teenager. The expectations after the introduction of insulin as a 'cure' for diabetes were not inevitably realized in all patients, and indeed it was commonly a difficult disease to manage. Good metabolic control could be obtained by rigid attention to detail: 4–6 injections per day (even of relatively impure insulin), meticulous attention to diet, obsessive monitoring of diabetes and regular sustained exercise.

However, many patients did not achieve the desired outcome and medical practitioners began to suggest that bad control implied bad patients. In my view, this attitude has remained since those early days, with the onus of failure being placed on the patient—despite the obvious inability of any diabetes management regimen to replicate the intricate homeostatic mechanisms that regulate normal metabolism.

Unnatural insulin is delivered to an inappropriate site (peripheral circulation, instead of into the hepatic portal system), at the wrong time (i.e. without direct feedback control with pancreatic glucose concentration) and at the wrong doses (very high peripheral insulin levels are needed to achieve useful concentrations at the liver).

Brittle diabetes

At the extreme of the spectrum of bad control are a small number of patients who suffer not only generally high blood glucose concentration but also wide metabolic swings: frequent episodes of hypoglycaemia (often nocturnal) and hospital admissions for diabetic ketoacidosis (DKA). They became known as having 'brittle' diabetes, a term first used in textbooks on diabetes in the 1920s (see Chapter 10). More recently, Tattersall defined the state as 'patients whose lives are constantly disrupted by episodes of hyperglycaemia or hypoglycaemia, whatever the cause' [28].

From the earliest descriptions, physicians tried to explain brittle diabetes in terms of intrinsic problems with the diabetes itself (abnormal counter-regulatory hormone reactions, pituitary abnormalities, coexisting diseases associated with diabetes) or abnormal reactions to the insulin injection (defective insulin absorption or excessive insulin degradation and high insulin antibody production). The 1970s and 1980s saw the introduction of home blood glucose monitoring, newer insulin preparations, continuous subcutaneous insulin infusion (CSII) and automatic machines such as the Biostator, and these advances triggered a series of investigations in the UK and the USA into brittle diabetes, attempting to unearth the responsible organic defect [29,30]. Interestingly, all of the groups began to describe a relatively homogeneous collection of patients who were being referred for investigation of extreme brittleness. These were nearly all young women ranging in age from late childhood into their early twenties. They were c-peptide negative, had poor glycaemic control and were often prescribed high doses of insulin, yet many were significantly overweight. Most had been referred to the investigating units for detailed study after several years of major difficulties in their home base. Detailed studies of these patients, particularly in the Newcastle [31] and Guy's group [32], and Schade's group in the USA [33], revealed a high incidence of marked behavioural abnormalities (factitious disease, malingering, communication disorders). All these groups concluded that poor concordance was an important cause of brittleness; the Guy's group after many years of searching for organic causes of brittle diabetes, stated firmly that 'the most likely cause of rapidly developing hyperglycaemia and ketosis in these patients remains insulin deficiency due to the patient interrupting insulin administration' [34].

For any centre that cares for young people with type 1 diabetes for several years, it is likely that at least one such case emerges—when the medical team often struggles to support such a difficult patient. As the understanding of brittle diabetes has evolved over the years, it is now time for a wider interpretation to be put in place. Tattersall's definition specifically mentions constant disruption. However, many teenagers fall into a broader description of brittleness, which would identify a greater number of patients. These patients suffer occasional (perhaps only one) life-threatening episodes of DKA and/or hypoglycaemia, but have periods of relative stability, although glycaemic control is usually poor. They may have overt behavioural problems and/or difficult home, school or relationship circumstances. The immediate cause of poor control is generally undertreatment with insulin.

Insulin omission

Insulin deficiency producing erratic control and subsequently brittle diabetes with episodes of DKA is most likely due to insulin omission. Manipulation and factitious insulin delivery have been seen in patients with the most severe psychological disturbance. Several case reports have been published of patients hiding insulin to induce hypoglycaemia, dilution of insulin for injection or infusion by pumps, and tampering with intravenous and intraperitoneal catheters [35]. As mentioned, most of these have come to light only after extensive hospital investigation.

More recently, insulin omission has emerged as a widespread and common phenomenon, which probably accounts for the vast majority of episodes of DKA in the older teenager known to have diabetes. This had long been suspected by clinicians, but direct evidence has only recently been forthcoming. Capillary blood glucose testing and glycated haemoglobin estimation in the 1980s confirmed the suboptimal control of many young people with diabetes, and poor concordance with the prescribed therapy regimens (insulin and diet) is an obvious explanation. However, as Steel so eloquently stated, 'there is a reluctance to believe that patients would deliberately cheat their doctor and after all "she is such a nice girl that she would never do anything like that" ' [36].

In our unit, Thompson examined the differences between young and older diabetic people presenting with DKA [37]. No specific cause (e.g. infection) was established in the majority of young cases and they responded dramatically to simple fluid and insulin therapy. It was possible to show that the cause of DKA in this group was omission of insulin, using the DARTS/MEMO (diabetes audit and research, Tayside, Scotland/medicines monitoring unit, University of Dundee) database as a direct measure of insulin prescription in the Tayside region. A unique identifier for each patient (the community health index, CHI) allowed accurate tracking of insulin

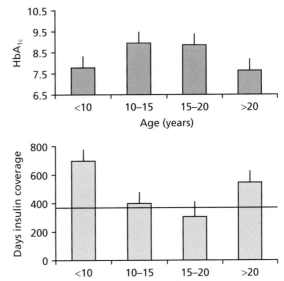

Fig. 9.3 Lack of concordance in collecting insulin prescriptions and influence on glycaemic control. Insulin omission in the middle teenage years is associated with poor HbA$_{1c}$ levels. Data from Morris *et al.* [38].

prescriptions in 90 young people with type 1 diabetes (aged under 25 years) [38]. In the older teenagers it was found that over 50% failed to collect all of their prescribed insulin over 1 year, and that 28% collected less than one-third of their insulin. A low collection rate of insulin was associated with a high overall poor control and a high admission rate for DKA (Fig. 9.3).

In the DIABAUD2 study, daily insulin dose (units/kg/day) increased with age. There was a considerable spread in dose with a significant proportion of patients prescribed >1.0 unit/kg/day; however, HbA$_{1c}$ remained disappointingly poor throughout. One interpretation is that more insulin is required to overcome the insulin resistance of adolescence, just to maintain (poor) control. Another is that insulin is continued to be prescribed by health workers in ever increasing doses, not realizing that the teenagers are not taking a significant percentage of their insulin dose. We favour the latter explanation. Moreover, the data from the DARTS/MEMO study and DIABAUD2 suggest that persisting poor control (HbA$_{1c}$ > 11% in our clinic) indicates insulin deficiency because the patient is taking less insulin than prescribed.

Insulin, weight and eating disorders

Diabetes, particularly for girls, is a battleground between the powerful effect insulin has on fat metabolism and the culturally unacceptable body images of excessive weight in modern society. The high doses of insulin frequently used to achieve as low a blood glucose level as possible may increase carbohydrate intake and body fat mass. Data from the Hvidore International Study Group confirm the excessive weight of older teenage girls with type 1 diabetes—a phenomenon in all clinics. For these girls excessive weight gain can become their major problem.

The failure to translate advice from the diabetes health professionals into self-management is not generally due to lack of knowledge: many studies have revealed that the understanding of diabetes is high among diabetic children and teenagers and their parents. Rather, it is the desire to exploit this information that is the key to concordance with the diabetes regimens [39]. Therefore, it is not surprising that many teenagers learn that insulin omission can be used effectively to keep their weight down.

At the same time it has been accepted that there is a higher incidence of eating disorders (anorexia nervosa, bulimia, binge eating) in diabetic youngsters, particularly girls [40]. Given that eating disorders are common in young people anyway, it is not surprising that they are commoner in diabetes, with its emphasis on diet as a treatment modality. The combination of insulin omission and erratic eating habits is potentially a powerful tool to reduce weight or keep weight steady—but obviously at the expense of poor glycaemic control. Many patients appear to find this acceptable even with the symptoms of hyperglycaemia and the risk of DKA.

Intercurrent diseases causing poor diabetic control

A sudden change in the stability of the diabetes may point to specific diseases associated with diabetes, which may lead to erratic glycaemic control. In the young, other autoimmune diseases are the most likely: thyroid antibodies have been reported in 10–50% of diabetic people under the age of 25 years [41], although clinical hypothyroidism or thyrrotoxicosis are rarer (<5%). Other diseases to be considered in any case of deteriorating control include asymptomatic coeliac and Addison's disease. Chronic infections (e.g. tuberculosis) do not seem to be particularly common in diabetes, although all children are prone to other general childhood illnesses that should be considered (infection, leukaemia, etc.).

Complications and the teenager with diabetes

The DCCT trial, along with several other clinical studies, confirmed the association between long-term suboptimal blood glucose control and the risk of microvascular complications. Persistently poor control in teenagers increases that risk considerably, and notably the development of malignant microvascular changes, particularly retinopathy. Not surprisingly, long-term diabetic complications are considerably commoner in adults with diabetes who have had a period of poor control in their teenage years. It is likely that the overall complication risk is falling in stable diabetic patients, but increasing in the poorly controlled cases. The latter also have a poorer quality of life and more complications in pregnancy; tragically, some die young from severe episodes of hypoglycaemia or DKA.

Gastric stasis due to autonomic neuropathy may be commoner than generally appreciated [42]. It is likely, however, that this is a secondary and reversible complication of poor glycaemic control rather than the primary cause of the brittleness of the diabetes itself. Improving control can reverse symptoms of bloating, abdominal pains and vomiting.

Recurrent hypoglycaemia

Frequent episodes of hypoglycaemia are part of the poor control seen in the teenage years. Hypoglycaemia alone with stable and acceptable glycaemic control ($HbA_{1c} < 8.5\%$) is seen frequently in children and young people. The hypoglycaemic attacks usually follow exercise or omission of food (especially in the young child), or may occur during periods of illness. Severe episodes, especially in association with poor glycaemic control and DKA, typify the picture of unstable adolescence in diabetes.

A separate factor to be considered in teenagers is alcohol abuse, which now affects girls as frequently as boys. Alcohol is particularly associated with severe nocturnal hypoglycaemia and some evidence suggests that some cases of the 'dead in bed' syndrome in young diabetic people may be alcohol-related.

Care strategies for the adolescent

The approach to poor glycaemic control in the adolescent with diabetes has to be made on two levels: first, to help the individual patient with erratic control and life-threatening episodes of hypoglycaemia and DKA; second, a more general approach to the effective delivery of diabetes care in an attempt to minimize the problem. At the root of both, we believe, is the lack of concordance with the diabetes regimens.

Diabetes therapy

As always, specific therapy should be tailored to the individual patient. Insulin, diet and exercise still remain the cornerstone of therapy as for all age groups, with advice not to smoke and to limit alcohol consumption. Pre-pregnancy advice about diabetes is essential. These elements have to be tailored to the person's rapidly changing lifestyle, education programme and social situation.

Can these aims be achieved in real life? They can in some; indeed, for some teenagers, aggressive treatment of their diabetes with multiple injections or insulin pumps, close control of carbohydrate intake and regular exercise is the preferred and desired option. Teenagers, like all people with diabetes, must be given the options and helped to make decisions with which they are comfortable. There is limited evidence about the effectiveness of insulin regimens other than conventional twice-daily injections, but our experience of more intensive regimens suggests that they are acceptable and achieve good results in some teenagers—provided that they are willing to adhere to the injection and monitoring regimen. Our system is to offer and try these regimens, while remaining willing to change frequently.

No specific insulin regimen, however, can be prescribed in isolation of a behavioural and social package: a social support network.

Behavioural and social therapy

The overt severely brittle patient requires detailed psychological and often psychiatric support and therapy. While there are often severe social and family problems, the patient's behaviour (malingering, factitious therapy, interference) may suggest a specific psychiatric problem: personality disorder, depression, schizophrenia, anorexia nervosa and bulimia. In the younger child with unstable diabetes and unusual occurrences (e.g. inexplicable infections), consideration should be given to psychiatric disorder in the *parent*, i.e. Münchausen syndrome by proxy.

Poor control is usually present over a considerable time and may reach a point where the diabetes team request professional psychiatric or psychological help; perhaps one general failing of our service is the reluctance to consider these approaches sooner. The desire to continue to investigate these cases for an organic cause, the manipulation and fabrication by the patients, and the lack of easily available psychiatric resources often significantly delay psychiatric treatment.

Less unstable patients with erratic symptoms and poor control can mostly be supported within the diabetes clinic and by the diabetes team. Many of these patients do not have overt psychiatric disorders; they are usually reacting to difficult periods in their life, often due to problems (e.g. divorce, alcoholism and drugs, unemployment, poor education) or emotional difficulties such as problems with relationships, school or work problems, general low self-esteem and difficulties in accepting and coping with the diabetes. Specific diabetes-related problems sometimes compound these difficulties, for example needle phobia, being overweight and fear of complications or hypoglycaemia.

Insulin omission has to be handled with care and compassion: stark confrontation is problematical and unhelpful. Explanation that insulin omission occurs very frequently, with no judgement attached, is in my experience accepted by many young people. Even if they deny omitting their insulin, working with the patient must continue. Support and frequent contact often encourage a return to the routine of diabetes. Lapses should not be viewed with despair; living with diabetes is a marathon, not a sprint, while many professionals move on and out of the patient's life. Young people often reject an aggressive, dictatorial approach. Constant encouragement, regular factual information and consistency of the messages are important. The patients should be seen frequently by the team members (physicians, dietitians and nurses) in a variety of environments. Consideration should be given to a multiple injection regimen (e.g. premeal fast-acting insulin with a isophane preparation before supper), although many will prefer a simple regimen of twice-daily injections. It may be an acceptable trade-off against the risk of later complications to aim for suboptimal control, perhaps with HbA_{1c} around 10% but with no episodes of DKA or hypoglycaemia for a few years.

For many patients, the discussions will be detailed and frequent. I prefer to include other family members, while respecting the independence of the teenager. Open and honest discussion is, in my opinion, more successful in the long run.

The general lack of concordance with the therapy regimens is a challenge for all involved in the care of young people with type 1 diabetes. Observations using methodology from social science have led me to the view that in an individualistic society, as in the UK, the empowerment given to young people (and acknowledged by adults) allows them to reject the rigours of the diabetes regimens. In a more egalitarian society, where a collective approach to support and direction is given, teenagers seem to accept the diabetes routine more as a matter of course. Novel strategies of care are required to overcome these difficulties in accepting the diabetes care plans.

For instance, the DCCT suggested strongly that the change to a more intensive regimen (4 or more daily insulin injections or insulin pump therapy) was the effector that achieved good glycaemic control, although it has been argued that the clinical support package (intensive medical follow-up, additional nursing, diabetic input and frequent contact) was the main factor responsible. The Hvidore Study demonstrated that there are centre differences in glycaemic control, particularly in teenagers. Further analysis of the data suggests that differences in the mean metabolic control of various centres operated early in the course of the disease, and therefore that the intensive therapy package for the management of diabetes is set in place from the early encounters with the diabetic child and teenager.

As mentioned above, factors not analysed in the DIABAUD2 survey (e.g. deployment of resources, organization of the clinical structure, strategies of care, clinical philosophy) appear to influence glycaemic control in individuals. These presumably operate differently in various centres. From discussion within the SSGCYD, the best centres probably have a policy of frequent contact (both medical and nursing), with formal advice at least monthly (more often if required), with a rapid 'troubleshooting' service, frequent changes in insulin regimen (with no fixed favourite) and the aim of a near-normal target for HbA_{1c} (<7.5%).

As part of the development of a social support network, discussions and specific advice about diabetes will need to be delivered outside the clinical setting. Observational evidence has highlighted the impact that peer pressure can have in a surrounding conducive to young people sharing their difficulties about diabetes. Several years of contact with young people through the Young Diabetes Project (Firbush Summer Camp and the Youth Diabetes Meeting) [43] has brought into focus the concerns of young people with diabetes; for many, these activities have been the only social support that they have received in trying to live with diabetes.

New possibilities exist through novel forms of communication. 'Cyberspace' has the potential for social support to be delivered to large numbers of patients—not only information about diabetes, but also support in the form of directives, reminders, challenges, etc. It is hoped that the world of the adolescent with diabetes will effectively become a smaller, and therefore a more comfortable place in the very near future.

Conclusions

This chapter has presented a view that adolescents with type 1 diabetes should be approached with an individualized diabetes management plan, leaning towards an intensive insulin regimen, and backed by psychological and psychiatric assessment and treatment if required. For individual patients, support, compassion and detailed attention is required over a lengthy period.

Novel care approaches need to be considered to encourage more teenagers to treat their diabetes aggressively, and these should incorporate the social structure necessary for concordance with the diabetes management strategies.

While accepting that not all teenagers with diabetes achieve good control, it is quite feasible in the majority.

References

1 The Diabetes Control and Complications Trial Research Group. The effect of intensive treatment of diabetes on the development and progression of long term complications in insulin dependent diabetes mellitus. *N Engl J Med* 1993; 329: 977–86.

2 Mortensen HB, Marinelli K, Norgaard K *et al.* and the Danish Study Group of Diabetes in Childhood. A nationwide cross-sectional study of urinary albumin excretion rate, arterial blood pressure and blood glucose control in Danish children with type 1 diabetes mellitus. *Diabet Med* 1990; 7: 887–97.

3 Rosilio M, Cotton JB, Wieliczko MC *et al.* Factors associated with glycaemic control. A cross-sectional nationwide study in 2579 French children with type 1 diabetes. The French Pediatric Diabetes Group. *Diabetes Care* 1998; 21: 1146–53.

4 Green SA on behalf of Scottish Study Group for the Care of the Young Diabetic. Factors influencing glycaemic control in young people with type 1 diabetes in Scotland. A population based study (Diabaud2). *Diabet Med* 1999; 16 (Suppl 1): 9.

5 Mortensen HB, Hougaard P. Comparison of metabolic control in a cross sectional study of 2873 children and adolescents with IDDM from 18 countries. The Hvidore Study Group on Childhood Diabetes. *Diabetes Care* 1997; 20: 714–20.

6 Dorchy H. Dorchy's recipes explaining the 'Intriguing efficacity of Belgian conventional therapy' [letter; comment]. *Diabetes Care* 1994; 17: 458–60.

7 Hindmarsh PC, Matthews DR, Silvio LDI, Kurtz AB, Brook CGD. Relation between height velocity and fasting insulin concentrations. *Arch Dis Childhood* 1988; 63: 665–6.

8 Dunger DB, Cheetham TD, Holly JMP, Matthews DR. Does recombinant insulin like growth factor (IGFI) have a role in the treatment of insulin-dependent diabetes mellitus during adolescence? *Acta Paediatr Suppl* 1993; 388: 49–52.

9 Green F, Khan F, Kennedy G *et al.* Syndrome X and endothelial function in children. *Diabet Med* 1999; 16 (Suppl 1): 5.

10 White E, Wilson AC, Greene SA *et al.* Body mass index centile charts to assess fatness of British children. *Arch Dis Childhood* 1995; 72: 38–41.

11 Pinhas-Hamiel O, Zeitler P. Type 2 diabetes in adolescents, no longer rare. *Pediatr Rev* 1998; 19: 434–5.

12 Gregory JW, Wilson AC, Greene SA. Obesity among adolescents with diabetes *Diabet Med* 1992; 9: 344–7.

13 Allen DA, Tennen H, McGrade BJ, Affleck G, Ratzan S. Parent and child perceptions of the management of juvenile diabetes. *J Pediatr Psychol* 1983; 8: 129–41.

14 Burroughs T, Harris MA, Pontious SL, Santiago JV. Research on social support in adolescents with IDDM. *Diabetes Educator* 1997; 23: 438–48.

15 Drotar D. Relating parent and family functioning to the psychological adjustment of children with chronic health conditions. *J Pediatr Psychol* 1997; 22: 149–66.

16 Hauser ST, Jacobson AM, Lavori P *et al.* Adherence among children and adolescents with insulin-dependent diabetes mellitus over a four-year longitudinal follow-up. *J Pediatr Psychol* 1990; 15: 527–42.

17 Anderson BJ, Auslander WF, Jung KC, Miller JP, Santiago JV. Assessing family sharing of diabetes responsibilities. *J Pediatr Psychol* 1990; 15: 477–92.

18 Anderson BJ, Ho J, Brackett J, Finkelstein D, Laffel L. Parental involvement in diabetes management tasks. *J Pediatr* 1997; 130: 257–65.

19 White K, Kolman ML, Wexler P, Polin G, Winter RJ. Unstable diabetes and unstable families. *Pediatrics* 1984; 73: 749–55.

20 Coleman JC. *The Nature of Adolescence*, 2nd edn. London: Routledge, 1990.

21 Montemayor R. The study of personal relationships during adolescence. *Personal Relationships During Adolescence*. London: Sage, 1994: 1–6.

22 Glasgow RE *et al.* Future directions for research on pediatric chronic disease management: lessons from diabetes. *J Pediatr Psychol* 1995; 20: 389–402.

23 La Greca AM. Peer influences in pediatric chronic illness: an update. *J Ped Psychol* 1992; 17: 775–84.

24 La Greca AM, Auslander WF, Greco P, Spetter D, Fisher EB Jr, Santiago JV. I get by with a little help from my family and friends: adolescents' support for diabetes care. *J Ped Psychol* 1995; 20: 449–76.

25 Skinner TC, Hampson SE. Social support and personal models of diabetes in relation to self-care and well-being in adolescents with type 1 diabetes mellitus. *J Adolescence* 1998; 21: 703–15.

26 Greene AC. *Health carers' and young peoples' conceptualisations of chronic illness: an anthropological interpretation of diabetes mellitus*. PhD Thesis. University St Andrews, Scotland, UK, 2000.

27 Greene AC, Tripaldi M, McKeirnan P, Morris A, Newton R, Greene SA. Promoting empowerment in young people with type 1 diabetes. *Diabet Med* 1999; 16 (Suppl 1): 20.

28 Tattersall RB. Brittle diabetes re-visited: the third Arnold Bloom memorial lecture. *Diabet Med* 1997; 14: 99–110.

29 Williams G, Pickup JC, Keen H. Continuous intravenous insulin infusion in the management of brittle diabetes: etiologic and therapeutic implications. *Diabetes Care* 1985; 8: 21–7.

30 Schade DS, Duckworth WC. In search of the subcutaneous insulin resistance syndrome. *N Engl Med* 1986; 315: 147–3.

31 Gill GV, Alberti KGMM. Outcome of brittle diabetes. *BMJ* 1991; 303: 285–6.

32 Williams G, Pickup JC. The natural history of brittle diabetes. *Diabetes Res* 1988; 7: 13–18.

33 Schade DS. Brittle diabetes: strategies, diagnosis and treatment. *Diabetes Metab Rev* 1988; 4: 371–90.

34 Williams G, Gill G, Pickup J. Brittle diabetes [letter]. *BMJ* 1991; 303: 714.

35 Gill G. The spectrum of brittle diabetes. *J R Soc Med* 1992; 5: 259–61.

36 Steel JM. 'Such a nice girl'. *Lancet* 1994; 344: 765–6.

37 Thompson CJ, Cummings F, Chalmers J, Newton RW. Abnormal insulin treatment behaviour: a major cause of ketoacidosis in the young adult. *Diabet Med* 1995.

38 Morris AM, Boyle DIR, McMahon AD *et al.* for the DARTS/MEMO Collaboration. Adherence to insulin treatment, glycaemic control and ketoacidosis in IDDM. *Lancet* 1997; 350: 1505–10.

39 Howells LAL, Wilson AC, Johnston M, Newton RW, Greene SA. Self-efficacy, problem solving and knowledge as predictors of glycaemic control in young people with type 1 diabetes: a cross-sectional and longitudinal study. *Hormone Res* 1998; 50: 119.

40 Steel JM, Young RJ, Lloyd GG, MacIntyre CCA. Abnormal eating attitudes in young insulin-dependent diabetics. *Br J Psychiatry* 1989; 1555: 515–21.

41 Neufelt M, Maclaren NK, Riley WJ *et al.* Islet cell and other organ specific antibodies in US Caucasians and Blacks with insulin dependent diabetes mellitus. *Diabetes* 1980; 8: 589–92.

42 Campbell IW, Heading RC, Tothill P, Buist TA, Exing DJ, Clarke BF. Gastric emptying in diabetic autonomic neuropathy. *Hormone Metab Res Suppl* 1980; 9: 81–6.

43 Davies RR, Newton RW. Progress in the Youth Diabetes Project. *Pract Diabetes* 1989; 6: 644.

10: Does brittle diabetes exist?

Geoffrey V. Gill

Introduction

The concept of 'brittle' diabetes has been used by diabetologists for decades to describe patients with unstable glycaemic control that appears to defy all normal management strategies. As such, it is clearly an essentially subjective concept, and therefore not surprisingly its frequency, causation and even its very existence are disputed. To compound the frustrations and confusions surrounding brittle diabetes, even its origin and meaning are now in considerable doubt. This chapter will review the development of brittle diabetes as a clinical concept, explore its characteristics and aetiological factors, and finally consider whether the syndrome is clinically useful or meaningful, and indeed whether it does in fact exist.

Historical aspects

Brittle diabetes must be unique as a clinical syndrome in that, until very recently, all articles describing the condition gave a reference to its origin that was entirely wrong! A random browse through my own files on the subject reveals 10 reports from Europe and North America between 1977 and 1997 [1–10], in which this 'original' reference was quoted (or more accurately, 'misquoted'). The reference is attributed to the American physician Rollin Woodyatt (1878–1953), writing in *Cecil's Textbook of Medicine* (quotations vary in page and edition, but are all in the 1930s when Woodyatt did indeed write the diabetes section). Schade in 1988 [11] first drew attention to the doubtful validity of the Woodyatt reference, and in 1991, Williams and colleagues also reported finding no details of brittle diabetes mentioned when these references were checked [12]. This was confirmed by a more extensive literature search by Tattersall [13], who in his sentinel paper on the subject in

1977 [1] took the reference from a report by Haunz in 1950 [14]. From there on, the misquotation became a 'self-replicating bibliographic virus' [12]!

The details recorded in this mythical reference are bizarre. As well as erroneous textbooks, editions and page numbers, a clearly quoted definition has frequently been quoted—'insulin-dependent diabetes whose control is so fragile that they are subject to frequent and precipitous fluctuations between hyperglycaemia and insulin reactions and in whom causes of instability have been excluded' [3]. The origin of this quotation has never been found, but there is no doubt that *fluctuations* of glycaemia were regarded as the hallmark of 'brittleness' in the 1930s and 1940s. Tattersall's researches [14] have revealed the earliest reference so far discovered mentioning brittle diabetes—Wilder's textbook of 1940 [15]. In this he describes patients who pass 'rapidly from the condition of hyperglycaemia, even with acidosis, to hypoglycaemia and back again'. He also states that 'Woodyatt has labelled them brittle cases'. It seems likely, therefore, that the 'brittle' label was coined by Woodyatt at some time in the 1930s, but that it was an oral rather than written description. Perhaps this story emphasizes the power of the oral historical tradition, and our current insistence that every medical term used nowadays must be backed up by an acceptable written reference.

Problems of definition

The 'Woodyatt' concept of brittleness has not stood the test of time. Rapid fluctuations between hyper- and hypoglycaemia as a cause of severe diabetic instability is now relatively uncommon [16–18]. This may be related to modern insulin regimens of at least two injections a day. In Woodyatt's time, there was a vogue for once-daily insulin, often with very long-acting preparations (such as impure bovine protamine-zinc insulin), and 'roller-coaster' glycaemic control was not uncommon.

Molnar in 1964 [19] attempted a redefinition but again concentrated on 'diabetic hyperlability' and fluctuations of control. Both the Woodyatt concept and Molnar's definition did, however, assume that brittleness only occurred in type 1 diabetes, and this has not been disputed since. The 'Woodyatt' and Molnar definitions, however, are problematic. Knowles considered that virtually all children and teenagers with type 1 diabetes were brittle by these definitions [20], and in 1997 Tattersall pointed out that their insistence on fluctuating control excluded patients with severe debilitating recurrent ketoacidosis [1]. He suggested that brittle diabetes be redefined as 'the patient whose life is constantly being disrupted by episodes of hypo- or

Table 10.1 Evolving concepts of brittle diabetes: all definitions assume that brittle diabetes occurs only in type 1 disease.

Author	Definition	Year
Woodyatt (reputed!)	Subject to precipitous fluctuations between hyperglycaemia and insulin reactions	?1930s
Molnar [19]	Diabetic hyperlability	1964
Tattersall [1]	Life constantly disrupted by hypo- or hyperglycaemia whatever the cause	1977
Schade [11]	Either incapacitated, or life disrupted more than three times per week, by repeated hypo- or hyperglycaemia	1988
Tattersall et al. [16]	At least three hospitalizations with either hypo- or hyperglycaemia in a 2-year period	1991
Gill et al. [18]	Severe glycaemic instability of any sort leading to life disruption and repeated and/or prolonged hospitalizations.	1996

hyperglycaemia whatever their cause' [1]. This definition has been widely accepted since, and by concentrating on life disruption as a qualifying criterion, and allowing any type of glycaemic instability, it has focused subsequent research on brittle diabetes in a more fruitful direction.

'Life disruption', however, is highly subjective, and it has been pointed out that regular insulin injections, a special diet and blood glucose monitoring could be considered life disrupting [21]! This has led to a search for 'tighter' definitions, although none have been entirely successful. Schade in 1988 considered that glycaemic instability should be totally incapacitating, or causing life disruptions at least three times weekly [12]. In 1991 Tattersall and colleagues [16], in studies of brittle diabetes outcome, attempted to introduce a quantitative element, though the number of required admissions was relatively low (Table 10.1). Finally, in 1996, Gill and colleagues [18] suggested the original 1997 Tattersall definition should be retained, but with the added requirement of recurrent and/or prolonged hospitalizations [18].

The evolution of brittle diabetes definitions is summarized in Table 10.1, and the search will continue, though it may be ultimately futile considering the problem and enigmatic features of the condition. Perhaps we are trying to be too pragmatic. Brittle patients tend to be well known to their care teams because they disrupt the lives of doctors and nurses, as well as their own! Even simple parameters such as the size and weight of their case notes may be as good a marker of brittleness as anything else (Fig. 10.1)!

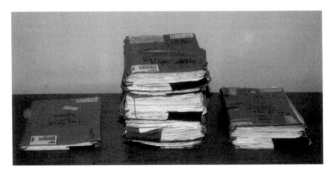

Fig. 10.1 Is definition that difficult? Spot the brittle diabetic!

Characteristics of brittle diabetes

The definition problems previously discussed make accurate epidemiological surveys difficult. However, recurrent hospital admissions do appear to be very much part of the modern brittle syndrome [17,22]. A study from Liverpool has attempted to assess national UK brittle diabetes prevalence using the augmented Tattersall definition requiring recurrent and/or prolonged hospitalizations [18]. The study involved a questionnaire survey of all UK diabetic clinics, and a 72% return was obtained. A total of 414 brittle diabetic patients were reported from an estimated total diabetic patient number of 354 824. There was a markedly higher rate of reporting from paediatric compared with adult clinics. The crude prevalence rate of brittle diabetes was 0.9 per 1000 total diabetic patients for adults, and 9.8 per 1000 for children. In terms of reporting clinics, this amounted to 1.4 per adult clinic and 0.5 per paediatric clinic. These figures are in surprising agreement with a 1985 prevalence 'guestimate' of 'perhaps between 1 and 5 per 1000' [3].

Perhaps more interesting than the prevalence estimates, this study provided interesting information on age distribution (Fig. 10.2). There was a marked peak in the second and third decades of life, and a smaller one between the ages of 55 and 70 years. The increased frequency of brittle diabetes in the young has been demonstrated in other smaller surveys [5,7,17,23]. The smaller problem of 'elderly brittle' diabetes has also been recorded [24–27]. Despite this 'second peak', the mean age of the total groups was still young (26 years), and there was a small but significant female excess. The study also confirmed earlier reports in confirming a remarkably stereotyped pattern of hospitalizations amongst brittle diabetic patients [16,17]. Their glycaemic instability 'polarizes' into three patterns (Fig. 10.3).

1 *Recurrent ketoacidosis (DKA).* The largest proportion of patients exhibit

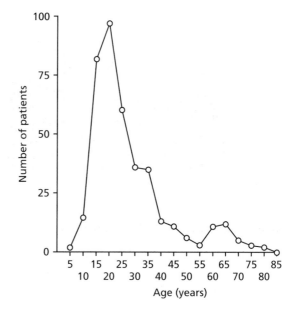

Fig. 10.2 Age distribution graph of 414 UK patients with brittle diabetes. From Gill *et al.* [18] with permission.

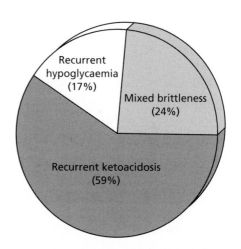

Fig. 10.3 Brittle diabetes—properties of patients with the three major metabolic syndromes of brittleness.

virtually pure hyperglycaemic instability, with over 90% of their admissions due to DKA [17]. The proportion of patients with this type of brittle diabetes has been estimated as 59% [18], and these patients are young (usually in their teens and twenties) and usually female (Table 10.2). These patients are often characterized by remarkable frequencies and lengths of admissions [5,7,23], and an 'impossibility' of control by standard means, which may lead to 'heroic' forms of therapy. These have included insulin infusion by subcutaneous [23],

Table 10.2 Characteristics of the major syndromes of brittle diabetes. Adapted from Gill *et al.* [18] with permission.

	Proportion (%)	Mean age (years)	Sex ratio (M : F)
Recurrent DKA	59	22	1 : 2.4
Mixed brittleness	24	28	1 : 1.9
Recurrent hypoglycaemia	17	34	1 : 1.1

intramuscular [23,28], intraperitoneal [29] and intravenous [30] routes. Even implantable insulin infusion pumps [31] and pancreatic transplantation [32] have been used in extreme cases.

2 *Recurrent hypoglycaemia.* A much smaller proportion of brittle diabetic patients show an opposite pattern of instability, with over 90% of admissions due to hypoglycaemia [17]. This category accounts for about 17% of total brittle patients, and they are generally older than those with recurrent DKA, and have approximately equal sex ratio (Table 10.2) [17,18,32]. Patients with recurrent hypoglycaemic brittle diabetes are less stereotyped than those with recurrent DKA. Though their mean age is older (34 vs 22 [18]), the range is much wider. Admission patterns are also variable, as are underlying causative factors [33].

3 *Mixed brittle diabetes.* This constitutes about 24% of the brittle syndrome (Table 10.2), and as the name suggests, these patients have no clear pattern of glycaemic instability [17,18]. Interestingly, in terms of mean age and sex distribution, they are in between the two extreme groups with recurrent DKA and recurrent hypoglycaemia (Table 10.2).

Aetiology—the 'organic' era (1978–85)

Theories on the causation of brittle diabetes have, like the origins of the term and its definition, been surrounded by controversy and debate. Much important early literature was until recently forgotten and considerable 'reinventing of the wheel' has taken place.

In the late 1970s and early 1980s, there was considerable interest and concern amongst British and American clinical diabetologists over what appeared to be the appearance of a new syndrome—young female type 1 diabetic patients with recurrent idiopathic attacks of DKA, and failure to achieve even moderate to poor glycaemic control on large doses of subcutaneous insulin. These patients were referred tertially to two centres in the UK,

London (Guy's Hospital) [24] and Newcastle (Freeman Hospital) [7,34], and one in the USA (Albuquerque in New Mexico) [35]. The clinical scenario was remarkably stereotyped—all patients were female and young (in the second and third decades of life), and were hospital dependent in terms of recurrent attacks of DKA. This was despite large doses of subcutaneously delivered insulin. The Newcastle series, for example [7], comprised 19 females of mean age 19 years (range 13–27). They were receiving a mean daily insulin dose of 144 units, and were a mean 130% of ideal body weight. The total group had experienced 410 episodes of DKA. The extent of hospitalization was remarkable—one of the patients having a continuous spell in hospital of over 2 years.

A vigorous search subsequently ensued to find an organic cause for this syndrome. Because the condition occurred exclusively in young women, an 'oestrogenic' hypothesis was briefly entertained. The London group noted an association between age of onset of 'brittleness' and menarche [23]. However, it could not be explained why physiological hormone profiles could induce such gross hyperglycaemia, or why only a small number of young female type 1 diabetic patients were affected. A more plausible explanation put forward was that subcutaneously delivered insulin may fail to be absorbed into the systemic circulation. In a poorly acknowledged report in 1978, Dandona and colleagues reported six patients with unstable type 1 diabetes, who were taking several hundreds of units of subcutaneous insulin daily, but who could be easily controlled on 50–60 units of insulin daily delivered intravenously. They postulated a subcutaneous insulin absorption defect, and over the next few years other series of patients were described with apparent 'subcutaneous insulin resistance' (as the phenomenon became known) [7,23,36]. As well as the intravenous route, intramuscular insulin also achieved improved glycaemia, with higher plasma free insulin levels, on modest doses of insulin, compared with subcutaneous delivery [28]. Increased enzymatic degradation at subcutaneous injection sites was considered a likely possible cause, and beneficial effects were reported of adding aprotinin (a protease inhibitor) to subcutaneous insulin [37]. Impaired subcutaneous blood flow was also suggested [38], and similar addition of prostaglandins was reported to be helpful [39]. In addition to 'subcutaneous insulin resistance', other potential biochemical abnormalities were explored. No consistent abnormalities in counter-regulatory hormone profiles were found [40], but disturbed patterns of some intermediary metabolites (notably hyperlactataemia) were found in brittle compared with 'stable' type 1 diabetic patients [40]. One patient was described with massive intravenous insulin resistance (this was occasionally noted in other patients [3]), and in whom there appeared to be excessive clearance of circulating insulin [41]. Taylor and colleagues in Newcastle investigated adipocyte insulin receptor status in a group of brittle patients and found reduced receptor affinity [42]. Some of these patients later resolved and became non-brittle; when repeat receptor studies were carried out, these had also normalized [43]. Finally, in an elegant study, Husband and colleagues explored the glycaemic and keton-aemic responses to insulin withdrawal in a group of brittle versus stable dia-betic patients. Four hours after cessation of intravenously delivered insulin, the brittle group showed significantly greater blood glucose and (in par-ticular) plasma ketone 'escape' compared with the stable group [44]. Plasma levels of insulin and counter-regulatory hormones were similar in both groups, and all patients were demonstrated to be C-peptide negative.

By the mid 1980s the 'syndrome of recurrent DKA' (if not other brittle subgroups) appeared to have a firm organic explanation on the basis of impaired absorption of subcutaneous insulin, with some patients demon-strating more complex postabsorptive abnormalities of insulin action.

Aetiology—the 'behavioural era' (1985 onwards)

Reports from the Newcastle and Albuquerque groups in late 1984 and 1985, however, suggested that a major (if not *the* major) reason for these patients' instability was self induced [3,34,45]. In a 1984 abstract report entitled 'Brittle diabetes—all in the mind' [45], Gill and colleagues described serious factitious behaviour including simple omission of insulin, deliberate damage to infusion pumps and cannulae, and dilution of pump insulin solutions by tap water. Such therapeutic interference was reported in more detail by the same group [3], and was found in at least half of the tertially referred group of 19 young females with recurrent DKA. No psychiatric abnormalities were found, and overt psychological morbidity was uncommon. In the same year, Schade and colleagues in Albuquerque, New Mexico, reported on 'Factitious brittle diabetes mellitus' [46], documenting similar treatment interference. Also in 1985, this group published a major paper entitled 'In search of the subcutaneous insulin resistance syndrome' [34]. This documented a large series of cases in whom they had performed standardized subcutaneous insulin absorption tests [6] under strictly controlled ('imprisonment tactics' [3]) conditions. In no case could they demonstrate a defect in insulin absorp-tion. Retrospectively, it has to be conceded that in none of the earlier studies suggesting subcutaneous insulin absorption were patients supervised so closely, and insulin injections may not have been given at all (at the time, most patients were 'self-treating' on the wards), or had been given from the patients' own supplies (likely to have been diluted). By the end of the 1980s, brittle diabetes—or at least the syndrome of recurrent DKA—was regarded as usually a self-induced problem related to psychosocial stress, and one reviewer commented that those studying the problem had 'emerged from the last decade battle-scarred but wiser!' [8]. To be fair, the degree of deception and self-induced risk undertaken by these patients was remarkable [45,46]. However, three lines of evidence available in the literature had gone unnoticed or ignored, and should have drawn attention to a factitious aetiology.

First, three reports between 1949 and 1956 had recorded patients with clinical features similar or identical to those described over 20 years later. In 1949, Rosen and Lidz reported 12 patients with type 1 diabetes and recurrent DKA, which was induced by 'abandonment of their insulin regime' [47]. In 1952, Hinkle and Wolf reported a series with mixed brittle behaviour again probably related to life stresses [48]. Finally, in 1956 Peck and Peck reported a single patient in whom frequent DKA admissions were self-induced to avoid family stress [49]. The second line of 'forgotten evidence' concerns pure hypoglycaemic brittleness, which is well known to be frequently self-induced. Reports of this condition have been described by Scarlett et al. [50], who also review a literature going back to the 1940s. The condition occurs particularly in young type 1 diabetic persons [51], and is widely known as 'factitious hypoglycaemia' [52]. The term was in use at the time of the 'organic search' for the cause of recurrent DKA. The final ignored literature was Tattersall's paper of 1977 redefining brittle diabetes [1], and a subsequent review 2 years later by Gale and Tattersall [2]. Four pages in the Tattersall paper are devoted to 'emotional causes', including a review of the Rosen and Lidz [47] and Peck and Peck [49] papers of 1949 and 1956, respectively. The section also includes a case history of a patient with classical factitious hypoglycaemia. In the 1979 review, 'deliberate manipulation, fecklessness, or kicks' is discussed, as well as the interesting term 'metabolic Münchausen's syndrome' [2].

The predominantly self-induced nature of much—if not most—brittle diabetes is now well recognized and confirmatory reports continue to appear. A patient who induced recurrent hypoglycaemia because of 'feeling high' whilst hypoglycaemic was recorded in 1999 [53]. Studies from Dundee in Scotland have compared insulin prescription and consumption in young type 1 diabetic patients, and found a significant discrepancy between prescribed and consumed insulin in 28% of patients, who had poorer glycaemic control and more admissions with DKA [54].

Remaining aetiological controversies

The relationship between psychosocial stress and brittle diabetes, though widely accepted, is not simple. In their 1949 paper, Hinkle and Wolf suggested that psychological stress directly led to glycaemic instability [48]. This supposed 'adrenaline effect' has a tenuous evidence base. Standardized psychological stress in type 1 diabetic patients does not significantly increase blood glucose or ketone levels [55], and experimentally induced hypercatecholaminaemia has mild effects only [56]. It is likely that psychological stress, adverse life events and chaotic lifestyles induce diabetic instability by impaired self treatment, decision making, or by direct interference with normal treatment.

Regardless of mechanisms, there is no doubt that psychological factors do adversely affect glycaemic control. Thus, HbA_{1c} levels are greater in patients with neuroticism [57], depression [58], poor motivation [59], low educational achievement [60] and family stress [61]. HbA_{1c} levels are also higher in young type 1 patients [62], and in female compared with male diabetic patients [63]. It can be seen that these characteristics are very typical of brittle diabetic patients (particularly those with recurrent DKA), and in this respect it may be that brittle diabetes represents the extreme end of a spectrum of adaptation difficulties to a complex chronic disease requiring significant self management. It may therefore not be surprising that chest physicians recognize a similar syndrome of 'brittle asthma' [64,65], and 'brittle Addison's disease' has also recently been described [66].

Simple escape from adverse life events may be too simplistic a motivation for some of the more extreme cases of brittle diabetes. The repeated induction of potentially life-threatening attacks of DKA or hypoglycaemia is often remarkable. Rosen and Lidz described their patients as 'self-destructive' and even 'borderline psychotic' [47]. Gale and Tattersall observed that such patients 'court repeated disaster because of sheer fecklessness rather than from any ulterior motive' [2]. Flexner and colleagues [67] described the whole bizarre clinical scenario as the 'Game of Sartoris', after an American novel of the same name which detailed the self-destructive demise of a southern US family [68]. There may be clues here from the non-diabetic psychiatric literature. Favazza and Conterio have written on 'female habitual self-mutilation' [69], and others have drawn attention to this phenomenon [70,71]. There may be analogies with anorexia nervosa here, and indeed some patients with recurrent DKA do seem to exhibit features of eating disorders [72]. Finally, Joseph has described a syndrome of 'addiction to near-death' [73],

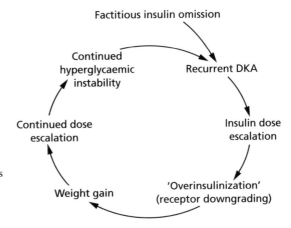

Fig. 10.4 The proposed 'vicious circle' of induced insulin resistance in factitious recurrent DKA.

in which she describes a 'very malignant type of self-destructiveness' which becomes 'in the nature of an addiction'. Finally, an almost universal feature of these patients is that they are 'nice girls' [74] and the true diagnosis is often delayed because family, nurses and doctors cannot believe that such behaviour is possible.

The above discussion on factitiously induced brittleness must not, however, be taken too far. There *are* organic causes for brittle diabetes. It is traditional in all such patients to review insulin systems, re-educate patients, search for occult infections and exclude endocrine syndromes of counter-regulatory hormone overproduction (e.g. phaeochromocytoma) [3,21]. In practice, such strategies are rarely productive. Coeliac disease, however, should be considered in 'mixed' or pure hypoglycaemic brittle diabetes [75,76]. Addison's disease or hypopituitarism can also cause exquisite insulin sensitivity and recurrent hypoglycaemia [2,77]. Hypoglycaemia unawareness [78] and nocturnal hypoglycaemia [79] should also be considered. Even in factitiously induced recurrent DKA, an 'organic phase' may ensue later due to iatrogenic escalation of insulin doses [7]. This can lead to an 'overinsulinization' syndrome with weight gain and reduced insulin sensitivity [79], which potentially sets up a vicious circle of continued hyperglycaemic instability (Fig. 10.4). There is evidence to support this hypothesis. Reversibly reduced insulin receptor affinity in patients with factitious DKA has been described [42,43], as well as genuine instances of insulin resistance [3,21,41]. Also, factitious behaviour at the time of presentation has not universally been recorded [7], and in one case a patient admitted to initially inducing DKA to escape sexual abuse, but after several episodes she could not regain control despite compliant behaviour [7]. It may be therefore that both organic and functional aetiologies for brittleness are not mutually exclusive.

Therapeutic dilemmas

The final dilemma with brittle diabetes concerns its management. Obviously, specific causes will require specific treatments (e.g. coeliac disease, hypoadrenalism, etc.), but in most cases no such diagnosis can be made. Follow-up studies have shown that with time most cases of brittleness resolve [16,80–82]. In the largest study (10 years follow-up) of 33 patients with severe recurrent DKA [82], 90% were 'non-brittle' at 10 years. However, this figure represents the proportion of *survivors*—five of the 26 traceable patients (19%) had died during the period, and of the rest there was an increased risk of complications (including pregnancy complications) compared with a control group. The study noted that resolution of brittleness often followed 'positive' life events such as stable relationships, marriage or employment. An expectant policy in these cases may be initially reasonable, but as time progresses without resolution, the increased risk of morbidity and mortality needs to be considered. In addition, these patients often become devoid of accessible peripheral veins due to recurrent cannulation, and even central veins may be thrombosed [7]. One of the deaths in the Liverpool follow-up series [82] was finally due to total lack of venous access. When situations such as this occur, various 'mechanistic interventions' have been tried (Table 10.3). These have been termed 'therapeutic mania' in the past, as they fail to address the real cause of instability, and may divert attention away from an underlying behavioural aetiology. However, at least some of the techniques have been apparently life saving, and have 'bought time' to await spontaneous resolution and/or to explore psychotherapeutic options.

Table 10.3 Possible management options for intractable brittle diabetes.

Mechanistic
Intravenous insulin infusion (IVII) [30]
Intraperitoneal insulin infusion (IPII) [29]
Implantable insulin pump (IV or IP) [31,83]
Pancreatic transplantation [32,84]

Psychological
Psychoanalysis [85]
Cognitive analytical therapy (CAT) [86]

All the 'mechanistic' options (Table 10.3) have significant risks—notably infection and catheter blockage for the insulin infusion techniques (including by implantable pump), and the problems of major surgery and lifelong immunosuppressant treatment with pancreatic transplantation. In that implantable pumps and pancreas transplants are not open to easy interference, they are probably the better options. Psychologically based therapies are obviously fundamentally more appropriate, but they are rarely highly effective. Cognitive analytical therapy (CAT) [86] is probably the most promising.

Finally, ethical dilemmas sometimes occur in the management of brittle diabetes. The confirmation of factitious instability may involve considerable covert detective work—such as C-peptide measurement during hypoglycaemic attacks [50], biochemical analysis of infusion fluids [45] and locker searches [7]. Most believe that such strategies can be justified in order to document therapeutic manipulation. The question then arises as to whether to confront the patient with this information. Again, most would agree to such a strategy, though the discussion should be frank and open, and not punitive and judgemental. Sadly, such confrontation rarely results in resolution of brittle instability, perhaps because of the 'addictive' nature of factitious behaviour [73], or the putative induced vicious cycle of overinsulinization [7,21] (Fig. 10.4).

Brittle diabetes—what's in a name?

Finally, we return to the title of this chapter—does brittle diabetes exist? The problem really lies with the unsatisfactory and mysterious term 'brittle'. In the past, it has been assumed that the term denotes a metabolically distinct form of diabetes, for which of course there is no evidence. However, provided no aetiological strings are attached to the label, the term usefully describes an extreme of chaotic diabetic control which defies normal treatment attempts. Even though its origin is obscure, the term 'brittle' is intrinsically attractive, and is certainly a popular one—as previously mentioned, the terms 'brittle asthma' [64,65] and 'brittle Addison's disease' [66] have also been adopted. The name really will not go away!

A further problem is the heterogeneous nature of brittle diabetes. Inside the broad spectrum, however, are two very distinct syndrome entities—'factitious hypoglycaemia' and the 'syndrome of recurrent DKA'—both with very stereotyped clinical characteristics, and both behaviourally based. The syndrome of recurrent DKA is still looking for an appropriate name. On the basis of its earliest comprehensive description, perhaps the 'Rosen–Lidz syndrome' [47] would be most appropriate? Diverse and difficult though the overall syndrome is, brittle diabetes is here to stay.

References

1 Tattersall R. Brittle diabetes. *Clin Endocrinol Metab* 1977; 6: 403–19.

2 Gale E, Tattersall R. Brittle diabetes. *Br J Hosp Med* 1979; 21: 589–97.

3 Gill GV, Walford S, Alberti KGGM. Brittle diabetes—present concepts. *Diabetologia* 1985; 28: 579–89.

4 Tattersall R. Brittle diabetes. *Br J Hosp Med* 1985; 291: 555–7.

5 Schade DS, Drumm DA, Duckworth WC, Eaton P. The etiology of incapacitating brittle diabetes. *Diabetes Care* 1985; 8: 12–20.

6 Schade DS, Eaton P, Drumm DA, Duckworth WC. A clinical algorithm to determine the etiology of brittle diabetes. *Diabetes Care* 1985; 8: 5–11.

7 Gill GV, Husband DJ, Walford S, Marshall SM, Home PD, Alberti KGGM. Clinical features of brittle diabetes. In: Pickup JC, ed. *Brittle Diabetes*. Oxford: Blackwell, 1985: 29–40.

8 Gill GV. Brittle diabetes. Current medical literature. *Diabetes* 1990; 7: 31–5.

9 Amiel SA. 'Brittle' diabetes. *BMJ* 1991; 303: 260–1.

10 Heller S. Brittle diabetes. *Diab Rev Int* 1995; 4: 3–5.

11 Schade DS. Brittle diabetes—strategies, diagnosis and treatment. *Diab Metab Rev* 1988; 4: 371–90.

12 Williams G, Gill GV, Pickup JC. Brittle diabetes. *BMJ* 1991; 303: 714.

13 Tattersall RB. Brittle diabetes revisited: the third Arnold Bloom Memorial Lecture. *Diabet Med* 1997; 14: 99–110.

14 Haunz EA. An approach to the problem of the brittle diabetic patient: a study of six cases. *JAMA* 1950; 142: 168–73.

15 Wilder RM, *Clinical Diabetes and Hyperinsulinism*. Philadelphia: WB Saunders, 1940: 100–1.

16 Tattersall R, Gregory R, Selby C, Kerr D, Heller S. Course of brittle diabetes: a twelve year follow-up. *BMJ* 1991; 302: 1240–3.

17 Gill GV. The spectrum of brittle diabetes. *J R Soc Med* 1992; 85: 259–61.

18 Gill GV, Lucas S, Kent LA. Prevalence and characteristics of brittle diabetes in Britain. *Q J Med* 1996; 89: 839–43.

19 Molnar GD. Observations on the aetiology and therapy of 'brittle' diabetes. *Can Med Assoc J* 1964; 90: 953–9.

20 Knowles HC. Brittle diabetes. In: Danowski TS, Hamwi TS, eds. *Diabetes Mellitus—Diagnosis, Treatment*. New York: American Diabetes Association, 1964, 109.

21 Gill G, Williams G. Brittle diabetes. In: Alberti KGGM, Zimmet P, DeFronzo RA, eds. *International Textbook of Diabetes Mellitus*, 2nd edn. Oxford: John Wiley, 1997: 1123–33.

22 Steel JM, Campbell IW. A personal experience of brittle diabetes, lessons learned and lessons still to learn. *Pract Diabetes Int* 1996; 13: 61–3.

23 Pickup J, Williams G, Johns P, Keen H. Clinical features of brittle diabetic patients unresponsive to optimised subcutaneous insulin therapy (continuous subcutaneous insulin infusion). *Diabetes Care* 1983; 6: 279–84.

24 Gale EAM, Dornan TL, Tattersall RB. Severe uncontrolled diabetes in the over-fifties. *Diabetologia* 1981; 21: 25–8.

25 Chapman J, Wright AD, Nattrass SM, Fitzgerald MG. Recurrent diabetic ketoacidosis. *Diabet Med* 1988; 5: 659–61.

26 Griffith DNW, Yudkin JS. Brittle diabetes in the elderly. *Diabet Med* 1989; 6: 440–3.

27 Benbow SJ, Walsh A, Gill GV. Brittle diabetes in the elderly—a UK study. *Diabet Med* 1997; 14 (Suppl 4): S3.

28 Pickup JC, Home PD, Bilous RW, Alberti KGGM, Keen H. Management of severely brittle diabetes by continuous subcutaneous and intramuscular insulin infusion: evidence for a defect in subcutaneous insulin absorption. *BMJ* 1981; 282: 347–50.

29 Pozza G, Spotti D, Micossi P *et al.* Long-term continuous intra-peritoneal insulin treatment in brittle diabetes. *BMJ* 1983; 286: 255–6.

30 Bayliss J. Brittle diabetes: long-term control with a portable, continuous intravenous insulin infusion system. *BMJ* 1981; 283: 1207–9.

31 Gill GV, Husband DJ, Wright PD *et al.* The management of severe brittle diabetes with 'Infusaid' implantable pumps. *Diabetes Res* 1986; 3: 135–7.

32 Du Toit DF, Heydenrych JJ, Coetzee AR, Weight M. Pancreatic transplantation in a patient with severe insulin resistance. *S Afr Med J* 1988; 73: 723–5.

33 Gill GV, Lucas S. Brittle diabetes characterised by recurrent hypoglycaemia. *Diabetes Metab* 1999; 25: 308–11.

34 Gill GV, Kent L, Williams G, Walford S, Alberti KGGM. An unusual case of relapsing brittle diabetes. *Pract Diabetes* 1995; 12: 38–9.

35 Schade DS, Duckworth WC. In search of the subcutaneous insulin resistance syndrome. *N Engl J Med* 1986; 315: 147–53.

36 Home PD, Massi-Benedetti M, Gill GV, Capaldo B, Shepherd GA, Alberti KGGM. Impaired subcutaneous absorption of insulin in 'brittle' diabetics. *Acta Endocrinol* 1987; 101: 414–20.

37 Friedenberg GR, White N, Cataland S, O'Dorisio TM, Sotos JF, Santiago JV. Diabetes responsive to intravenous but not subcutaneous insulin: effectiveness of aprotonin. *N Engl J Med* 1981; 305: 363–8.

38 Williams G, Pickup JC, Clark AJL, Bowcock S, Cooke E, Keen H. Changes in blood flow close to subcutaneous insulin injection sites in stable and brittle diabetics. *Diabetes* 1983; 32: 466–73.

39 Williams G, Pickup JC, Collins ACG, Keen H. Prostaglandin E_1 accelerates subcutaneous insulin absorption in insulin-dependent diabetic patients. *Diabet Med* 1984; 1: 109–13.

40 Massi-Benedetti M, Home PD, Gill GV, Burrin JM, Noy GA, Alberti KGGM. Hormonal and metabolic responses in brittle diabetic patients during feedback intravenous insulin infusion. *Diabetes Res Clin Prac* 1987; 3: 307–13.

41 Williams G, Pickup JC, Keen H. Massive insulin resistance apparently due to rapid decrease of circulating insulin. *Am J Med* 1987; 82: 1247–52.

42 Taylor R, Husband DJ, Marshall SM, Tunbridge WMG, Alberti KGMM. Adipocyte insulin binding and insulin sensitivity in 'brittle' diabetes. *Diabetologia* 1984; 27: 441–6.

43 Taylor R, Hetherington CS, Gill GV, Alberti KGMM. Changes in tissue insulin sensitivity in previously 'brittle' diabetes. *Horm Metab Res* 1986; 18: 493.

44 Husband DJ, Pernet A, Gill GV, Hanning I, Alberti KGMM. The metabolic response to insulin deprivation in idiopathic brittle diabetes. *Diabetes Res* 1986; 3: 193–8.

45 Gill GV, Walford S, Alberti KGMM. Brittle diabetes—all in the mind? *Diabetologia* 1984; 27: 279A.

46 Schade DS, Drumm DA, Eaton RP, Sterling WA. Factitious brittle diabetes. *Am J Med* 1985; 78: 777–84.

47 Rosen H, Lidz T. Emotional factors in the precipitation of recurrent diabetic acidosis. *Psychosom Med* 1949; 11: 211–15.

48 Hinkle LE, Wolf S. Importance of life stress in course and management of diabetes mellitus. *JAMA* 1952; 148: 513–20.

49 Peck FB, Peck FB. Tautologous diabetic coma—a behaviour syndrome. Multiple unnecessary episodes of diabetic coma. *Diabetes* 1956; 5: 44–6.

50 Scarlett JA, Mako MS, Reubenstein AH *et al.* Factitious hypoglycaemia. Diagnosis by measurement of serum C-peptide immunoreactivity and insulin-binding antibodies. *N Engl J Med*; 297: 1029–32.

51 Orr DP, Eccles T, Lawler R, Golden M. Surreptitious insulin administration in adolescents with insulin-dependent diabetes mellitus. *JAMA* 1986; 256: 3227–30.

52 Leading article. Factitious hypoglycaemia. *Lancet* 1978; i: 1293.

53 Cassidy EM, O'Halloran DJ, Barry S. Insulin as a substance of misuse in a patient with insulin-dependent diabetes mellitus. *BMJ* 1999; 319: 1417–18.

54 Morris AD, Boyle DIR, McMahon AD *et al.* Adherence to insulin treatment, glycaemic control, and ketoacidosis in insulin-dependent diabetes mellitus. *Lancet* 1997; 350: 1505–10.

55 Kemmar FW, Bisping R, Steingruber HJ *et al.* Psychological stress and metabolic control in patients with type I diabetes mellitus. *N Engl J Med* 1986; 314: 1078–84.

56 Pernet A, Walker M, Gill GV, Orskov H, Alberti KGMM, Johnston DG. Metabolic effects of adrenaline and noradrenaline in man: studies with somatostatin. *Diabet Metab* 1984; 10: 98–105.

57 Gordon D, Fisher SG, Wilson M, Fergus E, Paterson KR, Semple CG. Psychological factors and their relationship to diabetes control. *Diabet Med* 1993; 10: 530–4.

58 Mazze RS, Lucido D, Shamoon H. Psychological and social correlates of glycaemic control. *Diabetes Care* 1984; 7: 360–6.

59 Trigwell P, Grant PJ, House A. Motivation and glycaemic control in diabetes mellitus. *J Psychosom Res* 1997; 43: 307–15.

60 Lloyd CE, Wing RR, Orchard TJ, Becker DJ. Psychosocial correlates of glycaemic control: the Pittsburgh Epidemiology of Diabetes Complications (EDC) study. *Diabetes Res Clin Pract* 1993; 21: 187–95.

61 Vince R, McGrath M, Trudinger P. Family stress and metabolic control in diabetes. *Arch Dis Childhood* 1996; 74: 418–22.

62 Pound N, Sturrock NDC, Jeffcoate WJ. Age related changes in glycated haemoglobin in patients with insulin-dependent diabetes mellitus. *Diabet Med* 1996; 13: 510–13.

63 Strickland MH, Patan RC, Wales JK. Haemoglobin A_{1c} concentration in men and women with diabetes. *BMJ* 1984; 289: 733.

64 Turner-Warwick M. On observing patterns of airflow obstruction in chronic asthma. *Br J Dis Chest* 1977; 71: 73–86.

65 Ayres JG, Miles JF, Barnes PJ. Brittle asthma. *Thorax* 1998; 53: 315–21.

66 Gill GV, Williams G. Brittle Addison's disease: a new variation on a familiar theme. *Postgrad Med J* 2000; 76: 166–7.

67 Flexner CW, Weiner JP, Saudek CD, Dans PE. Repeated hospitalisations for diabetic ketoacidosis. The game of 'Sartoris'. *Am J Med* 1984; 76: 691–5.

68 Faulkner W. *Sartoris*. New York. Harcourt Brace, 1929.

69 Favazza AR, Conterio K. Female habitual self-mutilators. *Acta Psychiatr Scand* 1989; 79: 283–9.

70 Low G, Terry G, Duggan C, MacLeod A, Power M. Deliberate self-harm among female patients at a special hospital: an incidence study. *Health Trends* 1997; 29: 6–9.

71 McKerracher DW, Loughnane T, Watson RA. Self-mutilation in female psychopaths. *Br J Psychiatry* 1968; 114: 829–32.

72 Steel JM, Young RJ, Lloyd GG, Clarke BF. Clinically apparent eating disorders in young diabetic women associated with painful neuropathy and other complications. *BMJ* 1987; 284: 859–62.

73 Joseph B. Addiction to near death. *Int J Psycho-Analysis* 1982; 63: 449–56.

74 Steel JM. Such a nice girl. *Lancet* 1994; 344: 365–6.

75 Bhattacharyya A, Tymms DJ. Life-threatening hypoglycaemia due to previously unrecognised coeliac disease in a patient with type I diabetes mellitus. *Pract Diabetes Int* 1999; 16: 90–2.

76 Bradbury SL, Scarpello JHB. Recurrent hypoglycaemia as the presenting symptom of coeliac disease in a patient with type I diabetes. *Pract Diabetes Int* 1999; 16: 89–90.

77 Hardy KJ, Burge MR, Boyle PJ, Scarpello JHB. A treatable cause of recurrent severe hypoglycaemia. *Diabetes Care* 1994; 17: 722–4.

78 Hepburn DA, Patrick AW, Eadington DW, Ewing DJ, Frier BM. Unawareness of hypoglycaemia in insulin-treated diabetic patients: prevalence and relationship to autonomic neuropathy. *Diabet Med* 1990; 7: 711–17.

79 Rosenbloom AL, Clarke DW. Excessive insulin treatment and the Somogyi effect. In: Pickup JC, eds. *Brittle Diabetes*. Oxford: Blackwell, 1985: 103–31.

80 Williams G, Pickup JC. The natural history of brittle diabetes. *Diabetes Res* 1988; 7: 13–18.

81 Gill GV, Alberti KGMM. Outcome of brittle diabetes. *BMJ* 1991; 303: 285–6.

82 Kent LA, Gill GV, Williams G. Mortality and outcome of patients with brittle diabetes and recurrent ketoacidosis. *Lancet* 1994; 344: 778–81.

83 Dunn FL, Nathan DM, Scavini DM, Selam J-L, Wingrove TG. Long-term therapy of IDDM with an implantable insulin pump. *Diabetes Care* 1997; 20: 59–63.

84 Robinson ACJ, Pacy P, Kearney T *et al.* Pancreatic transplantation in 'brittle diabetes mellitus'—a case report. *Diabet Med* 1996; 13 (Suppl 7): S11.

85 Fonogy P, Moran GS. A psychoanalytical approach to the treatment of brittle diabetes in children and adolescents. In: Hodes M, Mooney S, eds. *Psychological Treatment in Disease and Illness*. London: Gaskell and the Society for Psychosomatic Research, 1993: 166–92.

86 Ryle A, Boa C, Fosbury J. Identifying the causes of poor self-management in insulin-dependent diabetes: the use of cognitive-analytic therapy techniques. In: Hodes M, Mooney S, eds. *Psychological Treatment in Disease and Illness*. London: Gaskell and the Society for Psychosomatic Research, 1993: 157–65.

11: How should hypoglycaemia unawareness be managed?

Simon R. Heller

Introduction

The inability to recognize impending hypoglycaemia is a common but often under-recognized complication of insulin-treated diabetes. It can devastate the lives of those affected, often leading to unemployment or the loss of a driving licence and also imposing huge strains on the whole family. This chapter will review the literature to establish the size of the problem and the circumstances which bring about its development. The competing hypotheses that have been proposed to explain its development will be discussed, and the work demonstrating how the syndrome can be reversed will be described. Finally, the speculation that hypoglycaemia unawareness might be preventable will be discussed.

Definitions of hypoglycaemia unawareness

Frier has defined hypoglycaemia unawareness as the 'inability to consciously perceive or discern the onset of hypoglycaemia' [1] and classified it as either normal, partial or absent [2]. However, one of the difficulties in agreeing a definition is that the level of awareness is not fixed. Some patients may be fully aware of hypoglycaemia during the day, but prone to severe episodes at night. A few may recognize hypoglycaemia most of the time and only suffer an occasional severe attack, while others always identify its onset although the strength of their warning symptoms is reduced. All these patients would be classified as partially aware yet their experiences are very different.

Most clinicians know patients with diabetes of many years' duration who have lost all ability to identify a low blood glucose. Frier has proposed the term 'chronic unawareness' to describe these individuals in contrast to those with 'acute' unawareness who lose warning signs after a period of tight glycaemic control. However, we have observed individuals who develop unawareness after a period of tight glycaemic control during pregnancy, and then never regain full symptomatic awareness even when their blood glucose control deteriorates and they stop experiencing hypoglycaemia.

Those with diabetes are not always reliable witnesses regarding their ability to recognize hypoglycaemia. When partners of patients with type 1 diabetes were questioned, a number who claimed complete awareness yet whose relatives reported frequent severe episodes, were identified [3]. Other workers have shown that individuals who believe they can recognize hypoglycaemia often fail to identify its onset during experimental hypoglycaemia [4]. Thus, estimates of the prevalence of unawareness based on patient questionnaires may underestimate its extent.

How common is hypoglycaemia unawareness?

Despite the potential difficulties obtaining reliable data, different studies have reported surprisingly similar numbers with hypoglycaemia unawareness. Unselected patient surveys indicate that the proportion of patients who report problems recognizing hypoglycaemia is around 20–25%. (Table 11.1) [2–6]. When hypoglycaemia unawareness was defined as a failure to develop symptoms during experimental hypoglycaemia, 26% of 43 patients were classified as unaware [4].

Table 11.1 Proportion of patients with type 1 diabetes suffering hypoglycaemia unawareness.

Study	Type of study	n	Patients with partial or total unawareness	
			Number	%
Hepburn et al. [2]	Epidemiological survey	302	70	23%
Mühlhauser et al. [5]	Epidemiological survey	523	129	25%
Pramming et al. [6]	Epidemiological survey	411	111	27%
Mokan et al. [4]	Physiological measurement during glucose clamp	43	11	26%

What causes hypoglycaemia unawareness?

The importance of the brain

The factor underlying the pathophysiology of hypoglycaemia unawareness is the metabolic dependence of cerebral tissue on glucose. The potential of the brain to utilize other fuels such as lactate and ketones during hypoglycaemia has been demonstrated experimentally [7,8], but during clinical episodes their concentration is probably too low to play a significant role. As blood glucose falls below 4 mmol/l and cerebral function is threatened, an array of physiological defences is activated in an attempt to return the glucose level to normal. These include the inhibition of insulin secretion, activation of the autonomic nervous system and the release of counter-regulatory hormones that increase hepatic glucose output and inhibit peripheral glucose uptake [9]. A detailed description of these responses is beyond the scope of this chapter and the reader is directed to other reviews [10]. However, the way in which hypoglycaemia is sensed and in particular activates autonomic responses needs further comment, because alterations in this pathway probably cause hypoglycaemia unawareness.

Different areas in the body have the capacity to respond to hypoglycaemia and generate a physiological response. The pancreatic β-cells react to hypoglycaemia by inhibiting insulin release [9] and there is also evidence that glucose concentration is monitored within the portal vein and modulates physiological defences to hypoglycaemia, perhaps during feeding [11]. However, recent experimental work, mostly in animals, suggests that glucose sensing responsible for initiating the major physiological response to hypoglycaemia is located within the hypothalamus.

Borg *et al.* have perfused the ventromedial hypothalamus (VMH) with 2-deoxy-glucose using microdialysis techniques to induce localized neuronal glucopenia [12]. This produced a counter-regulatory response, although perfusion of other areas of the brain had no effect. The same group have also perfused the VMH with glucose during systemic hypoglycaemia, which, by preserving glucose supply in this area, prevented an increase in counter-regulatory hormones [13]. Others have demonstrated glucose responsiveness in a proportion of hypothalamic neurones, with some responding to hyperglycaemia [14] and others to glucose lowering [15]. These neurones project to other areas concerned with pituitary–adrenal and peripheral sympathetic activation [16]. Thus, although more work is needed to clarify the physiology, it appears that hypoglycaemia is sensed in this region of the hypothalamus,

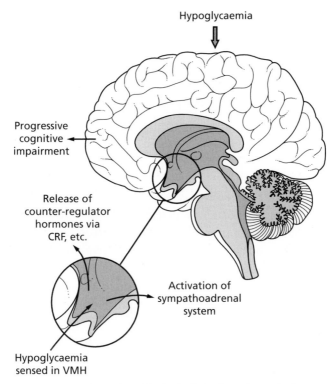

Hypoglycaemia

Progressive cognitive impairment

Release of counter-regulator hormones via CRF, etc.

Activation of sympathoadrenal system

Hypoglycaemia sensed in VMH

Fig. 11.1 Diagrammatic representation of the brain during hypoglycaemia demonstrating impaired cognitive function, sensing of hypoglycaemia in the ventromedial hypothalamus and subsequent activation of the autonomic nervous system and release of counter-regulatory hormones.

which then activates the autonomic nervous system and leads to release of counter-regulatory hormones. (Fig. 11.1) A failure of these neurones or pathways to respond to hypoglycaemia might prevent autonomic responses and produce hypoglycaemia unawareness.

Generation of symptoms and their relation to impaired cognition

Discharge of the autonomic nervous system not only releases adrenomedullary adrenaline (epinephrine) and noradrenaline (norepinephrine), but also activates peripheral physiological changes that alert patients to a falling glucose level and drives them to take action before cognitive ability is compromised. These symptoms (called autonomic or adrenergic) include sweating, tremor and palpitations. Other symptoms, for example loss of concentration and

Table 11.2 Symptoms of hypoglycaemia grouped by factor analysis after questioning of 295 patient with type 1 diabetes [17].

Autonomic	Neuroglycopenic	General malaise
Sweating	Confusion	Headache
Palpitations	Drowsiness	Nausea
Shaking	Odd behaviour	
Hunger	Speech difficulty	
	Incoordination	

blurring of vision, are the result of cerebral dysfunction due to neuroglycopenia but may also warn individuals that their blood glucose is low. Because neuroglycopenic symptoms represent a different pathophysiological process they are often recognized as separate group of symptoms by patients [17] (Table 11.2). The glucose concentrations at which these responses and different symptom groups develop, and their relationship to the threshold for cerebral dysfunction, are crucial to understanding the development of hypoglycaemia unawareness.

Experimental techniques such as the euglycaemic clamp have been used to establish the glycaemic thresholds for the different components of the response to hypoglycaemia. In normal subjects and diabetic patients who recognize hypoglycaemia, release of adrenaline (reflecting initial activation of the autonomic nervous system) occurs at a plasma glucose level of around 3.6 mmol/l [9]. If glucose is lowered further to 3.2 mmol/l, peripheral responses such as tremor or sweating start to develop, together with an increase in symptoms [18,19]. Cognitive ability starts to deteriorate at around 3 mmol/l and worsens as blood glucose falls [18,19]. This suggests that individuals who can identify hypoglycaemia, develop sufficient autonomic activation to generate symptoms before cognitive dysfunction supervenes, giving them time to take action to raise their blood glucose.

By contrast, patients with unawareness demonstrate a re-setting of the threshold for the onset of autonomic symptoms which are initiated at a lower glucose concentration, around 2.5 mmol/l [20,21]. Thus, because cerebral function worsens progressively as glucose falls and cognitive ability deteriorates, by the time patients develop autonomic symptoms, they are too cognitively impaired to behave appropriately. (Fig. 11.2) The hypothesis is based on relatively few studies and also rests on the assumption that the glycaemic threshold for autonomic activation may alter while that for cerebral dysfunction is relatively fixed [22]. Other data are less supportive, and indicate that

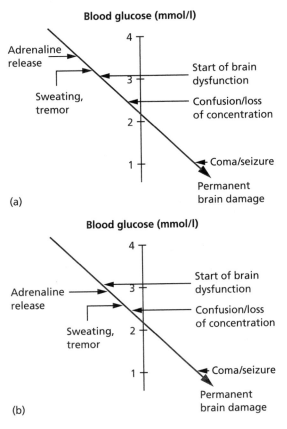

Fig. 11.2 (a) Representation of the glycaemic thresholds for the different components of the physiological response to hypoglycaemia in patients who are aware of hypoglycaemia. Thresholds of activation of autonomic symptoms and release of adrenaline are at a higher glucose level than those for cognitive impairment. (b) Glycaemic thresholds in patients with hypoglycaemia unawareness. Thresholds of activation of autonomic and adrenaline release are at a lower blood glucose than those for cognitive impairment.

the glucose threshold for cognitive dysfunction can also move [23]. Nevertheless, although further research is needed, this hypothesis fits the clinical description of hypoglycaemia unawareness and provides a useful theoretical framework to guide further research and new clinical approaches.

What factors are associated with hypoglycaemia unawareness?

This section concerns the clinical situations which are associated with hypoglycaemia unawareness and which are listed in Table 11.3. As discussed above, a factor common to all patients with hypoglycaemia unawareness is a diminished autonomic response to hypoglycaemia such that the glycaemic threshold is shifted to a lower concentration. Because autonomic activation is a crucial component of the physiological defence to hypoglycaemia, reduced responses are linked to attenuated rises in counter-regulatory hormones

Table 11.3 Clinical situations associated with hypoglycaemia unawareness.

Situation	Possible mechanisms
Long duration of diabetes	Unknown: Perhaps repeated hypoglycaemic damage to glucosensitive neurones
Tight metabolic control	Antecedent hypoglycaemia *possibly* leading to: Upregulation of neuronal glucose transport Cortisol surge with resulting impaired neurotransmission in key pathways Altered catecholamine sensitivity
Alcohol	Suppression of autonomic peripheral responses (tremor) Impaired cognition
Nocturnal episodes	Sleep preventing recognition of early symptoms Supine position impairing sympathoadrenal responses Sleep reducing sympathoadrenal responses
Children	Lack of abstract thought Prominence of behavioural change
Elderly	Prominence of impaired cognition Possible reduced autonomic response Reduced adrenergic sensitivity

particularly adrenaline. Thus, those with hypoglycaemia unawareness generally demonstrate reduced adrenaline responses during hypoglycaemia.

Long duration of diabetes

There are many reports of reduced hypoglycaemic warning signs in long-standing diabetes [24,25], but relatively few have calculated the proportion of those affected. These have confirmed a strong association between diabetes duration and unawareness. Pramming *et al.* [6] questioned 411 patients with type 1 diabetes and found that a greater proportion experienced hypoglycaemia without warning symptoms with increasing duration, from 20% at 10 years to 40% at 20 years. Around 50% of those with a duration of over 20 years reported alterations in hypoglycaemic symptoms.

How increased duration produces hypoglycaemia unawareness is unknown, although there are a number of potential causes. Autonomic neuropathy becomes more common with increased duration but other data, discussed below, suggests that its effect is minor. Because recurrent hypoglycaemia

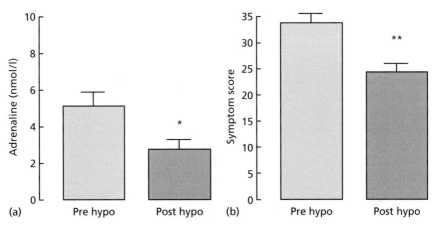

Fig. 11.3 Effect of antecedent hypoglycaemia. Peak responses of adrenaline (a) and hypoglycaemic symptom score (b) of nine normal subjects during experimental hypoglycaemia are shown before and after a 2-hour period of hypoglycaemia at 2.8 mmol/l. The peak response was measured at 2.5 mmol/l. Data from Heller and Cryer [27].

modifies the physiological response to hypoglycaemia, mild but repeated episodes might have a cumulative effect. Also because extremely severe hypoglycaemia can damage neural tissue, perhaps neurones, which detect hypoglycaemia, are sensitive to repeated insults. Resolution of these issues awaits further research.

The effect of tight glycaemic control and recurrent hypoglycaemia

In the 1980s, Amiel and colleagues showed that patients who improved their glycaemic control during intensive therapy developed impaired counter-regulatory and symptomatic responses to hypoglycaemia [26]. The defect appeared to be a resetting of thresholds of activation at a lower blood glucose but the mechanism was initially unclear. It now appears that this was caused by antecedent hypoglycaemia. We found that lowering glucose to around 3 mmol/l for 2 hours in normal subjects halved the adrenaline response and reduced symptoms during a further hypoglycaemic episode on the following day [27]. (Fig. 11.3) The same effect has been demonstrated in diabetic subjects, although its duration remains unclear [28]. Reduced responses have been observed for 7 days in normal subjects [29], although the effect may be shorter in those with diabetes [30]. It seems likely that antecedent hypoglycaemia contributes to defective responses during hypoglycaemia. Thus, repeated episodes may cause a viscious spiral of progressively impaired autonomic defences and eventual hypoglycaemia unawareness [31]. Antecedent hypoglycaemia may also reduce peripheral tissue sensitivity to adrenaline in patients with diabetes [32], but to what extent this contributes to hypoglycaemia unawareness is unclear.

The evidence that chronic hypoglycaemia in animals and humans increases both the expression of glucose transporters [33] and cerebral glucose uptake [34] suggests a possible pathophysiological mechanism. According to this hypothesis, those neurones responsible for initiating the autonomic response respond to antecedent hypoglycaemia by increasing glucose transporter expression and cellular glucose uptake. A subsequent episode of hypoglycaemia then fails to produce sufficient intraneuronal glycopenia to trigger a response, leading to diminished autonomic activation and hypoglycaemia unawareness. There are important weaknesses in the argument, however. Of most significance is the failure to demonstrate changes in glucose transporters following hypoglycaemia of short duration: periods of days or weeks are required in contrast to the major physiological changes produced by hypoglycaemia of a few hours.

Davis and colleagues have proposed an alternative mechanism based on clinical studies in non-diabetic subjects. A brief infusion of cortisol (to produce comparable plasma concentrations to those observed during insulin-induced hypoglycaemia) produces impaired counter-regulatory and sympathoadrenal responses to a subsequent hypoglycaemic challenge [35]. (Fig. 11.4)

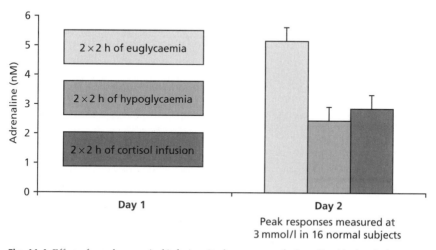

Fig. 11.4 Effect of antedent cortisol infusion. Peak responses of adrenaline (during the last 45 minutes) during experimental hypoglycaemia are shown following either two periods of clamped euglycaemia, hypoglycaemia or a cortisol infusion on the previous day. Data from Davis *et al.* [35].

In addition, they observed no impairment of hypoglycaemic physiological responses following antecedent hypoglycaemia in subjects with Addison's disease who cannot increase circulating cortisol [36]. Cortisol can suppress sympathetic neurotransmission and so might dampen the pathway of VMH sensing of hypoglycaemia and subsequent autonomic activation. The precise contribution of increases in cortisol to the pathogenesis of hypoglycaemia unawareness still needs to be established, but it could offer an opportunity for therapeutic intervention.

Sleep and problems of nocturnal hypoglycaemia

A problem for anyone with type 1 diabetes who keeps their glucose well controlled is the risk of nocturnal hypoglycaemia. This is partly due to the limitations of current insulin delivery and a long gap before the next meal, but is also due to other factors. Sleeping individuals will not respond to initial autonomic activation such as tremor, which would normally alert them during the day. Thus, by the time peripheral changes are intense enough to waken them, they may be too cognitively impaired to take action. In addition, a supine position rather than an upright posture reduces adrenaline and symptomatic responses to hypoglycaemia [37]. Finally, sleep itself suppresses the hypoglycaemic sympathoadrenal response [38]. The combination of all these factors may explain why biochemical nocturnal hypoglycaemia is so common, with reported rates of between 30% and 70%. To what extent repeated nocturnal episodes contribute to progressive loss of physiological defences and unawareness during hypoglycaemia is unknown.

Autonomic neuropathy

The development of hypoglycaemia unawareness has long been attributed to autonomic neuropathy [39]. Supporting evidence includes the association with long-duration diabetes, the frequent onset of autonomic neuropathy in diabetes and the importance of autonomic activation to hypoglycaemic symptoms. However, recent experimental work has challenged this assumption. Patients with hypoglycaemia unawareness and diminished adrenaline responses often have intact cardiovascular reflexes [18,40], the standard cardiac test of autonomic neuropathy. Furthermore, some patients with classical autonomic neuropathy exhibit a relatively normal endocrine and symptomatic response to experimental hypoglycaemia [2]. Bolli and colleagues have shown that those with established autonomic neuropathy may have an additional reduction in adrenaline during experimental hypoglycaemia [41]. However, overall it appears that autonomic neuropathy does not play a major role in generating hypoglycaemia unawareness. The term 'hypoglycaemia-associated autonomic failure' (HAAF) has been used to describe the specific failure of the hypoglycaemia-induced autonomic response that occurs after improved glycaemic control to distinguish the condition from classical autonomic neuropathy [42].

Other clinical associations

Young children with diabetes often fail to recognize the onset of hypoglycaemia, partly because they are incapable of abstract thought, but even in older children behavioural disturbance is a prominent symptom. The physiological basis for these observations is unclear.

Autonomic symptoms are also less prominent in elderly patients. This may be due to a diminished intensity of sympathoadrenal responses to hypoglycaemia and sensitivity to adrenaline [43] or a greater vulnerability of the ageing brain to neuroglycopenic dysfunction.

Alcohol reduces some of the peripheral hypoglycaemic responses (such as tremor) and also impairs the perception of hypoglycaemic symptoms [44]. Because it also inhibits gluconeogenesis, it presents particular hazards to diabetic patients prone to hypoglycaemia.

For many years, beta-blocking agents were considered to an important potential cause of hypoglycaemia unawareness due to inhibition of the peripheral sympathoadrenal response. However, experimental studies have demonstrated that overall symptom scores are unaltered by beta-blockers since other responses such as sweating (mediated by sympathetic cholinergic fibres) are increased [45]. Indeed, it has recently been proposed (backed by some preliminary data) that this effect might be exploited as a specific therapy for hypoglycaemia unawareness [46]. It is probably best to avoid nonselective agents since they also inhibit $beta_2$-mediated hepatic glucose release, but selective beta-blockers appear safe.

The risks of severe hypoglycaemia in patients with hypoglycaemia unawareness

The inability to recognize impending hypoglycaemia and its association with impaired adrenomedullary responses to hypoglycaemia implies that those affected will be prone to severe hypoglycaemia. This statement is supported by both retrospective and prospective studies, with reported increases in rates of severe hypoglycaemia of between three and six times compared to those with normal awareness [2,47]. It is also important to note that this level of risk applies to conventional treatment: these rates might rise higher in those undertaking intensive insulin therapy.

How can hypoglycaemia unawareness be reversed?

The exact cause of hypoglycaemia unawareness remains unknown. However, the observation that brief periods of hypoglycaemia can induce defects in physiological defences to subsequent episodes indicates that the mechanism is functional rather than structural, at least early on. It then follows that avoidance of hypoglycaemia might reverse these defects [27]. This hypothesis has now been tested in different centres.

Fanelli et al. studied eight patients with type 1 diabetes of relatively short duration with unawareness [48], who undertook a programme of hypoglycaemia avoidance. This consisted of a basal/bolus regimen with patients contacted daily and preprandial glucose targets of 7–8 mmol/l. Responses to hypoglycaemia were assessed at baseline, 2 weeks and 3 months later. These showed that the glucose thresholds for increases in autonomic symptoms and adrenaline moved from 2.3 and 2.8 mmol/l, respectively, to 3.1 and 3.5 mmol/l with some responses recovering within 2 weeks.

Cranston et al. studied 12 patients, with a long duration of diabetes and unawareness, of whom half had tight glycaemic control [49]. After baseline evaluation, a hypoglycaemia avoidance approach was undertaken, with multiple injections, frequent glucose monitoring and at least weekly contact with staff. The authors commented that substantial re-education was needed and that it generally took 3 months to achieve the goal of 3 weeks' total freedom from hypoglycaemia. Importantly, when patients were re-tested after the hypoglycaemia-free period, the glucose concentration at which cognitive dysfunction became impaired was unchanged at 2.8 mmol/l, while the level at which patients first noted symptoms had shifted from 2.3 mmol/l to 3.4 mmol/l. (Fig. 11.5) They also noted increased adrenaline, noradrenaline and growth hormone responses.

A similar design was used to study six patients [50], who remained in hospital for 3 days and underwent a hypoglycaemic challenge before continuing the programme at home. The authors found significant increases in symptoms within 3 days and comparable increases in autonomic symptoms to controls after 3–4 weeks. Interestingly, counter-regulatory responses,

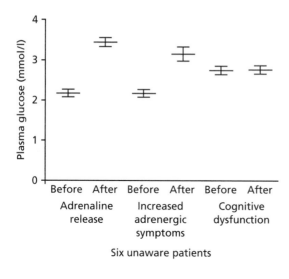

Fig. 11.5 Effect of hypoglycaemia avoidance on glycaemic thresholds of physiological responses to hypoglycaemia. Glycaemic thresholds for the release of adrenaline, increase in adrenergic symptoms and cognitive dysfunction measured before and after a period of hypoglycaemia avoidance. Data from Cranston *et al.* [49].

including adrenaline, failed to increase after hypoglycaemia avoidance. It is not clear why autonomic symptoms recovered in the absence of other signs of autonomic activation. This group have recently retested four of the six, 3 years later [51]. Increases in symptom scores during hypoglycaemia were slightly reduced compared to those at the end of the original programme, but were still higher than baseline. As the authors comment, this suggests that the patients may have continued to use skills acquired during the original study to avoid hypoglycaemia and maintain symptomatic awareness.

These studies demonstrate reversibility of hypoglycaemia unawareness, at least in part, over 2–3 months, even in those with longstanding unawareness. What is not reported is whether some patients were excluded due to a failure to prevent hypoglycaemia. Informal discussion indicates that this occurred in at least two of the studies. One of the centres which now offers a hypoglycaemia avoidance programme as a clinical service reports that up to 50% of those enrolled are unable to complete the course (personal communication).

Nevertheless, the following components appear important: frequent patient contact, multiple blood glucose testing including measurements at night, and strict glucose targets. HbA_{1c} rose in all the studies described above albeit insignificantly, although a more recent study reported reversal of unawareness at the expense of a significant increase in HbA_{1c} [52]. However, none of these represented a major deterioration in glycaemic control. In summary, hypoglycaemia unawareness appears to be reversible, even in those with diabetes of long duration. The approach is labour intensive but since it would probably involve only a few patients, could be within the scope of most units.

Is hypoglycaemia unawareness inevitable with tight glycaemic control?

The results of the Diabetes Control and Complications Trial (DCCT) and other studies of intensified insulin therapy indicate that the price to be paid for the benefits of a blood glucose close to normal is an increased risk of severe hypoglycaemia. Severe episodes in those conventionally treated affected around 10% in a year, a risk which rose threefold in those allocated to intensified treatment, and similar figures have been reported from other studies [53]. In the DCCT, 30% of severe episodes occurred without warning. It seems reasonable to conclude that the limitations of present insulin delivery coupled with the acquired pathophysiology of repeated hypoglycaemia inevitably produces considerable hypoglycaemia unawareness and severe episodes in those maintaining near normoglycaemia.

However, Berger and colleagues have challenged this assumption [54]. They have highlighted the considerable variation in rates of severe hypoglycaemia reported by different centres during the DCCT and suggest that the variation is not necessarily random or due to different individual characteristics of the patients in different centres. They propose that better training of patients to undertake intensive insulin therapy may lead to lower rates of severe hypoglycaemia and, by implication, less hypoglycaemia unawareness. Their published data appear to support their hypothesis. They have demonstrated long-lasting improvements in HbA_{1c} without major increases in rates of severe hypoglycaemia following a 5-day training programme which emphasized flexible eating, frequent blood glucose monitoring, carbohydrate counting and patient independence [55]. It is important to note that their definition of hypoglycaemia is narrower than that used in the DCCT but their premise that better skills-based training can produce less severe hypoglycaemia during intensive insulin therapy is provocative and seems worth pursuing.

How should glycaemic control be tightened to prevent hypoglycaemia unawareness?

All three groups who undertook programmes of hypoglycaemia unawareness reversal commented on how much work was involved, and that it could not

Frequent contact between patient and healthcare
professional
Regular blood glucose monitoring
Nocturnal blood glucose measurement
Avoidance of *all* hypoglycaemic episodes
Glucose targets which prevent biochemical hypoglycaemia

Table 11.4 Important features
of a hypoglycaemia avoidance
programme.

be used with large numbers. Much of this extra effort relates to frequent
one-to-one contact between the doctor and patient. The other essential components are frequent blood glucose monitoring and insulin dose adjustment
to achieve agreed glycaemic targets and avoid hypoglycaemia. (Table 11.4)
These are also the main features of the Berger course. It appears that the aims
of healthcare professionals encouraging tight control should be to develop the
skills of patients until they can adjust insulin dose and eating independently.

An alternative approach for which there is also experimental support is
the use of blood glucose awareness training (BGAT). The skills-based programme pioneered by Cox and colleagues teaches patients to identify their
blood glucose at all levels using symptoms, performance cues and moods.
They recently demonstrated preserved adrenaline responses to hypoglycaemia following intensive insulin therapy in patients who underwent this
training [56]. However, the training failed to reduce hypoglycaemic episodes
compared to controls.

Other factors are important. Because nocturnal hypoglycaemia is common, those undertaking intensive insulin therapy need to make occasional
measurements during the night. Bolli and colleagues have pointed out that
those with a HbA_{1c} level of below 6% are particularly likely to develop
impaired physiological defences to hypoglycaemia and hypoglycaemia
unawareness [57]. They have proposed an HbA_{1c} target of between 6% and
7%, which minimizes the risk of hypoglycaemia unawareness without
increasing vulnerability to microvascular complications.

The place of quick-acting insulin analogues in preventing or reversing
hypoglycaemia unawareness has yet to be determined, although there are
theoretical reasons why they may be useful. When used as part of a basal-
bolus regimen, fast-acting analogues reduce episodes of hypoglycaemia,
especially during the night in those with tight glycaemic control [58]. This did
not preserve endocrine or symptomatic responses to hypoglycaemia in one
controlled trial [59]. However, the question of whether rapid-acting analogues have additional benefits in reversing hypoglycaemia unawareness
needs to be tested in a formal study.

Table 11.5 Potential treatments for hypoglycaemia unawareness.	Caffeine Cortisol antagonists Drugs modulating neurotransmission Beta-blocking agents

A similar strategy but using an alternative approach involves continuous subcutaneous insulin infusion (CSII) at night [60]. This reduced hypoglycaemic episodes and improved counter-regulatory and symptomatic responses to hypoglycaemia in 14 patients with type 1 diabetes. The current high cost of insulin pumps has limited their general use but they may be useful to those with particular problems of nocturnal hypoglycaemia and unawareness.

Are there prospects of specific treatments for hypoglycaemia unawareness

There is no immediate prospect of specific pharmaceutical treatment for hypoglycaemia unawareness but some agents have sufficient theoretical and experimental support to merit further exploration of their clinical potential. (Table 11.5) Caffeine reduces cerebral blood flow and when administered before experimental hypoglycaemia produces a greater increase in both symptoms and catecholamines compared to placebo in both diabetic and non-diabetic subjects [61]. Whether these changes can be exploited to provide a useful specific therapy for hypoglycaemia unawareness needs to be established by ongoing clinical trials.

Another potential treatment might exploit the action of cortisol in inhibiting the counter-regulatory and symptomatic response to hypoglycaemia. Chronic cortisol antagonism is clearly undesirable but there is a theoretical rationale for investigating the effect of intermittent low-dose metyrapone in preventing or treating hypoglycaemia unawareness.

Finally, in time it may be possible to target the neurotransmitters concerned with generating the sympathoadrenal and symptomatic response to hypoglycaemia. However, it is too early to anticipate when such an intervention might prove sufficiently specific to preserve or increase physiological defences to hypoglycaemia.

Conclusions

Hypoglycaemia unawareness will remain a major barrier to the management of insulin-treated diabetes as long as insulin delivery systems remain imperfect. The exact pathogenesis is not clear, although it is clearly associated with long duration and recurrent hypoglycaemia. The ventromedial hypothalamus probably plays a critical role in the generation of symptoms and the development of the syndrome. The use of specific therapeutic agents to prevent or reverse unawareness is now a realistic long-term aim. However, at present a useful approach is to introduce skills-based training with glucose targets, which avoids biochemical symptomatic hypoglycaemia and maintains an HbA_{1c} level between 6% and 7%.

References

1 Frier BM. Hypoglycaemia in the diabetic adult. *Baillières Clin Endocrinol Metab* 1993; 7: 757–77.
2 Hepburn DA, Patrick AW, Eadington DW, Ewing DJ, Frier BM. Unawareness of hypoglycaemia in insulin-treated diabetic patients: prevalence and relationship to autonomic neuropathy. *Diabet Med* 1990; 7: 711–17.
3 Heller SR, Chapman J, McCloud J, Ward JD. Unreliability of reports of hypoglycaemia by diabetic patients. *BMJ* 1995; 310: 440.
4 Mokan M, Mitrakou A, Veneman T *et al.* Hypoglycemia unawareness in IDDM. *Diabetes Care* 1994; 17: 1397–403.
5 Mühlhauser I, Heinemann L, Fritsche E, Von Lennep K, Berger M. Hypoglycaemic symptoms and frequency of severe hypoglycaemia in patients treated with human and animal insulin preparations. *Diabetes Care* 1991; 14: 745–9.
6 Pramming S, Thorsteinsson B, Bendtson I, Binder C. Symptomatic hypoglycaemia in 411 type 1 diabetic patients. *Diabet Med* 1991; 8: 217–22.
7 Amiel SA, Archibald HR, Chusney G, Williams AJK, Gale EAM. Ketone infusion lowers hormonal responses to hypoglycaemia: evidence for acute cerebral utilization of a non-glucose fuel. *Clin Sci (Colch)* 1991; 81: 189–94.
8 King P, Kong MF, Parkin H *et al.* Intravenous lactate prevents cerebral dysfunction during hypoglycaemia in insulin-dependent diabetes mellitus. *Clin Sci (Colch)* 1998; 94: 157–63.
9 Schwartz NS, Clutter WE, Shah SD, Cryer PE. The glycemic thresholds for the activation of glucose counterregulation are higher than the threshold for symptoms. *J Clin Invest* 1987; 79: 777–81.
10 Cryer PE, Fisher JN, Shamoon H. Hypoglycemia. *Diabetes Care* 1994; 17: 734–55.
11 Hevener AL, Bergman RN, Donovan CM. Novel glucosensor for hypoglycemic detection localized to the portal vein. *Diabetes* 1997; 46: 1521–5.
12 Borg WP, Sherwin RS, During MJ, Borg MA, Shulman GI. Local ventromedial hypothalamus glucopenia triggers counter-regulatory hormone release. *Diabetes* 1995; 44: 180–4.
13 Borg MA, Sherwin RS, Borg WP, Tamborlane WV, Shulman GI. Local ventromedial hypothalamus glucose perfusion blocks counterregulation during systemic hypoglycemia in awake rats. *J Clin Invest* 1997; 99: 361–5.
14 Dunn-Meynell AA, Govek E, Levin BE. Intracarotid glucose selectively increases Fos-like immunoreactivity in paraventricular, ventromedial and dorsomedial nuclei neurons. *Brain Res* 1997; 748: 100–6.
15 Niimi M, Sato M, Tamaki M *et al.* Induction of Fos protein in the rat hypothalamus elicited by insulin-induced hypoglycemia. *Neurosci Res* 1995; 23: 361–4.
16 Pacak K, Palkovits M, Kopin IJ, Goldstein DS. Stress-induced norepinephrine release

in the hypothalamic paraventricular nucleus and pituitary-adrenocortical and sympathoadrenal activity: *in vivo* microdialysis studies. *Front Neuroendocrinol* 1995; 16: 89–150.

17 Deary IJ, Hepburn DA, MacLeod KM, Frier BM. Partitioning the symptoms of hypoglycaemia using multi-sample confirmatory factor analysis. *Diabetologia* 1993; 36: 771–7.

18 Heller SR, Macdonald IA, Herbert M, Tattersall RB. Influence of sympathetic nervous system on hypoglycaemic warning symptoms. *Lancet* 1987; ii: 359–63.

19 Mitrakou A, Ryan CM, Veneman T *et al.* Hierarchy of glycemic thresholds for counter-regulatory hormone secretion, symptoms and cerebral dysfunction. *Am J Physiol* 1991; 260: E67–74.

20 Heller SR, Macdonald IA. The measurement of cognitive function during acute hypoglycaemia: experimental limitations and their effect on the study of hypoglycaemia unawareness. *Diabet Med* 1996; 13: 607–15.

21 Hepburn DA, Patrick AW, Brash HM, Thomson I, Frier BM. Hypoglycaemia unawareness in type 1 diabetes: a lower plasma glucose is required to stimulate sympathoadrenal activation. *Diabet Med* 1991; 8: 934–45.

22 Maran A, Lomas J, Macdonald IA, Amiel SA. Lack of preservation of higher brain function during hypoglycaemia in patients with intensively-treated IDDM. *Diabetologia* 1995; 38: 1412–18.

23 Fanelli CG, Pampanelli S, Porcellati F, Bolli GB. Shift of glycaemic thresholds for cognitive function in hypoglycaemia unawareness in humans. *Diabetologia* 1998; 41: 720–3.

24 Lawrence RD. Insulin hypoglycaemia. Changes in nervous manifestations. *Lancet* 1941; ii: 602.

25 Balodimos MC, Root HE. Hypoglycaemic insulin reactions without warning symptoms. *JAMA* 1959; 171: 101–7.

26 Amiel SA, Sherwin RS, Simonson DC, Tamborlane WV. Effect of intensive insulin therapy on glycemic thresholds for counter-regulatory hormone release. *Diabetes* 1988; 37: 901–7.

27 Heller SR, Cryer PE. Reduced neuroendocrine and symptomatic responses to subsequent hypoglycemia after one episode of hypoglycemia in non-diabetic humans. *Diabetes* 1991; 40: 223–6.

28 Dagogo-Jack SE, Craft S, Cryer PE. Hypoglycemia-associated autonomic failure in insulin-dependent diabetes mellitus. *J Clin Invest* 1993; 91: 819–28.

29 George E, Harris N, Bedford C *et al.* Prolonged but partial impairment of the hypoglycaemic physiological response following short-term hypoglycaemia in normal subjects. *Diabetologia* 1995; 38: 1183–90.

30 George E, Marques JL, Harris ND *et al.* Preservation of physiological responses to hypoglycemia 2 days after antecedent hypoglycemia in patients with IDDM. *Diabetes Care* 1997; 20: 1293–8.

31 Cryer PE. Hypoglycaemia begets hypoglycaemia in IDDM. *Diabetes* 1993; 42: 1691–3.

32 Korytkowski MT, Mokan M, Veneman TF *et al.* Reduced beta-adrenergic sensitivity in patients with type 1 diabetes and hypoglycemia unawareness. *Diabetes Care* 1998; 21: 1939–43.

33 Kumagai. AK, Kang Y-S, Boado RJ, Pardridge WM. Upregulation of blood–brain barrier GLUT1 glucose transporter protein and mRNA in experimental chronic hypoglycaemia. *Diabetes* 1995; 44: 1399–404.

34 Boyle PJ, Nagy RJ, O'Connor AM *et al.* Adaptation in brain glucose uptake following recurrent hypoglycemia. *Proc Natl Acad Sci USA* 1994; 91: 9352–6.

35 Davis SN, Shavers C, Costa F, Mosqueda-Garcia R. Role of cortisol in the pathogenesis of deficient counterregulation after antecedent hypoglycemia in normal humans. *J Clin Invest* 1996; 98: 680–91.

36 Davis SN, Shavers C, Davis B, Costa F. Prevention of an increase in plasma cortisol during hypoglycemia preserves subsequent counter-regulatory responses. *J Clin Invest* 1997; 100: 429–38.

37 Hirsch IB, Heller SR, Cryer PE. Increased symptoms of hypoglycaemia in the standing position in insulin-dependent diabetes mellitus. *Clin Sci (Colch)* 1991; 80: 583–6.

38 Jones TW, Porter P, Sherwin RS *et al.* Decreased epinephrine responses to hypoglycemia during sleep. *N Engl J Med* 1998; 338: 1657–62.

39 Hoeldtke RD, Boden G, Shuman CR, Owen OE. Reduced epinephrine secretion and hypoglycemia unawareness in diabetic autonomic neuropathy. *Ann Intern Med* 1982; 96: 459–62.

40 Ryder REJ, Owens DR, Hayes TM, Ghatei MA, Bloom SR. Unawareness of hypoglycaemia and inadequate hypoglycaemic counterregulation: no causal relation with diabetic autonomic neuropathy. *BMJ* 1990; 301: 783–7.

41 Bottini P, Boschetti E, Pampanelli S *et al.* Contribution of autonomic neuropathy to reduced plasma adrenaline responses to hypoglycaemia in IDDM. *Diabetes* 1997; 46: 814–23.

42 Cryer PE. Iatrogenic hypoglycemia as a cause of hypoglycemia-associated autonomic failure in IDDM. A vicious cycle. *Diabetes* 1992; 41: 255–60.

43 Meneilly GS, Cheung E, Tuokko H. Altered responses to hypoglycaemia of healthy elderly people. *J Clin Endocrinol Metab* 1994; 78: 1341–8.

44 Kerr D, Macdonald IA, Heller SR, Tattersall RB. Alcohol intoxication causes hypoglycaemia unawareness in healthy volunteers and patients with Type 1 (insulin-dependent) diabetes. *Diabetologia* 1990; 33: 216–21.

45 Kerr D, Macdonald IA, Heller SR, Tattersall RB. Beta-adrenoceptor blockade and hypoglycaemia. A randomised, double-blind, placebo controlled comparison of metoprolol CR, atenolol and propranolol LA in normal subjects. *Br J Clin Pharmacol* 1990; 29: 685–93.

46 Chalon S, Berlin I, Sachon C, Bosquet F, Grimaldi A. Propranolol in hypoglycemia unawareness. *Diabet Metab* 1999; 25: 23–6.

47 Gold AE, MacLeod KM, Frier BM. Frequency of severe hypoglycemia in patients with type I (insulin dependent) diabetes with impaired awareness of hypoglycemia. *Diabetes Care* 1994; 17: 697–703.

48 Fanelli CG, Epifano L, Rambotti AM *et al.* Meticulous prevention of hypoglycaemia normalizes the glycemic thresholds of most of neuroendocrine responses to, symptoms of, and cognitive function during hypoglycemia in intensively treated patients with short-term IDDM. *Diabetes* 1993; 42: 1683–9.

49 Cranston I, Lomas J, Maran A, Macdonald IA, Amiel SA. Restoration of hypoglycaemia awareness in patients with long-duration insulin-dependent diabetes. *Lancet* 1994; 344: 283–7.

50 Dagogo-Jack SE, Rattarasarn C, Cryer PE. Reversal of hypoglycemia unawareness, but not counterregulation, in IDDM. *Diabetes* 1994; 43: 1426–34.

51 Dagogo-Jack S, Fanelli CG, Cryer PE. Durable reversal of hypoglycaemia unawareness in type 1 diabetes. *Diabetes Care* 1999; 22: 866–7.

52 Liu D, McManus RM, Ryan EA. Improved counter-regulatory hormonal and symptomatic responses to hypoglycemia in patients with insulin-dependent diabetes mellitus after 3 months of less strict glycemic control. *Clin Invest Med* 1996; 19: 63–82.

53 The Diabetes Control and Complications Trial (DCCT). *N Engl J Med* 1993; 329: 683–9.

54 Berger M, Mühlhauser I. Implementation of intensified insulin therapy: a European perspective. *Diabet Med* 1995; 12: 201–8.

55 Bott S, Bott U, Berger M, Mühlhauser I. Intensified insulin therapy and the risk of severe hypoglycaemia. *Diabetologia* 1997; 40: 926–32.

56 Kinsley BT, Weinger K, Bajaj M *et al.* Blood glucose awareness training and epinephrine responses to hypoglycemia during intensive treatment in type 1 diabetes. *Diabetes Care* 1999; 22: 1022–8.

57 Pampanelli S, Fanelli C, Lalli C *et al.* Long-term intensive insulin therapy in IDDM. Effects on HbA_{1c}, risk for severe and mild hypoglycaemia, status of

counterregulation and awareness of hypoglycaemia. *Diabetologia* 1996; 39: 677–86.

58 Heller SR, Amiel SA, Mansell P. Effect of the fast-acting insulin analog lispro on the risk of nocturnal hypoglycemia during intensified insulin therapy. *Diabetes Care* 1999; 22: 1067–611.

59 Heller SR, Amiel SA, Macdonald IA, Tattersall RB. Does insulin lispro preserve the physiological defences to hypoglycaemia during intensive insulin therapy? *Diabetologia* 1998; 41 (Suppl 1): A241.

60 Kanc K, Janssen MM, Keulen ET *et al.* Substitution of night-time continuous subcutaneous insulin infusion therapy for bedtime NPH insulin in a multiple injection regimen improves counter-regulatory hormonal responses and warning symptoms of hypoglycaemia in IDDM. *Diabetologia* 1998; 41: 322–9.

61 Debrah K, Sherwin RS, Murphy J, Kerr D. Effect of caffeine on recognition of and physiological responses to hypoglycaemia in insulin-dependent diabetes. *Lancet* 1996; 347: 19–24.

12: Is multiple injection therapy the treatment of choice in type 1 diabetes?

Maureen M. J. Janssen and Robert J. Heine

Introduction

Treatment with human regular (short-acting) insulin before each meal, in combination with one or two daily injections of NPH insulin (multiple injection therapy, MIT), is generally recommended as the treatment of choice for patients with type 1 diabetes mellitus [1]. In this chapter, the rationale for this recommendation is discussed. An important role in this discussion is played by the Diabetes Control and Complications Trial (DCCT); multiple injection therapy was one of the two treatment regimens applied in the intensive arm of this trial. The DCCT proved that intensive insulin therapy, as compared to conventional insulin therapy, caused a significant and sustained reduction in HbA_{1c} level [2], resulting in a retardation of both the onset and the progression of the microvascular complications of diabetes [2]. It may be argued, however, that multiple injection therapy itself was not an important contributor to these benefits, as conventional and intensive insulin therapy differed in a number of additional respects, including blood glucose self-monitoring frequency and treatment goals. The same argument applies to the principal drawback of intensive insulin therapy observed in the DCCT, an increase in the frequency of severe hypoglycaemia. In addition to overall glycaemic control and frequency of hypoglycaemia, the effects of multiple injection therapy on nocturnal glycaemic control and flexibility of lifestyle are discussed in this chapter. At the end of the chapter a summary of the effects of multiple injection therapy and other currently available insulin injection regimens on different treatment outcomes is presented.

Historical perspective of insulin injection treatment

The history of insulin injection treatment started in January 1922 in Toronto

General Hospital, when a 14-year-old boy suffering from diabetes was the first human to receive an injection of the insulin extract prepared by Banting, Best and Collip [3]. The discovery of insulin caused a spectacular change in the treatment of type 1 diabetes, which at the time consisted of undernutrition or 'starvation therapy' [4]. Insulin production was taken up rapidly: by October 1923 insulin was available in North America and Europe [3]. These first insulin preparations were very impure, acid extracts of ox or pork pancreas [5]. Injections, which were given at least once but usually a few times a day, had to be followed by a meal after about 15 minutes [4].

Apart from improvements in the purity of available preparations, the first major progress in insulin therapy was the development of insulin with protracted action. In 1936, Hagedorn and colleagues produced an insulin preparation with delayed absorption from the subcutaneous tissue by combining insulin with protamine. A modification of this protracted insulin resulted, in 1946, in the production of isophane insulin or NPH (neutral protamine Hagedorn) [5,6]. A similar principle was applied for the production of the zinc or lente insulins in 1951. The protracted effect of these last insulins is obtained by adding small amounts of zinc at neutral pH, resulting in an amorphous zinc insulin precipitation [7]. Insulin action can be prolonged even further by altering the physical state from amorphous to crystalline zinc insulin particles (ultralente) [5]. An important advantage of these longer-acting insulin preparations was that they could spare patients the discomfort of multiple daily injections of (short-acting) insulin. Until about 1979, when the introduction of continuous subcutaneous insulin infusion brought the first notion of intensified insulin treatment [8], many patients were treated with one daily injection of lente insulin [5]. Isophane insulin was used for the production of biphasic (premixed) insulin preparations, with a wide range of proportions of short-acting and intermediate-acting insulin. The most widely used combination, a 30/70% mixture of short-acting and NPH insulin, was developed for twice-daily insulin injection therapy [9]. Both NPH and lente insulins are used as basal insulin during multiple injection therapy.

Originally, all insulin preparations were derived from bovine or porcine insulin. The main disadvantage of these insulins was their immunogenicity, causing the formation of insulin antibodies [5]. The production of human insulin has been feasible since about 1980, either by semisynthetic conversion of porcine insulin or by recombinant DNA techniques [9]. Recombinant DNA technology has been exploited even further for the production of 'insulin analogues', modified insulin preparations with improved pharmacokinetic properties [10,11]. The first short-acting analogue available for clinical use, insulin lispro, has a reduced tendency to self-associate and therefore is absorbed more rapidly from the subcutaneous tissue than regular insulin [12,13]. Long-acting insulin preparations with improved pharmacokinetic profiles are currently under development [10].

Pharmacokinetics of currently available insulin preparations

An overview of the action profiles of the most commonly used insulin preparations is given in Table 12.1. It should be noted that these figures represent average time-courses. The pharmacokinetic profile of injected insulin depends mainly on the rate of absorption from the subcutaneous tissue. This rate is influenced not only by the chemical composition of the insulin preparation, but also by a large number of additional factors, including the anatomical injection site, insulin dose, temperature, exercise and massage of the injection site [14–16]. Both for regular and for NPH insulin, the coefficients of variation for the time until 50% of a standard insulin dose is absorbed are about 25% within and 50% between subjects [14]. Due to a shorter transit time through the subcutaneous tissue, the absorption of monomeric insulins is influenced to a lesser degree by external factors. The variability in serum insulin concentrations after subcutaneous injection with insulin lispro has been shown to be only 9.9%, vs 23.8% with regular insulin [17]. The variability in the rate of absorption of subcutaneously injected insulin is an important issue, as it contributes to the fluctuations of diurnal blood glucose profiles in type 1 diabetic patients [14].

Table 12.1 Action profiles of commonly used insulin preparations.

Insulin preparation	Onset of action (h)	Peak effect (h)	Action duration (h)	Origin
Regular	0.2–0.5	1.0–3.0	6.0–10.0	Human, animal
Short-acting analogue	< 0.5	0.5–1.5	4.0–5.0	Analogue
Isophane (NPH)	1.0–2.0	4.0–6.0	12.0–16.0	Human, animal
Lente	1.0–2.0	4.0–8.0	12.0–16.0	Human
	1.0–3.0	5.0–10.0	10.0–24.0	Animal
Ultralente	2.0–3.0	4.0–8.0	14.0–20.0	Human
	2.0–4.0	6.0–12.0	16.0–28.0	Bovine

Insulin injection regimens

In healthy, non-diabetic subjects there is an accurate closed-loop feedback between the arterial plasma glucose concentration and the secretion of insulin from the β-cells of the pancreas. Insulin secretion consists of two components: a steady basal insulin secretion and a rapid insulin response following the ingestion of meals [18]. In Fig. 12.1 the normal profile of insulin secretion is compared with the pharmacokinetic profiles of three commonly used insulin injection regimens: twice-daily therapy with a mixture of regular and NPH insulin, therapy with mixed insulin before breakfast, regular insulin before dinner and NPH insulin at bedtime, and multiple injection therapy with regular and NPH insulin. Continuous subcutaneous insulin infusion (CSII) is discussed in Chapter 13.

Twice-daily therapy with a fixed mixture of regular and NPH insulin is a simple regimen, with the short-acting insulin component to cover breakfast and dinner and the intermediate-acting insulin to cover basal insulin requirements and lunch. While requiring only two injections a day, an important drawback of this regimen is the limited flexibility it provides in timing and size of meals. The most important disadvantage, however, is related to the control of nocturnal blood glucose levels. As NPH insulin is injected before dinner, plasma insulin concentrations tend to peak between midnight and 3 AM, when basal insulin requirements are low, and then start to decrease towards the morning, when basal insulin requirements are increasing [19]. This may lead to the combination of hypoglycaemia during the early night and high blood glucose levels before breakfast. A possible solution is to split the evening dose of mixed insulin into an injection of regular insulin before dinner and an injection of NPH at bedtime. Multiple injection therapy with injections of regular insulin before each meal and NPH at bedtime allows greater flexibility in timing and size of meals. With this regimen, basal insulin supply during the daytime is covered partly by the regular insulin injections [18].

A modification of the multiple injection treatment regimen has become available after the introduction of the short-acting insulin analogue lispro. Insulin lispro has been shown to provide better postprandial glycaemic control than human regular insulin [20]. However, when applied in a multiple injection regimen with insulin lispro before meals and NPH insulin at bedtime, insulin lispro treatment is associated with a rise in blood glucose levels before dinner, due to the shorter duration of action in comparison to human regular insulin [21]. In Fig. 12.2 the serum insulin and blood glucose profiles

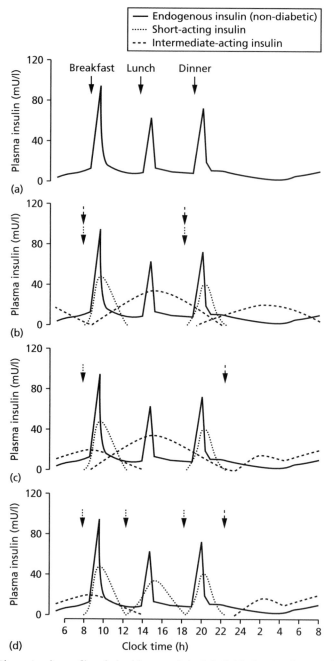

Fig. 12.1 Plasma insulin profiles of a healthy, non-diabetic individual eating three meals a day (a), compared with three different insulin treatment regimens for type 1 diabetes patients: twice-daily insulin therapy (b), treatment with a mixture of regular and NPH insulin at breakfast, regular insulin before dinner and NPH at bedtime (c) and multiple injection therapy with regular insulin before meals and NPH insulin at bedtime (d). Adapted from Amiel [18] with permission.

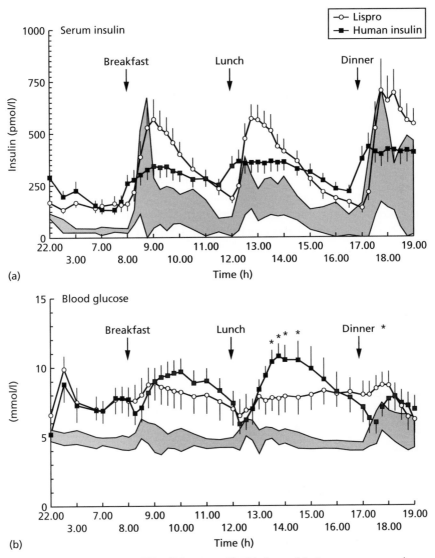

Fig. 12.2 Serum insulin (a) and blood glucose profiles (b) observed during a cross-over study with human regular insulin and insulin lispro in 12 type 1 diabetic patients. Results were obtained during in-hospital, three-meal test periods. The shaded area represents the data from six non-diabetic control subjects (mean ± SD). The white circles represent insulin lispro administration; the black squares represent human regular insulin administration. Adapted from Jacobs *et al.* [21] with permission.

of a cross-over study with human regular insulin and insulin lispro are shown as observed during in-hospital three-meal test periods. The increase in blood glucose levels observed when the interval between meals exceeds about 4 hours may be prevented by combining the premeal insulin lispro injections with variable proportions of intermediate-acting insulin, a regimen referred to as optimized basal bolus therapy [22].

Conventional versus intensive insulin therapy

Multiple injection therapy and CSII are sometimes referred to as 'intensive insulin therapy'. In a large clinical trial into the effects of glycaemic control on microvascular complications, the Diabetes Control and Complications Trial (DCCT), multiple injection therapy or CSII was applied in the intensive insulin therapy arm while twice-daily therapy was applied in the conventional insulin therapy arm [2]. The term 'intensive insulin therapy' is misleading, as it implies that it is the insulin regimen itself that intensifies glycaemic control [23]. In reality, however, in this trial intensive and conventional treatments differed in a number of additional respects, including treatment targets, education, blood glucose self-monitoring frequency, number of follow-up visits and availability of diabetes care providers. Indeed, intensive insulin therapy in the DCCT may be viewed as a comprehensive behavioural change programme [24]. Therefore, the term 'intensive insulin therapy' should not be used when referring to CSII or multiple injection therapy, but should be reserved for the comprehensive intervention programme employed to improve glycaemic control.

Benefits and drawbacks of multiple injection therapy

The effects of multiple injection treatment as part of intensified insulin therapy and twice-daily insulin treatment as part of conventional insulin therapy have been studied in two large randomized trials, the Stockholm Diabetes Intervention Study (SDIS) [25] and the DCCT [2]. In both trials HbA_{1c} was around 2% lower during intensive insulin therapy than during conventional therapy [26]. As discussed above, however, intensive and conventional insulin therapy differed in a number of additional factors, including treatment goals and self-monitoring frequency. Thus, the contribution of the insulin regimens per se to the difference in glycaemic control cannot be derived from these studies. Only a few small studies have investigated the effects of multiple injection therapy and twice-daily insulin therapy on glycaemic control under

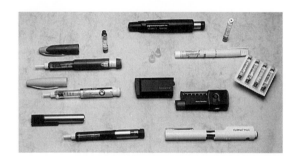

Fig. 12.3 A selection of the insulin pen injectors currently available for clinical use.

comparable treatment conditions [23–29]. In a cross-over study of already reasonably well-controlled type 1 diabetes patients, the mean HbA_{1c} level during multiple injection therapy was $8.1 \pm 0.4\%$ vs $7.6 \pm 0.4\%$ during twice-daily treatment with a mixture of short-acting and intermediate-acting insulin. This difference was not statistically significant [28]. Also, in the other studies of multiple injection therapy vs twice-daily therapy no differences in glycaemic control were observed [23,27,29]. It may therefore be concluded that multiple injection therapy in itself does not improve glycaemic control. There is some evidence that CSII provides better glycaemic control than thrice-daily insulin therapy [30]. However, in other studies no differences in glycaemic control were observed between CSII and twice-daily insulin therapy [31] or multiple injection therapy (Chapter 13) [32]. As for optimized basal bolus therapy with insulin lispro, some studies have demonstrated an improvement of glycaemic control in comparison to multiple injection therapy with human regular insulin [33,34].

Multiple injection therapy allows for a more flexible lifestyle than twice-daily insulin therapy, which requires a relatively stable diet with three meals and a set number of snacks a day. However, the freedom associated with multiple injection therapy should not be overestimated, as large variations in food intake and insulin dosages are likely to result in fluctuating blood glucose levels. This may explain why in some patients a deterioration of glycaemic control is observed after switching from twice-daily to multiple injection therapy [35]. Multiple injection therapy may also be considered more convenient to use than CSII, an advantage which has become even more marked after the introduction of the practical and very popular insulin pen injectors [36]. A large selection of insulin pen injectors is currently available for clinical use (Fig. 12.3).

An alarming side-effect of intensive insulin therapy observed in the DCCT was a threefold increase in the frequency of severe hypoglycaemia

[37]. This observation was confirmed in a meta-analysis combining data of 14 randomized trials of intensive and conventional insulin therapy [26]. This analysis also revealed that the risk of severe hypoglycaemia was related to HbA_{1c} decrease.

The increased risk of severe hypoglycaemia during intensive insulin therapy was only seen with a relative HbA_{1c} reduction in relation to baseline HbA_{1c} level of 8% or more. By contrast, the risk of severe hypoglycaemia decreased with a reduction of less than 8%, possibly because of a better distribution of the daily insulin dose with either CSII or multiple injection therapy. Also for the DCCT results, detailed statistical analyses have been performed to determine the relationship between the increased risk of severe hypoglycaemia during intensive insulin therapy and the improvement of glycaemic control [37]. These demonstrated that the increased risk of hypoglycaemia was related not only to HbA_{1c}, but also to the intensive insulin therapy *per se*. This could be interpreted as evidence of an association between multiple injection therapy and CSII with severe hypoglycaemia risk, or alternatively, as indicating a link between the pursuit of normoglycaemia and risk of severe hypoglycaemia. The latter explanation is supported by a population-based study of type 1 diabetic patients, which identified patients' determination to reach normoglycaemia as a predictor of severe hypoglycaemic episodes [38]. In the latter study, no relationship was detected between frequency of severe hypoglycaemia and mode of insulin treatment. A number of other studies, however, have demonstrated that CSII confers a lower risk of severe hypoglycaemia than multiple injection therapy (Chapter 13) [39,40]. There is also some evidence that multiple injection treatment with insulin lispro before meals causes a reduction in the frequency of severe hypoglycaemia [41], which is likely to result from a reduced risk of nocturnal hypoglycaemia due to an increase in blood glucose levels starting about 4–5 hours after dinner [42]. No data on the risk of severe hypoglycaemia during optimized basal bolus therapy with insulin lispro are available.

Concerning glycaemic control as well as the risk of severe hypoglycaemia, results from the DCCT do not allow a direct comparison of twice-daily therapy with either multiple injection therapy or CSII. In a study comparing multiple injection therapy and twice-daily insulin therapy under comparable treatment conditions, no difference in the frequency of symptomatic hypoglycaemia was observed [28]. Taken together, there is no firm evidence that multiple injection therapy is associated with a higher risk of severe hypoglycaemia than twice-daily insulin therapy. As discussed above, there is some evidence that CSII confers a lower risk of severe hypoglycaemia than

Table 12.2 Frequencies of severe hypoglycaemia during intensive insulin therapy reported in different large-scale studies: frequency of severe hypoglycaemia (SH) is expressed as number of episodes per 100 patient-years.

Study	Patient number	Study design	Definition SH	SH frequency
Reichard et al. [25]	44	Randomized, controlled One centre Prospective evaluation SH	Hypoglycaemia requiring assistance of another person	110
DCCT [37]	711	Randomized, controlled Multicentre Prospective evaluation SH	Hypoglycaemia requiring assistance of another person	61.2
Bott et al. [45]	636	Observational, uncontrolled Multicentre Prospective evaluation SH	Hypoglycaemia requiring glucagon or i.v. glucose	17
Pampanelli et al. [44]	112	Observational, uncontrolled One centre Retrospective evaluation SH	Hypoglycaemia requiring assistance of another person	1

multiple injection therapy. The main factor determining risk of hypoglycaemia appears to be the level of glycaemic control. However, some authors challenge the notion that intensified glycaemic control necessarily causes a high risk of severe hypoglycaemia [43]. In a number of studies, very low frequencies of severe hypoglycaemia have been reported in intensively treated type 1 diabetic patients [44,45]. Table 12.2 gives an overview of the frequencies of severe hypoglycaemia observed in a number of large-scale studies, some of which are uncontrolled. The large differences in hypoglycaemia frequency observed may be partly explained by differences in definition and assessment of severe hypoglycaemia. Another factor explaining the variation may be related to local differences in patient education and diabetes care policies. These differences are so large, however, that they call for further investigation.

An important consideration when comparing the benefits and drawbacks of the different insulin treatment regimens available is the control of nocturnal glycaemia. In healthy, non-diabetic subjects, insulin requirements have been shown to decrease shortly after midnight, remain stable for a couple of hours and then increase between 6.00 and 8.00 in the morning [19]. The latter phenomenon, referred to as the 'dawn phenomenon', probably results from a reduced insulin sensitivity of the liver induced by the secretion of growth hormone earlier in the night [19,46]. Despite these variations in insulin sensitivity, plasma glucose concentrations remain perfectly stable overnight in non-diabetic subjects due to the closed-loop feedback between the arterial plasma glucose concentration and the secretion of insulin by the pancreas [46]. During twice-daily insulin therapy and multiple injection therapy, nighttime insulin requirements are provided by intermediate-acting or long-acting insulin preparations. These preparations have a peak effect at 3–5 hours after injection, followed by rapidly waning insulin concentrations about 6–8 hours after injections [19] (Table 12.1). It follows from the normal physiology outlined above that this pharmacokinetic profile is in fact very unsuitable for nocturnal glycaemic control and favours the occurrence of hypoglycaemia in the early night and hyperglycaemia in the early morning [19]. The mismatch between insulin requirements and insulin supply is aggravated during twice-daily therapy, where the injection of basal insulin (mixed with regular insulin) is given before dinner [18]. However, even when basal insulin is injected at bedtime, by splitting the evening dose of regular and basal insulin or by switching to multiple injection therapy, nocturnal glycaemic control is still far from ideal. During multiple injection therapy high frequencies of (asymptomatic) nocturnal hypoglycaemia have been observed [47].

The risk of nocturnal hypoglycaemia is a complicating factor in the

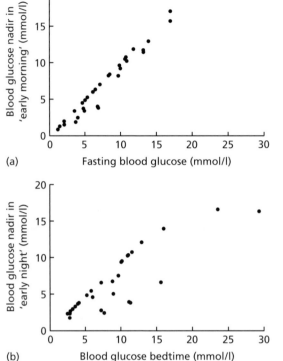

(a)

(b)

Fig. 12.4 Association between fasting blood glucose concentration and blood glucose nadir in the early morning (a) and between bedtime blood glucose concentration and blood glucose nadir in the early night (b). Adapted from Vervoort *et al.* [47].

management of strict glycaemic control, as strong associations have been observed between strict control of the fasting and bedtime blood glucose levels with the blood glucose nadirs in the early morning and early night, respectively [47] (Fig. 12.4). CSII provides better overnight glycaemic control than multiple injection therapy, as the low insulin depot of CSII results in a lower variability of absorption [19]. In addition, variable infusion rates may be employed to provide for changing insulin requirements [19]. In future, better nocturnal glycaemic control may also become possible by the development of basal insulin analogues with improved pharmacokinetic properties. The ideal basal insulin analogue should have a slow onset of action, no peak effect, a total duration of action of longer than 24 hours and a low intrasubject coefficient of variation of effect [11].

The elusive goal of truly good glycaemic control

In the DCCT, very strict intensive treatment goals were formulated (premeal blood glucose values of 3.9–6.7 mmol/l, postprandial values below 10 mmol/l and HbA_{1c} results within the normal range, i.e. below 6.05%). The difficulty involved in reaching these goals is illustrated by the fact that even in the intensive arm of the DCCT less than 5% of patients actually maintained an average HbA_{1c} below 6.05%. In clinical practice, even less ambitious HbA_{1c} targets appear difficult to attain. In addition, 'truly good' glycaemic control cannot be defined on the basis of HbA_{1c} targets only, but requires an acceptable frequency of biochemical hypoglycaemia. The increased frequency of severe hypoglycaemia during intensive insulin therapy in the DCCT indicates that 'truly good' glycaemic control was probably rare. There are two reasons why near-normal glycaemic control appears to be an elusive goal. The first reason relates to the imperfect nature of currently available subcutaneous insulin therapy. The second reason is that the self-management behaviours required to control blood glucose levels are very demanding. For example, it has been estimated that four to seven home blood glucose measurements a day are required to achieve good glycaemic control [18]. Although no data are available on the subject, it may be speculated that during multiple injection therapy, due to the more physiological insulin profile provided, less effort is required than during twice-daily therapy to attain a certain degree of glycaemic control. However, the main factor determining the effort associated with self management is probably the degree to which the patient wishes to bring glycaemic control to non-diabetic levels.

Conclusions

Table 12.3 summarizes the effects of multiple injection therapy and other currently available insulin injection regimens based on human regular insulin on the different treatment outcomes discussed. Insulin treatment regimens based on short-acting insulin analogues are not included in this table as treatment recommendations in this area, including mode and importance of optimized basal insulin administration, are rapidly changing by ongoing research. There is some evidence to suggest that CSII is superior to multiple injection therapy with regard to hypoglycaemia risk.

Multiple injection therapy may be preferred over twice-daily therapy as it allows for a more flexible lifestyle. Depending on the desired degree of glycaemic control, however, all regimens put great demands on patients with regard to self regulation. An important consideration is the control of nocturnal glycaemia. While multiple injection therapy provides a better nocturnal glycaemic control than twice-daily therapy, the most optimal control of nocturnal

Table 12.3 Overview of first choice and second choice insulin injection regimens based on human regular insulin for the different treatment goals discussed in this chapter.

	First choice	Second choice	Remarks
Patient convenience	BID	TID	
Flexible lifestyle	MIT	CSII	
Strict glycaemic control	–	–	No firm evidence that any of the treatment regimens is superior
(Severe) hypoglycaemia risk	CSII	–	No firm evidence that MIT is superior to BID or TID
Nocturnal hypoglycaemia risk	CSII	MIT TID	

BID, twice-daily therapy with a mixture of regular and NPH insulin; CSII, continuous subcutaneous insulin infusion; MIT, multiple injection therapy; TID, treatment with a mixture of regular and NPH insulin before breakfast, regular insulin before dinner and NPH insulin at bedtime.

glycaemia with the lowest risk of nocturnal hypoglycaemia can be provided by CSII. Twice-daily insulin regimens, preferably with splitting of the evening dose of regular and NPH insulin, may be very convenient for patients with a relatively stable life pattern who achieve satisfactory glycaemic control using this treatment. On the other side of the spectrum, multiple injection therapy may not provide sufficient glycaemic control for some patients. These patients are better off with CSII, in particular if nocturnal glycaemic control is a problem and fasting blood glucose levels are very unstable. More than any other medical treatment insulin injection treatment is to a large extent a tailor-made therapy, depending on the specific requirements of a particular patient. This situation has not changed since the introduction of the fast-acting insulin analogues, which have been shown to improve postprandial glycaemic control and have a lower variability in absorption from the subcutaneous tissue, but present new problems with regard to the supply of basal insulin. Possibly, a new outlook on insulin injection therapy will become possible after the introduction of new basal insulin analogues with more physiological activity profiles. Of equal importance, however, is further research into the medical and behavioural components of intensive insulin therapy that determine good glycaemic control [48], as this may help to replicate the success of the DCCT and explain the large differences in HbA_{1c} and hypoglycaemia frequency between different studies and different diabetes centres.

References

1 European Diabetes Policy Group 1998. A desktop guide to Type 1 (insulin-dependent) diabetes mellitus. *Diabet Med* 1999; 16: 253–66.

2 The Diabetes Control and Complications Trial Research Group. The effect of intensive treatment of diabetes on the development and progression of long-term complications in insulin-dependent diabetes mellitus. *N Engl J Med* 1993; 329: 977–86.

3 Bliss M. *The Discovery of Insulin.* Edinburgh: Paul Harris Publishing, 1983.

4 Tattersall RBA. Force of magical activity: the introduction of insulin treatment in Britain 1922–26. *Diabet Med* 1995; 12: 739–55.

5 Brange J. *Galenics of Insulin Preparations.* Heidelberg: Springer-Verlag, 1987.

6 Krayenbühl C, Rosenberg T. Crystalline protamine insulin. *Rep Steno Mem Hosp Nord Insulinlab* 1946; 1: 60–73.

7 Hallas-Møller K. The lente insulins. *Diabetes* 1956; 5: 7–14.

8 Tamborlane WV, Sherwin RS, Genel M, Felig P. Reduction to normal of plasma glucose in juvenile diabetes by subcutaneous administration of insulin with a portable pump. *N Engl J Med* 1979; 300: 573–8.

9 Heine RJ. The insulin dilemma: which one to use? In: Krall LP, Alberti KGMM, Turtle JR, eds. *World Book of Diabetes in Practice*, Vol. 3. Amsterdam: Elsevier, 1988.

10 Lee WL, Zinman B. From insulin to insulin analogs: progress in the treatment of type 1 diabetes. *Diabetes Rev* 1998; 6: 73–88.

11 Galloway JA, Chance RA. Approaches to insulin analogues. In: Marshall SM, Home P D, eds. *The Diabetes Annual.* Amsterdam: Elsevier Science, 1994.

12 Dimarchi RD, Chance RE, Long HB, Shields JE, Slieker LJ. Preparation of insulin with improved pharmacokinetics relative to human insulin through consideration of structural homology with insulin like growth factor I. *Horm Res* 1994; 41 (Suppl. 2): 93–6.

13 Howey DC, Bowsher RR, Brunelle R, Woodworth JR. (Lys (B28), Pro (B29)-human insulin. a rapidly absorbed analogue of human insulin. *Diabetes* 1994; 43: 396–402.

14 Binder C, Lauritzen T, Faber O, Pramming S. Insulin pharmacokinetics. *Diabetes Care* 1984; 7: 188–99.

15 Koivisto VA. Various influences on insulin absorption. *Neth J Med* 1985; 28 (Suppl 1): 25–8.

16 Linde B. Dissociation of insulin absorption and blood flow during massage of a subcutaneous injection site. *Diabetes Care* 1986; 9: 570–4.

17 Antsiferov M, Woodworth JR, Mayorov A, Ristic S, Dedov I. Within patient variability in postprandial glucose excursion with lispro insulin analog compared with regular insulin. *Diabetologia* 1995; 38: A190.

18 Amiel SA. Insulin injection treatment and its complications. In: Pickup J, Williams G, eds. *Textbook of Diabetes.* Oxford: Blackwell Science, 1996.

19 Bolli GB, Perriello G, Fanelli CG, De Feo P. Nocturnal blood glucose control in type 1 diabetes mellitus. *Diabetes Care* 1993; 16 (Suppl 3): 71–89.

20 Anderson JH Jr, Brunelle RL, Koivisto V *et al.*, the Multicenter Insulin Lispro Study Group. Reduction of postprandial hyperglycemia and frequency of hypoglycemia in IDDM patients on insulin-analog treatment. *Diabetes* 1997; 46: 265–70.

21 Jacobs MAJM, Keulen ETP, Kanc K *et al.* Metabolic efficacy of preprandial administration of Lys (B28), Pro (B29) human insulin analog in IDDM patients. *Diabetes Care* 1997; 20: 1279–86.

22 Bolli GB, Di Marchi RD, Park GD, Pramming S, Koivisto VA. Insulin analogues and their potential in the management of diabetes mellitus. *Diabetologia* 1999; 42: 1151–67.

23 Home PD. Intensive insulin therapy in clinical practice. *Diabetologia* 1997; 40: S83–7.

24 Lorenz RA, Bubb J, Davis D *et al.* Changing behavior. Practical lessons from

the Diabetes Control and Complications Trial. *Diabetes Care* 1996; 19: 648–52.

25 Reichard P, Bengt-Yngve N, Rosenquist U. The effect of long-term intensified insulin treatment on the development of microvascular complications of diabetes mellitus. *N Engl J Med* 1993; 329: 304–9.

26 Egger M, Davey Smith G, Stettler C, Diem P. Risk of adverse effects of intensified treatment in insulin-dependent diabetes mellitus: a meta-analysis. *Diabet Med* 1997; 14: 919–28.

27 Small M, Macrury S, Boal A, Paterson KR, Maccuish AC. Comparison of conventional twice daily subcutaneous insulin administration and a multiple injection regimen (using the Novopen) in insulin-dependent diabetes mellitus. *Diabetes Res* 1988; 8: 85–9.

28 Houtzagers CMGJ, Berntzen PA, Van Der Stap H *et al.* Efficacy and acceptance of two intensified conventional insulin therapy regimens: a long-term crossover comparison. *Diabet Med* 1989; 6: 416–21.

29 Haakens K, Hanssen KF, Dahl-Jorgensen K, Vaaler S, Aagenaes O, Mosand R. Continuous subcutaneous insulin infusion (CSII), multiple injections (MI) and conventional insulin therapy (CT) in self-selecting insulin-dependent diabetic patients. A comparison of metabolic control, acute complications and patient preferences. *J Int Med* 1990; 228: 457–64.

30 Home PD, Capaldo B, Burrin JM, Worth R, Alberti KGMMA. Crossover comparison of continuous subcutaneous insulin infusion (CSII) against multiple insulin injections in insulin-dependent diabetic subjects: improved control with CSII. *Diabetes Care* 1982; 5: 466–71.

31 Calabrese G, Bueti A, Santeusiano F *et al.* Continuous subcutaneous insulin injection treatment in insulin-dependent diabetic patients: a comparison with conventional optimized treatment in a long term study. *Diabetes Care* 1982; 5: 457–65.

32 Schiffrin A, Belmonte MM. Comparison between continuous subcutaneous insulin infusion and multiple injections of insulin.

A one-year prospective study. *Diabetes* 1982; 31: 255–64.

33 Del Sindaco P, Ciofetta M, Lalli C *et al.* Use of the short-acting insulin analogue lispro in intensive treatment of Type I diabetes mellitus: importance of appropriate replacement of basal insulin and time-interval injection–meal. *Diabet Med* 1998; 15: 592–600.

34 Lalli C, Ciofetta M, Del Sindaco P *et al.* Long-term intensive treatment of Type I diabetes with the short-acting insulin analogue lispro in variable combination with NPH insulin at mealtime. *Diabetes Care* 1999; 22: 468–77.

35 Hardy KJ, Jones KE, Gill GV. Deterioration in blood glucose control in females with diabetes changed to a basal-bolus regimen using a pen-injector. *Diabet Med* 1991; 8: 69–71.

36 Murray DP, Keenan P, Gayer E *et al.* A randomised trial of the efficacy and acceptability of a pen injector. *Diabet Med* 1988; 5: 750–4.

37 The Diabetes Control and Complications Trial Research Group. Hypoglycemia in the Diabetes Control and Complications Trial. *Diabetes* 1997; 46: 271–86.

38 Mühlhauser I, Overmann H, Bender R, Bott U, Berger M. Risk factors of severe hypoglycaemia in adult patients with Type I diabetes—a prospective population based study. *Diabetologia* 1998; 41: 1274–82.

39 Eichner HL, Selam JL, Holleman CB, Worcester BR, Turner DS, Charles MA. Reduction of severe hypoglycemic events in type I (insulin dependent) diabetic patients using continuous subcutaneous insulin infusion. *Diabetes Res* 1988; 8: 189–93.

40 Bode BW, Steed RD, Davidson PC. Reduction in severe hypoglycemia with long-term continuous subcutaneous insulin infusion in type 1 diabetes. *Diabetes Care* 1996; 19: 324–7.

41 Holleman F, Schmitt H, Rottiers R, Rees A, Symanowski S, Anderson JH and the Benelux–UK Insulin Lispro Study Group. Reduced frequency of severe hypoglycemia and coma in well-controlled IDDM patients treated with

insulin lispro. *Diabetes Care* 1997; 20:
1827–32.

42 Ahmed ABE, Home PD. The effect of the
insulin analog lispro on nighttime blood
glucose control in type 1 diabetic patients.
Diabetes Care 1998; 21: 32–7.

43 Mühlhauser I, Santiago JV, Bolli GB. The
frequency of severe hypoglycaemia during
intensive insulin therapy. *Diab Nutr
Metab* 1988; 1: 77–88.

44 Pampanelli S, Fanelli C, Lalli C *et al.*
Long-term intensive insulin therapy in
IDDM. Effects on HbA$_{1c}$, risk for severe
and mild hypoglycaemia, status of
counterregulation and awareness of
hypoglycaemia. *Diabetologia* 1996; 39:
677–86.

45 Bott S, Bott U, Berger M, Mühlhauser I.
Intensified insulin therapy and the risk of
severe hypoglycaemia. *Diabetologia*
1997; 40: 926–32.

46 Bolli GB, De Feo P, De Cosmo S *et al.*
Demonstration of a dawn phenomenon in
normal human volunteers. *Diabetes*
1984; 33: 1150–3.

47 Vervoort G, Goldschmidt HMG, Van Doorn
LG. Nocturnal blood glucose profiles in
patients with type 1 diabetes mellitus on
multiple (≥4) daily insulin injection
regimens. *Diabet Med* 1996; 13: 794–9.

48 Glasgow RE, Fisher EB, Anderson BJ
et al. Behavioral science in diabetes.
Contributions and opportunities.
Diabetes Care 1999; 22: 832–43.

13: Is insulin pump treatment justifiable?

John C. Pickup

Introduction

The notion of delivering insulin to diabetic patients by an infusion pump arose in the 1970s [1–8], as evidence accumulated that diabetic microangiopathy was most likely the consequence of many years of poor glycaemic control [9]. To test this hypothesis definitively it would be necessary radically to improve diabetic control over long periods of time and observe the effect on diabetic complications. It was thought that one logical way of accomplishing this would be to mimic the multirate insulin delivery of the non-diabetic person—constant low-level basal secretion and mealtime boosts of insulin— by controlled infusion from an electromechanical pump. The first studies used a portable pump to infuse insulin intravenously over some days [1], a technique which is limited in duration and general application by the risks of thrombosis and septicaemia with the intravenous route. However, the development of continuous subcutaneous insulin infusion (CSII) in 1977–78 [7,8] and its subsequent evaluation and refinement [10–12] provided a safe and highly effective means of maintaining many years of near normoglycaemia in the majority of type 1 diabetic subjects.

CSII was used in several of the first randomized and controlled prospective research trials testing the effect of strict glycaemic control on the progress of diabetic microangiopathy, such as the Kroc [13], Steno [14] and Oslo [15] studies. Its research use is particularly well demonstrated, of course, in the Diabetes Control and Complications Trial (DCCT) [16], where CSII was used as one form of intensive therapy (with multiple insulin injections). However, almost from the start of evaluating CSII as a research tool, several physicians started using insulin pumps as a form of routine therapy in selected type 1 diabetic patients. Its use in this way was well established by the early 1980s [12] and has continued in several countries, encouraged by the development of smaller, more reliable pumps with microprocessor control of infusion rates and appropriate alarm systems in the event of malfunction. Moreover, health insurance and national diabetes associations in some countries such as the USA and Germany have accepted that the costs of insulin pumps and supplies can be covered by insurance ('normal funding mechanisms'), when CSII is prescribed by a physician and undertaken according to recommended guidelines [17]. In the USA, more than 70 000 people with diabetes are being treated by CSII.

In other countries such as the UK where the costs are not usually met by the National Health Service, only a few hundred insulin pumps are in use. Here, there has been vigorous debate extending over some 20 years about the place of CSII in routine diabetes management, the evidence of its cost effectiveness in comparison with modern injection treatment, whether there are proven indications for its use and how pump programmes should be funded. It is on these issues that this chapter is focused. The procedures for managing patients on CSII and general reviews of its pharmacokinetics, effectiveness and complications can be found elsewhere [18–20].

Shortly after the first research studies began of insulin infusion from a portable pump worn on the outside of the body, a number of groups started investigating the feasibility of managing diabetes by totally implanted insulin pumps [21–23]. Possible advantages were seen to include placing the pump out of site, where it would be less likely to be damaged, and with easy access to central venous and especially intraperitoneal insulin delivery. Pharmacokinetic studies showed that insulin absorption from the peritoneal cavity was more rapid than after subcutaneous injection [24], and much of it occurred into the portal blood stream [25]. Intraperitoneal insulin is thus directed in a more physiological manner to the liver, perhaps reducing the peripheral hyperinsulinaemia seen with most or all subcutaneous regimens, with their theoretical risk of promoting atherosclerosis [26]. The high cost of implantable pumps, their relative invasiveness and several technical problems have so far limited the number of such pumps to some hundreds of patients. But implanted pump technology is likely to improve further, and we should therefore consider the present and possible future place of implantable insulin infusion pumps (IIP) in diabetes management.

Continuous subcutaneous insulin infusion

Costs

CSII is more costly, both in monetary terms and in terms of the demands placed on the patient and medical staff. In the UK, there are two currently available pumps for CSII and both cost about £2000. The MiniMed (model 508) insulin infusion pump has a lifetime estimated by the company of 7 years and the Disetronic H-Tron V-100 is supplied as a two-pump set, each of which has a programmed 2-year lifetime. Supplies include batteries, delivery cannulae and pump syringes, the cost of which are currently about £15 per week for either pump.

It is debatable to what extent CSII is more demanding than the modern intensive insulin injection regimens, which themselves call for extensive education, motivation, frequent monitoring and skilled healthcare professionals. Pump patients must also be willing, motivated and capable of undertaking CSII and its monitoring procedures, particularly frequent home blood glucose testing. Comprehensive education programmes for CSII include pump operation, understanding the effect of exercise and sport and how to adjust insulin rates during these activities, bathing procedures, instructions for action in case of hypoglycaemia, hyperglycaemia, intercurrent illness, ketonuria and pump breakdown.

Quality of glycaemic control in type 1 diabetes during CSII

But if we accept that CSII is expensive and demanding, its use in routine diabetes management, as opposed to research, depends on the evidence that it has advantages compared to modern, optimized multiple insulin injection therapy (MIT). Early studies showed the marked improvement in control which is possible with CSII and established it as a form of intensive insulin treatment, but the comparison was with conventional (non-optimized) injection regimens [8,10,14].

In subsequent trials of CSII versus MIT [15,16,27–35], the overall quality of control as judged by glycated haemoglobin percentage or mean blood glucose concentration has been found to be either broadly comparable during treatment by CSII or MIT, or slightly better on pump therapy. However, it is worth emphasizing that interpretation of these comparative studies is difficult because patients who chose (in non-randomized trials) or agree to be allocated CSII (in so-called randomized trials) may differ in many ways from the general diabetic population. They might, for example, be more compliant, cooperative and motivated and more likely to do well on CSII, or they might have suffered especially troublesome diabetic control on injections and have unusually difficult diabetes, and be more likely to do badly on CSII.

Unfortunately, there are no large-scale, long-term randomized studies

Table 13.1 Randomized trials of CSII vs MIT.

Study	Patients (no.)†	Duration CSII (months)	Mean blood glucose, (mmol/l)		Glycated Hb (%)	
			MIT	CSII	MIT	CSII
Schiffrin and Belmonte [27]	16	6	6.5 ± 2.3	6.3 ± 2.3	8.4 ± 0.5	8.2 ± 0.5
Reeves et al. [28]	10	2	5.9 ± 0.2‡	6.4 ± 0.4	9.0 ± 0.4	9.0 ± 0.4
			6.5 ± 0.4§		9.0 ± 0.5	
Home et al. [29]	10	2.5	9.3 ± 0.9	7.1 ± 0.6**	11.7 ± 0.6	10.0 ± 0.7**
Dahl-Jørgensen et al. [15]	15	24	6.4 ± 0.3	5.3 ± 0.3	9.1 ± 0.4	8.7 ± 0.3
Marshall et al. [30]	12	6	9.1 ± 0.8‖	5.2 ± 0.4	9.0 ± 0.4	9.2 ± 0.5
Saurbrey et al. [31]	21	5	8.7 ± 0.4	7.6 ± 0.2*		

*$P < 0.05$, **$P < 0.03$.
† Patients = number on CSII.
‡ Twice-daily short-acting and lente.
§ Ultralente + multiple short-acting insulin.
‖ Mean fasting blood glucose.

comparing CSII and MIT in type 1 diabetic subjects. One of the longest dura-tion, but with small patient numbers, is the Oslo study [15], where 45 type 1 diabetic subjects were randomly assigned to MIT, CSII or conventional injec-tion therapy (15 in each group). After 2 years, both the mean blood glucose level (5.3 ± 0.3 mmol/l vs 6.4 ± 0.3, mean ± SD, CSII vs MIT) and glycated haemoglobin (8.7 ± 0.3 vs 9.1 ± 0.4%) were similar in the two intensively treated groups (Table 13.1). Several other studies involving from five to 21 patients randomized to CSII or MIT for up to 6 months have also shown that mean blood glucose concentration and glycated haemoglobin are similar or slightly less during pump therapy compared to that during MIT [27–31]. These studies are too small or of too short a duration to make conclusions about the comparative frequency of serious hypoglycaemia or ketoacidosis.

Non-randomized studies comparing CSII and MIT predominate (Table 13.2) and generally involve large numbers of subjects (>50) treated for more than 1 year [32–35]. In the DCCT, for example, over the mean study dura-tion of 6.5 years, 124 patients used CSII for more than 90% of the time, 147 used both CSII and MIT and 284 were treated by MIT for most of the time [16,36]. Glycated haemoglobin was similar during CSII and MIT, though about 0.2–0.4% lower on CSII ($P < 0.001$) (Fig. 13.1).

Hypoglycaemia in type 1 diabetes during CSII

The frequency of severe hypoglycaemia (resulting in coma or seizure) or ketoacidosis in the DCCT was modestly higher on pump therapy than MIT.

Table 13.2 Non-randomized trials of CSII vs MIT.

Study	Patients (no.)†	Duration CSII (yr)	Glycated Hb (%)	
			MIT	CSII
Knight *et al.* [32]	63	2	10.9 ± 2.1	9.8 ± 1.9
DCCT [16]	124	6.5	7.0^*	6.8
Bode *et al.* [33]	55	3.1	7.7 ± 1.5	7.4 ± 1.2
Haardt *et al.* [34]	60	?	$9.3 \pm 0.2^{**}$	8.6 ± 0.2
Boland *et al.* [35]	25	1	8.3 ± 1.3	7.5 ± 0.9

$^*P < 0.05, ^{**}P < 0.0$.
Patients = number on CSII.

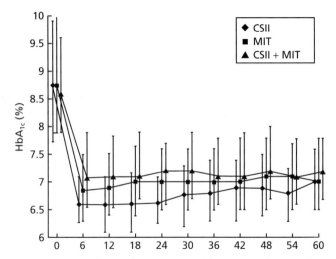

Fig. 13.1 Median HbA_{1c} in the three intensive insulin treatment groups of the Diabetes Control and Complications Trial—CSII, MIT and mixed CSII and MIT. Bars represent from 25th to 75th percentiles. From DCCT Research Group [36] with permission from the American Diabetes Association.

It should be noted, however, that the DCCT patients who were at high risk of hypoglycaemia, and thus potentially those who may benefit most from CSII, were excluded after the initial feasibility study. Several other non-randomized studies now indicate that hypoglycaemia on injection therapy is markedly reduced by CSII therapy.

In the study carried out by Bode *et al.* [33], 55 subjects who had been receiving MIT for at least 1 year before switching to CSII had comparable control on the two therapies—glycated haemoglobin 7.7% vs 7.4% (MIT

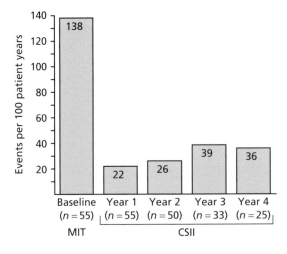

Fig. 13.2 Frequency of severe hypoglycaemic events in 55 type 1 diabetic subjects treated by MIT (baseline) and then by CSII. From Bode *et al.* [33] with permission from the American Diabetes Association.

vs CSII, NS)—though the incidence of severe hypoglycaemia was dramatically less on CSII (Fig. 13.2). Patients with a history of severe hypoglycaemia and/or hypoglycaemia unawareness were included, but not identified as a separate group in the analysis. The rate of ketoacidosis was the same in the two groups. It is worth noting that two case reports from other workers describe patients with hypoglycaemia unawareness and recurrent severe hypoglycaemia during MIT where the frequency of hypoglycaemia was reduced after instituting CSII, despite an unchanged glycated haemoglobin level [37].

The lower frequency of hypoglycaemia during CSII is confirmed in a recent study in which 25 adolescents chose CSII and 50 chose MIT [35]. HbA_{1c} improved with both treatments and was similar at 6 months (7.7 ± 1.0 vs 8.1 ± 1.0%, CSII vs MIT), though good control appeared to be easier to maintain with CSII, as the HbA_{1c} after 12 months was significantly lower with pump therapy (7.5 ± 0.9 vs 8.3 ± 1.3%, $P = 0.003$). Despite the lower HbA_{1c}, the rates of all hypoglycaemic events requiring assistance or resulting in coma were reduced by nearly 50% in the CSII group. Ketoacidosis was not different in the two groups.

In an early study, Knight *et al.* [32] reported on 99 patients who chose CSII and 169 who chose MIT (Table 13.2); though the glycated haemoglobin was again lower during CSII (9.8 ± 1.9 vs 10.9 ± 2.1%), the rate of hypoglycaemia was similar at 0.16 episodes of coma/patient/year for each therapy.

Finally, in a retrospective analysis of 60 type 1 diabetic patients in France [34], there was a slight but significant reduction in glycated haemoglobin on

CSII compared to MIT (8.6 ± 0.2 vs 9.3 ± 0.2%, $P < 0.01$) but again a clear reduction in the incidence of severe hypoglycaemia (1.5 ± 0.9 vs 6.6 ± 2.9 episodes per year, $P < 0.05$). Ketoacidosis was not different during CSII and injection treatment.

Further improvement in glycaemic control with CSII using monomeric insulin

The quickly absorbed monomeric insulin analogue, lispro, is now considered by most physicians experienced in pump therapy to be the insulin of choice for CSII. A number of randomized, crossover studies comparing lispro with regular human insulin for CSII [38–41] have shown that pump treatment with lispro results in improved glycated haemoglobin and blood glucose levels, particularly postprandial glucose values, either without increasing the frequency of hypoglycaemia [39] or with some reduction [38].

It can be concluded that although all forms of intensive insulin therapy probably increase the risk of hypoglycaemia relative to non-optimized regimens, in many patients the frequency of major hypoglycaemia may be markedly less during pump treatment, particularly when lispro is used as the pump insulin.

Glycaemic control in type 2 diabetes during CSII

There is little experience of CSII in type 2 diabetes [42–44] and it is not usually considered a management option in this category of patients [45]. However, there are indications that it can improve control in those poorly controlled on oral agents or insulin injections [43], and more research is needed.

The 'dawn phenomenon'

The dawn phenomenon, defined as a rising blood glucose concentration in the few hours before breakfast, resulting in fasting hyperglycaemia, was a topic of considerable interest in the 1980s. Although fasting hyperglycaemia as part of the 24-hour rhythm in blood glucose levels has been known to occur in diabetic patients for at least 70 years [46–48], it was highlighted again by Schmidt et al. in 1981 [49]. These authors described increases of up to 15.3 mmol/l in injection-treated type 1 diabetic subjects between the nocturnal nadir of blood glucose concentration and the prebreakfast value.

Many of the patients with the dawn phenomenon were shown to have declining plasma insulin concentrations during the night and therefore waning of the previous evening's delayed-action insulin injection seems a major contributor to the pathogenesis of the hyperglycaemia. Several workers have proposed moving the evening intermediate-acting insulin injection from before the evening meal to bedtime to extend its action and reduce fasting hyperglycaemia [27,50,51].

The other major influence on the causation of the dawn phenomenon is a decrease in prebreakfast insulin sensitivity caused by nocturnal growth hormone surges [52,53], the biological effects of which may coincide with falling plasma insulin levels.

Rather confusingly, Geffner *et al.* [54] reported that a large proportion of patients (nine of 15) treated by single basal-rate CSII experienced a marked dawn phenomenon (mean nadir to prebreakfast increase 7.9 mmol/l), which was contrary to early experiences with CSII where a dawn phenomenon was considered rare. We found, for example, that less than 1% of 103 24-hour blood glucose profiles during CSII in 41 type 1 diabetic patients had a dawn increase >5 mmol/l [55]. This discrepancy may be accounted for by the fact that the basal insulin infusion rate was relatively low in the study of Geffner *et al.* and increasing the rate from 23.00 hours by 18–68% significantly reduced fasting hyperglycaemia [54]. Later studies also showed that a dawn phenomenon was marked when the basal rate was low (0.75 units/h) but was abolished when the rate was increased by about 50% from shortly before midnight [56].

Modern insulin infusion pumps have the capacity to preprogramme automatic infusion rate changes throughout the day, which allows the rate to be increased by about 50–100% during the night, say between 03.00 and 09.00 hours, and thus minimize any dawn phenomenon. In fact, most patients do not benefit from multiple basal rate changes and can be managed with just 1–3 infusion rates throughout the day.

In considering whether CSII is the only or best approach to avoiding the dawn phenomenon, it should be noted that strategies exist for minimizing prebreakfast hyperglycaemia with insulin injection regimens, including moving the evening injection of isophane or lente insulin to bedtime to prolong its action, as mentioned above [27,50,51]. However, the peak of intermediate-acting insulin at about 4–6 hours after injection, produces a risk of nocturnal hypoglycaemia. In a recent study, Kanc *et al.* [57] showed that substitution of bedtime isophane with night-time CSII for 2 months reduced the total number of hypoglycaemic episodes in type 1 diabetic subjects.

Another alternative to CSII for the management of the dawn phenomenon might be one of the new long-acting insulin formulations made by protein engineering techniques, which are soluble in the vial but precipitate after injection into the subcutaneous tissue. The first of these, insulin glargine (Aventis), has an essentially peakless activity profile after injection, with a plateau of activity from about 4–8 h [58]. Incorporation of glargine as the delayed-action insulin in regimens significantly lowers prebreakfast blood glucose levels in comparison with regimens based on isophane. However, there is as yet no information on glargine-based regimens vs CSII.

Brittle diabetes

The type of brittle diabetes characterized by recurrent episodes of ketoacidosis, apparently high insulin requirements and disrupted lifestyle is not usually improved by CSII [59,60]. If CSII has a use in brittle diabetes it is chiefly as an investigative tool to exclude management errors of injection timing and dosage during conventional treatment. The syndrome seems to occur most frequently in adolescent females [60]. The aetiology has been much discussed and investigated (see Chapter 10), and a large proportion have psychological and social problems [60]; they are often suspected of deliberately interfering with their treatment [61,62]. Indeed, pump therapy offers additional opportunities for malefaction such as inverting or removing batteries, as well as practices such as dilution of insulin and eating binges which have been detected in brittle diabetic patients receiving insulin injections. There are some notable exceptions of patients with recurrent ketoacidosis who have been improved by CSII—Blackett [63] described four adolescent girls with brittle diabetes where the total number of admissions to hospital per year was reduced from 29 to five and the HbA_{1c} from 13.5% to 11.9% after 1 year of CSII. In general, it is not advisable to persist in these cases when there is no initial improvement on pump treatment.

True resistance to subcutaneously injected insulin is rare [64], but Meier et al. [65] have described a 35-year-old woman with longstanding type 1 diabetes who did not have a significant blood glucose response over 4 hours to the subcutaneous injection of 20 units of regular short-acting insulin, but where severe hypoglycaemia occurred after this period. Normal intravenous insulin sensitivity suggested delayed absorption of insulin from the subcutaneous site. A 2-day trial of CSII using the monomeric insulin, lispro, normalized blood glucose levels, though CSII using regular insulin resulted in hyperglycaemia and ketonuria.

Brittle lifestyle

From the earliest days of CSII, it has been said that pumps should be especially suitable for those with an erratic, unpredictable lifestyle, because the maintained basal infusion and easily adjustable mealtime insulin boosts should make it possible to delay or omit meals and yet keep stable control. While this is almost certainly true, and questionnaires of patient likes and dislikes during CSII confirm that flexibility of insulin dosage and mealtimes is a frequently cited positive feature in many active people [66], there are no formal trials comparing diabetic control during MIT and CSII in such circumstances.

Patient preference

In countries such as the USA and Germany where the cost of CSII is borne by health insurance, a large number of type 1 diabetic patients are being treated by CSII because they have chosen this as their preferred form of optimized insulin therapy. It should be considered, therefore, whether patient preference is an acceptable indication for CSII, and in this respect it is valuable to review attitudes to an alternative form of technology-driven intensive therapy: insulin pens. Unlike CSII, there is no evidence that glycaemic control or the frequency of hypoglycaemia is better with pens than with insulin delivered by needle and syringes [67], and pen use depends on patients choosing a method which is easier, more convenient and less painful. Physicians presumably sanction pen use because it is safe, because patient enthusiasm may encourage the use of multiple injections and better control and because there are no significant cost implications. It should be considered that CSII is at least as effective as MIT in achieving near-normoglycaemia, has advantages over injection therapy in some patients such as those with frequent hypoglycaemia, a marked dawn phenomenon or an erratic lifestyle, and is as safe as MIT if proper procedures are followed. If cost implications are set aside, it is difficult to deny it to patients who chose it, except on the grounds that a centre has little or no experience in the technique or is unable or unwilling to provide the support staff to teach and monitor treatment. In such circumstances, patients can be referred to an experienced pump centre.

Implantable insulin pumps

Some hundreds of patients with type 1 or type 2 diabetes have now been treated with an implantable insulin infusion pump (IIP). The three devices which have been used in most studies in the last decade are the Infusaid, MiniMed and Siemens Promedos pumps, with insulin delivery into the peritoneal cavity or intravenously.

Glycaemic control in type 1 diabetes during IIP

There are no large-scale, long-term randomized trials comparing the quality of glycaemic control achieved with IIP and intensive subcutaneous insulin therapy. In one small-scale trial, Selam *et al.* [68] randomly allocated 21 type 1 diabetic subjects to either IIP (Infusaid IP or IV) or intensive SC therapy with either CSII or MIT for 6 months. Glycaemic control was similar on the two treatments (HbA$_{1c}$ 7.5 ± 0.4 vs 7.8 ± 0.4%, MIT/CSII vs IIP, NS), and there were no hypoglycaemic episodes in either study group, but the standard deviation of blood glucose values, a measure of glycaemic fluctuations, was less in the IIP-treated subjects.

Other studies of implanted pumps and intensive subcutaneous therapy are not randomized, and IIP treatment has been compared with previous controls on MIT and/or CSII. Large numbers of patients have been evaluated in the EVADIAC (Evaluation dans le Diabète du Traitement par Implants Actifs) group of seven French centres which follow a common protocol for implanted pump studies [69,70]. In reports of 224 EVADIAC type 1 diabetic patients using Infusaid, MiniMed and Siemens pumps IP for 1–40 months, HbA$_{1c}$ was less during IIP treatment than CSII/MIT (7.4 ± 1.8 vs 6.8 ± 1.0%, $P < 0.001$). In this study, severe hypoglycaemia was also less with IIP (15.2 vs 2.5 episodes per 100 patient-years, $P < 0.001$) [69,70].

The Implantable Insulin Pump Trial Study Group is undertaking a US- and Italy-based multicentre evaluation of IIP [71,72]. In the most recent report of 76 patients [72], after an average 40 months of pump therapy with the Infusaid device IP or IV, blood glucose control was slightly improved on IIP (HbA$_{1c}$ 7.9 ± 1.5 vs 7.3 ± 1.3%, MIT/CSII vs IIP, $P < 0.05$). There was no difference in control during IV or IP pump therapy. As with the EVADIAC study, severe hypoglycaemia was reduced during IIP (33 vs 4 episodes per 100 patient years, $P < 0.003$).

Glycaemic control in type 2 diabetes during IIP

The only randomized controlled trial of IIP in type 2 diabetes is that of Saudek *et al.* [73]. Here, 59 patients were allocated to IIP (MiniMed IP) and 62 to MIT for 1 year. Glycaemic control was similar during the two treatments

(HbA$_{1c}$ 7.5 ± 0.8 vs 7.3 ± 0.8, MIT vs IIP, NS), but both the standard deviation of blood glucose concentration and mild hypoglycaemia were less during IIP than on MIT. The frequency of severe hypoglycaemia, not a common event during treatment of type 2 diabetes, was not different on the two treatments.

Complications of implanted pump therapy

The frequency of complications with IIP, mainly insulin underdelivery and implantation site problems, is still reasonably high, despite many years' experience with the technique [74–76]. Underdelivery is characterized by deterioration in control and the need for increased insulin dosages. It is caused by either microaggregation of insulin in the pumping mechanism which results in gradual reduction in insulin flow, or catheter blockage, which results in more rapid insulin deficiency. Catheters become occluded by fibrin clots at the end of the catheter or by omental encapsulation. A less common complication, associated with intravenous insulin delivery is venous thrombosis. So-called pump pocket problems include haematoma, local infection, skin erosion, abdominal pain and pump migration. Pump failures can be due to electronic and mechanical problems and premature battery depletion.

Research is active in reducing IIP complications, such as by improved non-aggregating insulin formulations and pump and catheter materials, but at the moment the moderately high frequency of complications is clearly a hindrance to the routine use of IIP.

Implanted insulin pumps and subcutaneous insulin resistance

A few patients with 'idiopathic' brittle diabetes who are apparently resistant to large doses of subcutaneously administered insulin but relatively sensitive to intravenous insulin have been successfully managed over some months by an IIP [77,78]. The case described by Campbell and Irsigler [73] is typical:

An 18-year-old girl with type 1 diabetes had been well controlled for 5 years on 44 units of subcutaneously injected insulin but then developed resistance to subcutaneous insulin administered by both injection and CSII. In the period 1979–82 she spent approximately 1 year in hospital, with 24 admissions for ketoacidosis. Up to 4000 units/day of insulin were given, though there was almost constant hyperglycaemia and ketosis (HbA$_{1c}$ 21.9%, reference range 5.1–9.3%). Intravenous insulin sensitivity was near normal, with reasonable control on a basal intravenous infusion of 2 units/h and 12 units at mealtimes.

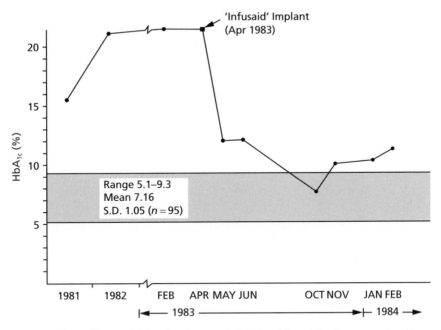

Fig. 13.3 Glycated haemoglobin values in a type 1 diabetic subject with subcutaneous insulin resistance during treatment with subcutaneous insulin (before April 1983) and after implantation of an Infusaid pump with intravenous insulin delivery. From Campbell and Irsigler [77] with permission.

In 1983, an Infusaid single-rate pump was implanted in the right pectoral region with catheter insulin delivery into the superior vena cava. Glycaemic control and insulin requirements improved dramatically, with a mean ± SD plasma glucose concentration of 6.2 ± 3.6 mmol/l and HbA_{1c} 7.8% (Fig. 13.3). The patient was well controlled after 10 months and returned to work.

As discussed above, the cause of insulin resistance in patients such as this is usually unclear. Accelerated insulin degradation by the subcutaneous tissue has been excluded in almost all [60], and most are suspected of deliberately interfering with their own treatment. It is possible that the success of IIP simply lies in the inaccessibility of the pump to tampering.

Summary and conclusions

CSII is a safe and effective form of intensive insulin treatment for type 1 diabetes. In most type 1 diabetic subjects average glycaemic control (HbA_{1c} and mean blood glucose concentration) is similar to or slightly better than that achieved with multiple insulin injection regimens. However CSII has a number of distinct advantages over MIT, most notably the frequency of hypoglycaemia is often less. Because of the ability to maintain a constant delivery of insulin during the night and to increase the infusion rate at a preset time during the night, prebreakfast glycaemic increases (the dawn phenomenon) can be minimized. Similarly, nocturnal hypoglycaemia during injection therapy, caused by the peak of insulinaemia from evening injection of delayed acting insulin, can be avoided by employing the basal infusion of CSII. Subjects with an erratic lifestyle who delay or omit meals probably find it easier to maintain good control with CSII. More studies are needed of CSII in type 2 diabetes before recommendations can be made about its usefulness in this category of patient.

Because CSII is more expensive and complex in its procedures than injection treatment it is probably sensible to restrict its use to two main classes of patient.

• Subjects who have failed in using intensive insulin injection regimens to achieve good control because of frequent hypoglycaemia, a marked dawn phenomenon or erratic lifestyle.

• Subjects who prefer CSII as their intensive treatment and in whom funding mechanisms are in place to support pump use, for example health insurance, patient or private funds.

All diabetic subjects considered for CSII must be willing and capable of undertaking the procedure and must be approved, instructed and supervised by physicians and healthcare professionals experienced in the technique.

Implanted insulin pumps also produce strict glycaemic control, which is similar to or slightly better than that possible with multiple injections or CSII using regular short-acting insulin regimens. Fluctuations of blood glucose are less than with intensive regimens based on regular short-acting insulin; hypoglycaemia may also be less frequent but data is based on non-randomized studies. There are no trials comparing IIP to CSII using insulin lispro which itself reduces glycaemic oscillations. A few rare cases of brittle diabetes characterized by extreme resistance to subcutaneous insulin are markedly improved by IIP.

At present, the high cost of IIP, the relative invasiveness of the procedure and the significant remaining technical problems outweigh the advantages of strict glycaemic control, except in a few patients with life-threatening brittle diabetes, where IIP can be considered as a therapeutic option. The real impact of IIP may come in the future when reliable *in vivo* glucose sensors are available that can be linked to the pump to form a closed-loop system. Progress with implantable and non-invasive glucose sensors is increasingly rapid [79,80], with (at the time of writing) two commercial devices having US Food and Drug Administration approval or conditional approval. Though it seems a long way off, with improvements in insulin formulation, biocompatibility of materials, refinements in pump technology and features to ensure safety of closed-loop insulin delivery, a completely implanted artificial pancreas might one day be a practicable management option for selected diabetic patients.

References

1 Slama G, Hautecouvature M, Assan R, Tchobroutsky G. One to five days of continuous insulin infusion on seven diabetic patients. *Diabetes* 1974; 23: 732–8.

2 Deckert TL, Lørup B. Regulation of brittle diabetes by a preplanned infusion programme. *Diabetologia* 1976; 12: 573–9.

3 Hepp KD, Renner R, Funcke HJ, Mehnert H, Haerten R, Kresse H. Glucose homeostasis under continuous intravenous insulin therapy in diabetes. *Horm Metab Res* 1977; 7 (Suppl): 72–6.

4 Genuth S, Martin P. Control of hyperglycemia in adult diabetics by pulsed insulin delivery. *Diabetes* 1977; 26: 571–81.

5 Service FJ. Normalisation of plasma glucose of unstable diabetes: studies under ambulatory fed conditions with pumped intravenous insulin. *J Lab Clin Med* 1978; 91: 480–9.

6 Irsigler K, Kritz H. Long-term continuous intravenous insulin therapy with a portable regulating apparatus. *Diabetes* 1979; 28: 196–203.

7 Pickup JC, Keen H, Parsons JA, Alberti KGMM. The use of continuous subcutaneous insulin infusion to achieve normoglycaemia in diabetic patients. *Diabetologia* 1977; 13: 425A.

8 Pickup JC, Keen H, Parsons JA, Alberti KGMM. Continuous subcutaneous insulin infusion: an approach to achieving normoglycaemia. *BMJ* 1978; 1: 204–7.

9 Tchobroutsky G. Relation of diabetic control to development of microvascular complications. *Diabetologia* 1978; 15: 143–52.

10 Tamborlane WV, Sherwin RS, Genel M, Felig P. Reduction to normal of plasma glucose in juvenile diabetes by subcutaneous administration of insulin with a portable infusion pump. *N Engl J Med* 1979; 300: 573–8.

11 Pickup JC, Keen H, Viberti GC *et al.* Continuous subcutaneous insulin infusion in the treatment of diabetes mellitus. *Diabetes Care* 1980; 3: 290–300.

12 Mecklenburg RS, Benson JW, Becker NM *et al.* Clinical use of the insulin infusion pump in 100 patients with type 1 diabetes. *N Engl J Med* 1982; 307: 513–18.

13 Kroc Collaborative Study Group. Blood glucose control and the evolution of diabetic retinopathy and albuminuria. *N Engl J Med* 1984; 311: 365–72.

14 Lauritzen T, Frost-Larson K, Larsen HW, Deckert T. Effect of 1 year of near-normal blood glucose levels on retinopathy in insulin-dependent diabetes. *Lancet* 1983; i: 200–4.

15 Dahl-Jørgensen K, Bringhman-Hansen O, Hanssen KF *et al.* Effect of near-normoglycaemia for two years on progression of early diabetic retinopathy and neuropathy: the Oslo Study. *BMJ* 1986; 293: 1195–9.

16 The Diabetes Control and Complications Trial Research Group. The effect of intensive treatment of diabetes on the development and progression of long-term complications in insulin-dependent

diabetes mellitus. *N Engl J Med* 1993; 329: 977–86.

17 American Diabetes Association. Continuous subcutaneous insulin infusion. *Diabetes Care* 2000; 23 (Suppl 1): 90.

18 Pickup JC. Alternative forms of insulin delivery: continuous subcutaneous insulin infusion. In: Pickup JC, Williams G, eds. *Textbook of Diabetes*, 2nd edn. Oxford: Blackwell Science, 1997: 34.1–12.

19 Fakas-Hirsch R, Hirsch IB. Continuous subcutaneous insulin infusion: a review of the past and its implementation for the future. *Diabetes Spectrum* 1994; 7: 80–138.

20 Kaufman FR, Halvorson M, Miller D, Mackenzie M, Fisher KF, Pitukcheewanont P. Insulin pump therapy in type 1 pediatric patients; now and into the year 2000. *Diab Metab Res Rev* 1999; 15: 338–52.

21 Buchwald H, Barbosa J, Varco RL *et al.* Treatment of a type II diabetic by a totally implantable insulin infusion device. *Lancet* 1981; i: 1233–5.

22 Irsigler K, Kritz H, Hagmuller G *et al.* Long-term continuous intraperitoneal insulin infusion with an implantable remote controlled insulin infusion device. *Diabetes* 1981; 30: 1072–5.

23 Schade DS, Eaton RP, Sterling WE *et al.* A remotely programmable insulin delivery system: successful short-term implantation in man. *JAMA* 1982; 247: 1848–53.

24 Schade DS, Eaton RP, Friedman NM, Spencer WJ. Normalisation of plasma insulin profiles with intraperitoneal insulin infusion in diabetic man. *Diabetologia* 1980; 19: 35–9.

25 Schade DS, Eaton RP, Davis T *et al.* The kinetics of peritoneal insulin absorption. *Metabolism* 1981; 30: 149–55.

26 Stout RW. Insulin and atheroma: 20 year perspective. *Diabetes Care* 1990; 13: 631–54.

27 Schiffrin A, Belmonte MM. Comparison between continuous subcutaneous insulin infusion and multiple injections of insulin. *Diabetes* 1982; 31: 255–64.

28 Reeves ML, Seigler DE, Ryan EA, Skyler JS. Glycemic control in insulin-dependent diabetes mellitus. Comparison of outpatient intensified conventional therapy with continuous subcutaneous insulin infusion. *Am J Med* 1982; 72: 673–80.

29 Home PD, Capaldo B, Burrin JM, Worth R, Alberti KGMM. A crossover comparison of continuous subcutaneous insulin infusion (CSII) against multiple insulin injections in insulin-dependent diabetic subjects: improved control with CSII. *Diabetes Care* 1982; 5: 466–71.

30 Marshall SM, Home PD, Taylor R, Alberti KGMM. Continuous subcutaneous insulin infusion versus injection therapy: a randomized cross-over trial under usual diabetic clinic conditions. *Diabet Med* 1987; 4: 521–5.

31 Saurbrey N, Arnold-Larson SM, Møller-Jensen B, Kühl C. Comparison of continuous subcutaneous insulin infusion with multiple insulin injections using the NovoPen. *Diabet Med* 1988; 5: 150–3.

32 Knight G, Boulton AJM, Drury J, Ward JD. Long term glycaemic control by alternative regimens in a feasibility study of continuous subcutaneous insulin infusion. *Diabetes Res* 1986; 3: 355–8.

33 Bode BW, Steed RD, Davidson PC. Reduction in severe hypoglycemia with long-term continuous subcutaneous insulin infusion in type 1 diabetes. *Diabetes Care* 1996; 19: 324–7.

34 Haardt MJ, Berne C, Dorange C, Slama G, Selam J-L. Efficacy and indications of CSII revisited: the Hôtel Dieu cohort. *Diabet Med* 1997; 14: 407–8.

35 Boland EA, Grey M, Oesterle A, Fredrickson L, Tamborlane WV. Continuous subcutaneous insulin infusion. A new way to lower risk of severe hypoglycemia, improve metabolic control, and enhance coping in adolescents with type 1 diabetes. *Diabetes Care* 1999; 22: 1779–84.

36 Diabetes Control and Complications Trial Research Group. Implementation of treatment protocols in the Diabetes Control and Complications Trial. *Diabetes Care* 1995; 18: 361–76.

37 Hirsch IB, Farkas-Hirsch R, Cryer PE. Continuous subcutaneous insulin

infusion for the treatment of diabetic patients with hypoglycemic unawareness. *Diabet Nutr Metab* 1991; 4: 41–3.

38 Melki V, Renard E, Lassman-Vague V *et al.* Improvement of HbA_{1c} and blood glucose stability in IDDM patients treated with lispro insulin analogue in external pumps. *Diabetes Care* 1998; 21: 977–81.

39 Renner R, Pfützner A, Trautman M, Harzer O, Sauter K, Landgraf R. Use of insulin lispro in continuous subcutaneous insulin infusion treatment. *Diabetes Care* 1999; 22: 784–8.

40 Schmauss SK, König A, Landgraf R. Human insulin analogue [LYS(B28), PRO(B29)]: the ideal pump insulin? *Diabet Med* 1998; 15: 247–9.

41 Zinman B, Tildesley H, Chiasson J-L, Tsui E, Strack T. Insulin lispro in CSII. Results of a double-blind crossover study. *Diabetes* 1997; 46: 440–3.

42 Dupré J, Champion M, Rodger NW. Advances in insulin delivery. *Baillières Clin Endocrinol Metab* 1982; 11: 525–48.

43 Jennings AM, Lewis KS, Murdock S, Talbor JF, Bradley C, Ward JD. Randomised trial comparing continuous subcutaneous insulin infusion and conventional insulin therapy in type II diabetic patients poorly controlled with sulphonylureas. *Diabetes Care* 1991; 14: 738–44.

44 Valensi P, Moura I, Paries J, Perret G, Attali JR. Short-term effects of continuous subcutaneous insulin infusion treatment on insulin secretion in non-insulin-dependent overweight patients with poor glycaemic control despite maximal oral anti-diabetic treatment. *Diabetic Metab* 1997; 23: 51–7.

45 Koivisto VA. Insulin therapy in type II diabetes. *Diabetes Care* 1993; 16 (Suppl 3): 29–39.

46 Gerritzen F. The 24-hour rhythm in diabetes. *Acta Med Scand* 1942; 111: 212–18.

47 Mollenstrom J. The treatment of diabetes with reference to the endogenous periodicity of the carbohydrate metabolism. *Acta Med Scand* 1934; 59: 145–61.

48 Hopman R. Insulinbehundlung unter Berucksichtigund des 24-Stunden-Rhythmus des Diabetes Mellitus. *Acta Med Scand Suppl* 1940; 108: 143–55.

49 Schmidt MI, Hadji-Georgopoulos A, Rendell M, Margolis S, Kowarski A. The dawn phenomenon, an early morning glucose rise: implications for diabetic intraday blood glucose variation. *Diabetes Care* 1981; 4: 579–85.

50 Francis AJ, Home PD, Hanning I, Alberti KGMM, Tunbridge WMG. Intermediate acting insulin given at bedtime: effect on blood glucose concentrations before and after breakfast. *BMJ* 1983; 286: 1173–6.

51 Peterson CM, Jovanovic LB, Brownlee M, Jones RL, Cerami A. Closing the loop: practical and theoretical. *Diabetes Care* 1980; 3: 318–21.

52 Campbell PJ, Bolli G, Cryer PE, Gerich JE. Pathogenesis of the dawn phenomenon in patients with insulin-dependent diabetes mellitus. *N Engl J Med* 1985; 312: 1473–9.

53 Perriello G, De Feo P, Fanelli C, Santeusanio F, Bolli G. Nocturnal spikes of growth hormone secretion cause the dawn phenomenon in type 1 (insulin-dependent) diabetes mellitus by decreasing hepatic (and extrahepatic) sensitivity to insulin in the absence of insulin waning. *Diabetologia* 1990; 33: 52–9.

54 Geffner ME, Frank HJ, Kaplan SA, Lippe BM, Levin SR. Early-morning hyperglycemia in diabetic individuals treated with continuous subcutaneous insulin infusion. *Diabetes Care* 1983; 6: 135–9.

55 Bending JJ, Pickup JC, Collins ACG, Keen H. Rarity of a marked dawn phenomenon in diabetic subjects treated by continuous subcutaneous insulin infusion. *Diabetes Care* 1985; 8: 28–3.

56 Koivisto VA, Yki J, Järvinen H, Helve E, Sirkka-Liisa K, Pelkonen R. Pathogenesis and prevention of the dawn phenomenon in diabetic patients with CSII. *Diabetes* 1986; 35: 78–82.

57 Kanc K, Janssen MMJ, Keulen ETP *et al.* Substitution of night-time continuous subcutaneous insulin infusion therapy for

bedtime NPH insulin in a multiple injection regimen improves counterregulatory hormonal responses and warning symptoms of hypoglycaemia in IDDM. *Diabetologia* 1998; 41: 322–9.

58 Bolli GB, Di Marchi RD, Park GD, Pramming S, Koivisto VA. Insulin analogues and their potential in the management of diabetes mellitus. *Diabetologia* 1999; 42: 1151–67.

59 Pickup JC, Home PD, Bilous RW, Keen H, Alberti KGMM. Management of severely brittle diabetes by continuous subcutaneous and intramuscular insulin infusions: evidence for a defect in subcutaneous insulin absorption. *BMJ* 1981; 282: 347–50.

60 Pickup J, Williams G, Johns P, Keen H. Clinical features of brittle diabetic patients unresponsive to optimised subcutaneous insulin therapy (continuous subcutaneous insulin infusion). *Diabetes Care* 1983; 6: 279–84.

61 Schade DS, Drumm DA, Duckworth WC, Eaton RP. The etiology of incapacitating, brittle diabetes. *Diabetes Care* 1985; 8: 12–20.

62 Schade DS, Drumm DA, Eaton RP, Sterling WA. Factitious brittle diabetes mellitus. *Am J Med* 1985; 78: 777–84.

63 Blackett PR. Insulin pump treatment for recurrent ketoacidosis in adolescence. *Diabetes Care* 1995; 18: 881–2.

64 Schade DS, Duckworth WC. In search of the subcutaneous-insulin-resistance syndrome. *N Engl J Med* 1986; 315: 147–53.

65 Meir M, Brand J, Standl E, Schnell O. Successful treatment with insulin analog lispro in IDDM with delayed absorption of subcutaneously applied human regular insulin and complicated intraperitoneal insulin infusion. *Diabetes Care* 1998; 21: 1044–5.

66 Pickup JC, Keen H, Viberti GC, Bilous RW. Patient reactions to long-term outpatient treatment with continuous subcutaneous insulin infusion. *BMJ* 1981; 282: 766–8.

67 Anonymous. Insulin pen: mightier than the syringe? *Lancet* 1989; i: 307–9.

68 Selam J-L, Raccah D, Jeandidier N, Lozano JL, Waxman K, Charles MA. Randomised comparison of metabolic control achieved by intraperitoneal insulin infusion with implantable pumps versus intensive subcutaneous insulin therapy in type 1 diabetic patients. *Diabetes Care* 1992; 15: 53–69.

69 Broussolle C, Jeandidier N, Hanaire-Broutin H. French experience of implantable insulin pumps. *Lancet* 1994; 343: 514–15.

70 Hanaire-Broutin H, Broussolle C, Jeandidier N *et al.* Feasibility of intraperitoneal insulin therapy with programmable implantable pumps in IDDM. *Diabetes Care* 1995; 18: 388–92.

71 Selam J-L, Micossi P, Dunn FL, Nathan DM. Clinical trial of programmable implantable insulin pump for type 1 diabetes. *Diabetes Care* 1992; 15: 877–85.

72 Dunn FL, Nathan DM, Scavini M, Selam J-L, Wingrove TG. Long-term therapy of IDDM with an implantable insulin pump. *Diabetes Care* 1997; 20: 59–63.

73 Saudek CD, Duckworth WC, Giobbie-Huder A *et al.* Implantable insulin pump vs multiple-dose insulin for non-insulin-dependent diabetes mellitus. A randomized clinical trial. *JAMA* 1996; 276: 1322–7.

74 Renard E, Baldet P, Picot M-C *et al.* Catheter complications associated with implantable systems for peritoneal insulin delivery. *Diabetes Care* 1995; 18: 300–6.

75 Renard E, Bouteleau S, Jacques-Apostol D *et al.* Insulin underdelivery from implanted pumps using peritoneal route. *Diabetes Care* 1996; 19: 812–17.

76 Scavini M, Galli L, Reich S, Eaton RP, Charles MA, Dunne FL. Catheter survival during long-term insulin therapy with an implanted pump. *Diabetes Care* 1997; 20: 610–13.

77 Campbell IW, Irsigler K. Subcutaneous insulin resistance: treatment by implantable device. In: Pickup JC, ed. *Brittle Diabetes.* Oxford: Blackwell Science, 1985: 289–300.

78 Wood DF, Goodchild K, Guillou P, Thomas DJ, Johnston DG. Management

of 'brittle diabetes' with a preprogrammable implanted insulin pump delivering intraperitoneal insulin. *BMJ* 1990; 301: 1143–4.

79 Pickup J, McCartney L, Rolinski O, Birch D. *In vivo* glucose sensing for diabetes management: progress towards non-invasive monitoring. *BMJ* 1999; 319: 1289.

80 Pickup J. Sensitive glucose sensing in diabetes. *Lancet* 2000; 355: 426–7.

14: Is there a role for sole transplantation of the pancreas (without kidney) in type 1 diabetes?

Robert A. Sells and David E. R. Sutherland

Introduction

Sole pancreas transplantation is, to say the least, contentious, and has for some time been a battleground between internists and surgeons. To point out the bone of contention simply: physicians, by and large, believe that careful glycaemic control using multiple insulin injections and glucose monitoring is likely to be able to reduce the progression of secondary microangiopathic complications of type 1 diabetes [1]. Yet a small percentage of diabetic patients still develop severe hypoglycaemia, recurrent ketoacidosis or have progressive visceral and neural complications despite strict glycaemic control. However, the surgical view (coloured no doubt by the remarkable improvement in patient survival and quality of life following a simultaneous pancreas/kidney transplant) is that we are currently achieving good enough results with sole pancreas transplantations in diabetes without renal failure to justify, in their view, pre-emptive pancreas transplant alone. Criticism from the other side highlights the invasiveness and expense of the procedure, the surgical and nephrological complications of immunosuppression in an immunologically compromised group of patients, and our ignorance of long-term success.

If sole pancreas transplantation were ever to be implemented on a large scale in type 1 diabetes (which is only likely to occur when and if islet transplantations become feasible), the immediate challenge would be to distinguish those patients who will develop rapidly progressive microangiopathy and serious complication (and who would thus qualify for a transplant) from those (the majority) who will live reasonably healthy lives for decades, with reasonable glycaemic control, on insulin treatment.

This debate is likely to be resolved by closer collaboration between physicians and surgeons. Agreement is needed that with rigorous patient selection,

224

adequate standards of surgery and scrupulously designed immunosuppression, the operation is as safe as continuing insulin therapy, and gives a high chance of preventing microangiopathic complications. This optimistic theme will be developed in this chapter.

Patient selection

Those potentially suitable for this operation are diabetic persons with severe hypoglycaemia unawareness, or patients in whom there have been failed attempts at intensified insulin therapy for metabolic control [2]. They should not have reversible comorbid risk factors such as recidivist smoking, heart failure or severe hypertension. Experience of simultaneous pancreas/kidney (SPK) transplantation in dialysis patients has demonstrated the serious risk of postoperative myocardial infarction and stroke, which should be excluded initially by routine nuclear ventriculography with stress and, if necessary, coronary angiography [3]. During the earlier, cyclosporin era of pancreas transplants alone (PTA), 6% at 1 year and 31% at 5 years required dialysis or renal transplantation, partly due to the nephrotoxic nature of the immunosuppressives. Although modern immunosuppression is not associated with this complication, patients for sole pancreas transplants should have a preoperative creatinine clearance of at least 80 ml/min to minimize this risk [2], although other workers find that a clearance of 40 ml/min is satisfactory [4]. The severity of proteinuria is an important determinant of success in avoiding diabetic nephropathy following pancreas transplantation. It is significant that stabilization or reversal of diabetic nephropathy more than 5 years after the operation is maintained in patients whose median urinary albumin level was only 103 mg/day prior to transplantation [5].

Patients should also be examined for peripheral vascular disease, retinopathy and neuropathy in addition to full cardiac investigations. This is because type 1 diabetic patients on dialysis and who are candidates for SPK transplantation commonly have occult critical coronary artery disease masked by the absence of angina, in addition to widespread atherosclerosis. In this group, rigorous cardiac screening is of proven benefit in SPK and this improved selection, combined with up-to-date immunosuppression, has produced a startling improvement in patient and graft survival, even in this disadvantaged group. It is likely therefore that the diabetic patient with normal renal function and minimally damaged arteries runs a much smaller operative risk [6].

The operation

There has been debate over whether the whole organ or a segmental pancreas transplant should be used routinely, how the exocrine secretion should be drained safely, and whether the venous effluent from the pancreatic graft should drain into the portal or the systemic circulations.

Cadaver pancreases are usually transplanted as a whole, *en bloc*, with a duodenal segment which is used to drain exocrine secretions. Most grafts are removed at multiorgan retrieval: when the liver is procured, the blood supply to the pancreas may be reconstituted with a Y graft of donor iliac artery to join the splenic and superior mesenteric arteries to the external iliac or common iliac artery of the recipient. Pelvic placement of the graft requires 'heterotopic' drainage of the pancreatic venous blood into the iliac vein. Since 1984, drainage of exocrine secretion has been detected by joining the duodenum to the bladder; gratuitously this technically safe procedure allows the postoperative monitoring of pancreas function and early detection of rejection by measuring urinary amylase. However in the mid 1990s, it became clear that up to 25% of bladder-drained patients develop intractable cystitis and acidosis, and straightforward enteric drainage to an adjacent loop of small bowel is becoming much more common. More effective immunosuppression has led to a reduction in pancreas transplant rejection. Thus, some think the loss of amylasuria as a prediction of early graft failure is outweighed by the lack of urological and metabolic complications using a bowel anastomosis. However, a recent Registry analysis of all cases done in the USA between 1996 and 1999, showed graft survival rates are still significantly higher for bladder- than for enteric-drained pancreas transplants alone [7]. For bladder-drained cases ($n = 98$) the 1-year insulin-independent rate was 78%, while for enteric drainage ($n = 73$) it was only 63% ($P < 0.05$). The same difference was seen for pancreas after kidney transplantation, another form of solitary pancreas transplantation in which kidney function cannot be used as a surrogate marker to detect rejection in the pancreas graft because the two organs are from different donors and the immune responses to the two organs are not linked. For pancreas after kidney transplants during 1996–99, the 1-year insulin independence rate was 81% for recipients of bladder-drained grafts ($n = 238$) and 68% for recipients of enteric-drained grafts ($n = 156$). By contrast, for simultaneous pancreas and kidney transplants from the same donor (renal graft function can be used as a surrogate marker for rejection that would effect both organs), the 1-year insulin independence rates were similar for recipients of bladder- ($n = 1203$) and enteric-

($n = 1170$) drained grafts, 85% and 84%, respectively. Thus, for pancreas transplants alone, bladder drainage may still be preferable to detect early rejection, and then later, if the chronic problems mentioned above develop, the graft can be converted to enteric drainage (required in approximately 10% of the cases reported to the Registry for 1996–97) [7].

A minority of sole pancreas recipients develop significant postoperative hypoglycaemia [8] due to hyperinsulinaemia and transient symptomatic postprandial hyperglycaemia. A solution would be to drain the pancreatic vein directly into the portal circulation. Stratta [9] has reported a prospective randomized controlled trial of 30 patients (15 with systemic-vein, exocrine bladder drainage and 15 with portal vein, exocrine enteric drainage) which will allow long-term comparison of the two procedures in terms of metabolic stability and graft survival. Technically the operations appear to be equally successful but results after long-term follow-up are not yet available.

In the Registry data [7] most pancreas transplantations in which the venous effluent was portally drained have been done simultaneously with the kidney, with 1-year insulin independence rates similar to those in which enteric exocrine drainage was combined with systemic venous drainage, 83% ($n = 194$) and 84% ($n = 937$), respectively.

The technical results of this operation have improved steadily as surgical teams have gone through their 'learning curves', and as the complications of immunosuppression have become less. Technical failures accounted for 30% of graft loss in the precyclosporin era, 14% during the cyclosporin era and 0% in the tacrolimus era ($P = 0.001$) [2]. Leakage at the crucial duodenal anastomosis, causing intra-abdominal complications, has similarly decreased to 8% compared to 37% in the precyclosporin era.

Another option that should be mentioned in a chapter on pancreas transplantation is the use of living donors for segmental grafts [10]. Living donors are now used for all organ transplantations except the heart. Of the nearly 13 000 pancreas transplantations reported to the International Pancreas Transplant Registry, approximately 1% have been segmental grafts from a living donor [7]. The largest experience is at the University of Minnesota, where through the end of 1999, 112 had been done including 51 pancreas transplants alone, 32 pancreas after kidney transplants and 29 simultaneous pancreas and kidney transplants [11]. Most of the solitary pancreas transplantations were done in the late 1970s and 1980s when the results of cadaver pancreas transplantation were not as good as today because of a higher rejection rate. During this period the 1-year graft survival rate for technically successful solitary pancreas transplants was 63% vs 55% for cadaver solitary pancreas transplantations. During the 1990s, the majority of living donor pancreas transplantations have been carried out simultaneously with a kidney, with a 1-year pancreas graft survival rate of 86%, at least as good as with cadaver organs [11]. Uraemic diabetics with simultaneous pancreas and kidney transplantations from living donors have the advantage of pre-empting the need for dialysis or the long waiting time for a cadaver kidney, and allowing the recipient to become insulin independent as well as dialysis free with one operation. For pancreas transplants alone the main advantage of a living donor has been the lower rejection rate, as well-matched pancreases have been available. When all pancreases from cadaver donors are used, there will be an incentive to do living donor segmental donor pancreas transplants alone to alleviate the shortage of organs as well.

Prevention of graft rejection

The prevention of rejection is crucial to good long-term survival. Early results from the International Pancreas Transplant Registry (IPTR) have demonstrated that pancreas transplants alone have a higher rejection rate than simultaneous pancreas kidney grafts. It was thought that was due to the lack of endogenous immunosuppression associated with chronic uraemia.

Using tacrolimus-based immunosuppression (with anti-T-cell antibody induction therapy, prednisone and mycophenolate mofetil (MMF) or azathioprine triple therapy), pancreas rejection episodes have been reduced or appear to be more easily reversed, with an actuarial graft survival rate of 66% at 4 years for pancreas transplant alone done in the mid 1990s reported from Minneapolis [2].

Anti-T-cell induction therapy is now used routinely in more than two-thirds of pancreas transplant recipients [7], and is associated with improved graft survival. Although no data have yet been published comparing induction vs non-induction treatment in a prospective randomized study, the latest US Registry data [7] shows that for 1996–99 bladder-drained pancreas transplants alone in recipients given an anti-T-cell agent for induction and tacrolimus and MMF for maintenance immunosuppression ($n = 50$), the insulin independence rates over time were not significantly different from those for similarly treated pancreas after kidney transplant recipients ($n = 107$) or simultaneous pancreas kidney transplant recipients ($n = 331$) at 1 year (83%, 86% and 87%, respectively) (Fig. 14.1).

Single-centre studies reveal that 'biopsy directed' adjustment of immunosuppression results in substantially improved graft survival and acceptably

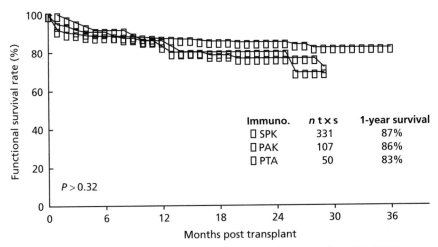

Fig. 14.1 Pancreas graft functional survival (insulin-independence) rates for 1996–99 US cadaver bladder-drained (BD) transplants by category in recipients given anti-T-cell agents for induction and tacrolimus + MMF for initial maintenance immunosuppression. Note no significant differences in outcome for solitary pancreas vs simultaneous pancreas kidney transplants. Adapted from Gruessner and Sutherland [7] with permission.

low infection rates of 90% at 1 year [12,13]. A single-centre study from Minneapolis [2] in 225 solitary pancreas transplants has shown that HLA matching has a significant impact on graft survival and pancreas graft loss due to rejection: graft survival at 1 year for zero HLA mismatches was 90% and for four to six mismatches, it was 47% ($P < 0.01$). The bulk of the graft failures in the poorly matched recipients was due to rejection. Two mismatches on the HLA-B or DR loci were associated with a significantly higher graft loss due to rejection than a 0 or 1 mismatch on each HLA locus. Multivariate analysis showed that B locus incompatibility was most significant. Optimizing HLA compatibility in pancreas transplant recipients is problematical; since these are mostly restricted to the DR3 or DR4 class II genotype, the waiting time for a reasonably well matched pancreas graft may be prolonged. It remains to be seen whether the superior immunosuppression achieved with FK-506 and MMF, without HLA matching, can produce the same excellent results as those which are currently being achieved with SPK transplantations [14].

Results

The results of pancreas transplants alone can be gathered from single-centre reports [2] or the Registry data [7]. The Registry shows that nearly all pancreas transplants alone have been reported from the USA. There was a remarkable improvement in early graft function rates during the last decade of the twentieth century. For pancreas transplants alone reported for 1987–89 ($n = 46$), the 1-year insulin independence rate was only 50% while for 1996–97 cases ($n = 100$) it was 69%. For 1996–99 cases in which the recipients were given modern immunosuppression (anti-T cell for induction, and tacrolimus/MMF for maintenance), the 1-year insulin independence rate was 83% for bladder-drained grafts.

It is not known what the 10-year insulin independence rate will be with this immunosuppressive regimen. However, if one takes the 1987–89 cases that were functioning at 1 year, 60% were still functioning at 10 years. Thus, even if the chronic rejection rate does not change, we can predict that the 10-year insulin independence rates for pancreas transplants being done today will be at least 50%. Pancreas transplant alone patient survival rates are much higher than graft survival rates, because the patient can return to insulin if rejection occurs. According to the Registry, 1-year patient survival rates for 1987–89 cases was 93% and for 1996–99 cases it was 97%. Most of the deaths that have occurred following a pancreas transplant have been cardiovascular in nature and it appears that the actual mortality risk of doing a pancreas transplantation is extremely low.

Whether there is actually a survival advantage of adding the pancreas is difficult to determine, because no randomized prospective studies have been carried out. However, data cited below indicates that for uraemic recipients of simultaneous pancreas/kidney transplants, the long-term survival is better than in those who receive only a kidney transplant. For solitary pancreas transplants, there is some data in neuropathic patients showing that a pancreas transplant alone improves survival rates. According to Navarro et al. [15], more than 30% of diabetic patients with grade 2 neuropathy are dead 5 years after the diagnosis of neuropathy is made, while for patients with a similar degree of neuropathy who underwent pancreas transplant alone, only 10% were dead 5 years later.

We shall have to wait several years for the results from long-term graft and patient survival data using FK-506/MMF-based immunosuppressive regimens. However, messages are coming through from the 10-year data on survival after SPK transplantation that simultaneous pancreas transplantation with a kidney reduces the mortality rate in diabetic patients, compared with those who receive a kidney alone. In a case-controlled study, Tyden et al. [14] compared the outcome of 14 SPK transplantations at 10 years with 12 (control) diabetic patients who received kidneys alone. The control group had been accepted for SPK transplantation, but received only a kidney graft either because a pancreas was not available, or the pancreas graft had been lost in the first year from a technical complication or rejection. Follow-up was for 10 years in all patients. Three of 14 SPK patients died, compared with 12 of 15 'kidney alone' transplant patients. It seems that this is the nearest we can get to a prospective randomized study comparing SPK with kidney transplant alone in type 1 diabetes with renal failure. Such a trial has been suggested [16] but was rejected on ethical grounds because of the proven advantage of SPK transplantations in improved quality of life. But as improved longevity is conferred on diabetic patients with end-stage renal disease by the addition of a pancreas transplant, it seems very likely that similar benefits will accrue from sole pancreas transplantation in problematical diabetes without renal failure. Autonomic neuropathy was also shown to be significantly improved in the Tyden paper [14]; as early mortality is linked to the severity of autonomic neuropathy [16], one might predict that a similar reduction in mortality might be seen after pancreas transplant alone.

The effect on secondary complications and quality of life

Most pancreas transplantions alone have been done in patients in whom complications of diabetes already exist, although not as advanced as in those who also need a kidney transplantation. Because the leading indication for a pancreas transplant alone has been hypoglycaemic unawareness, this implies the presence of at least autonomic neuropathy. Even if the neuropathy does not improve, at least the situation is improved, as severe hypoglycaemia is unlikely in a pancreas transplant recipient, because exogenous insulin is not administered and an overdose cannot occur.

For diabetic recipients in whom the objective is prevention or treatment of secondary complications, it has been shown that successful pancreas transplantation can reverse microscopic lesions of diabetic nephropathy [5] and that neuropathy can at least stabilize if not improve [16–18]. Although a series of pancreas transplantations done very early after the onset of diabetes has not been carried out, it would be predicted that secondary complications would not develop in recipients of successful grafts, given the data from the DCCT [1]. However, in this situation the lack of diabetic complications might be undone by the emergence of immunosuppressive complications or non-immunosuppressive side-effects of the immunosuppressive drugs used to prevent rejection. An examination of the diabetic literature and the immunosuppressive literature simply indicates that both routes have the potential for chronic complications to occur, but whether the incidences are the same or different or whether the complications have equivalent morbidity or not is difficult to determine. In the absence of a randomized prospective trial, it is just as reasonable for a diabetic patient to choose to undergo pancreas transplantation as it is to choose remaining diabetic. The current diabetic management regimen is difficult. Ideally at least four fingersticks a day for blood sugar monitoring and four insulin injections, 50 needlesticks a week, 2500 needlesticks a year and 25 000 over a decade. Even if such a regimen is followed faithfully, there is no guarantee that control will be adequate to prevent secondary complications. Thus, we can see why it would be tempting for a diabetic to take the transplant/oral immunosuppression route.

If antirejection regimens are developed that are truly tolerogenic, that is immunosuppressive and non-immunosuppressive side-effects are eliminated, then the only deterrent to pancreas transplantation would be the major surgery required [18]. This may be solved by islet transplantation [19]. Islet transplant research has been ongoing for nearly 30 years; until recently only 8% of recipients remained insulin-free at one year [20]. However, in a landmark publication [21], Shapiro *et al.* describe 100% survival of islet grafts, 4–15 months post-intraportal infection, in 7 patients treated with steroid-free, non-nephrotoxic, anti-rejection prophylaxis. Confirmation of this work will confirm the principle and practice of the procedure, for which the demand will surely be considerable.

The first decade of the twenty first century should see a resurgence of clinical islet transplant trials, and if successful, this approach will replace pancreas transplantation and indeed has potential for widespread application, the only limit being the shortage of donors for allografts. To achieve insulin independence by transplantation in the majority of type 1 diabetics will almost certainly require the application of porcine islet xenografts. Whether methods to consistently prevent rejection of xenografts are developed before other approaches, such as β-cell regeneration and thwarting of autoimmunity are developed for clinical application, remains to be seen. It could be one of the exciting races of the new millennium. In the interim, we should apply today's technology to treat today's patients and pancreas transplant alone should be in the armamentarium of every diabetologist.

References

1 DCCT Research Group. Diabetes control and complications trial (DCCT): the effect of intensive treatment of diabetes on the development and progression of long-

term complications in IDDM. *N Engl J Med* 1993; 329: 977–86.

2 Gruessner RWG, Sutherland DER, Najarian JS, Dunn DL, Gruessner AC. Solitary pancreas transplantation for non-uraemic patients with labile insulin-dependent diabetes mellitus. *Transplantation* 1997; 64: 1572–7.

3 Schweitzer EJ, Anderson L, Kuo EC *et al.* Safe pancreas transplantation in patients with coronary artery disease. *Transplantation* 1997; 63: 1294–9.

4 Stratta RJ, Taylor RJ, Gill IS. Pancreas transplantation: a managed cure approach to diabetes. *Curr Prob Surg* 1996; 33: 709–808.

5 Fioretto P, Steffes NW, Sutherland DER, Goetz FC, Mauer M. Reversal of lesions of diabetic nephropathy after pancreas transplantation. *N Engl J Med* 1998; 339: 69–75.

6 Sells RA. Cardiovascular complications following renal transplantation. *Transplantation Rev* 1997; 11: 111–26.

7 Gruessner AC, Sutherland DER. Analyses of pancreas transplant outcomes for United States cases reported to the United Network for Organ Sharing (UNOS) and non-US cases reported to the International Pancreas Transplant Registry (IPTR). In: Cecka JM, Terasaki PI, eds. *Clinical Transplants.* Los Angeles: UCLA Tissue Typing Laboratory, 1999.

8 Redmon JB, Teuscher AU, Robertson RP. Hypoglycemia after pancreas transplantation. *Diabetes Care* 1998; 21: 1944–50.

9 Stratta RJ. In: Hakim NS, Stratta RJ, Dubernard JM, eds. *Pancreas Transplantation in the 1990s.* International Congress and Symposium Series no 232. London: Royal Society of Medicine, 1998: 101–20.

10 Gruessner AC, Sutherland DER. Pancreas transplantation in the United States (US) and non-US as reported to the United Network for Organ Sharing and the International Pancreas Transplant Registrar. In: Cecka JM, Terasaki PI, eds. *Clinical Transplants 1996. Los Angeles: UCLA Tissue Typing Laboratory*, 1997: 47–67.

11 Bartlett ST, Schweitzer EJ, Johnson LB. Equivalent success of simultaneous pancreas–kidney and solitary pancreas transplantation: a prospective trial of Tacrolimus immunosuppression with percutaneous biopsy. *Ann Surg* 1996; 224: 440–9.

12 Drachenberg CB, Papadimitriou JC, Klassen EK *et al.* Evaluation of pancreas transplant needle biopsy; reproducibility and revision of histological grading system. *Transplantation* 1997; 63: 1579–86.

13 Jordan ML, Shapiro R, Gritsch HA *et al.* Long-term results of pancreas transplantation and the tacrolimus immunosuppression. *Transplantation* 1999; 67: 266–72.

14 Tyden G, Bolinder J, Solders G, Brattstrom C, Tibell A, Groth C-G. Improved survival in patients with insulin dependent diabetes mellitus and end stage diabetic nephropathy, 10 years after combined pancreas and kidney transplantation. *Transplantation* 1999; 67: 645–8.

15 Navarro X, Kennedy WR, Loewenson RB, Sutherland DER. Influence of pancreas transplantation on cardio-respiratory reflexes, nerve conduction and mortality in diabetes mellitus. *Diabetes* 1990; 39: 802–6.

16 Pyke DA. A critique of pancreas transplantation. *Clin Transplant* 1990; 4: 235.

17 Gruessner AC, Sutherland DER. Analyses of pancreas transplant outcomes for United States cases reported to the United Network for Organ Sharing (UNOS) and non-US cases reported to the International Pancreas Transplant Registry (IPTR). In: Cecka JM, Terasaki PI, eds. *Clinical Transplants 1999. Los Angeles: UCLA Tissue Typing Laboratory*, 2000.

18 Navarro X, Kennedy WR, Aeppli D, Sutherland DER. Neuropathy and mortality in diabetes: influence of pancreas transplants. *Muscle Nerve* 1996; 19: 1009–16.

19 Hering BJ, Ricordi C. Islet transplantation in type 1 diabetes: results,

research priorities and reasons for optimism. *Graft* 1999; 2: 12–27.

20 Breudel M, Hering B, Schulz A, Bretzel R. *International Islet Transplant Registry Report*. Giessen, Germany: University of Giessen, 1999: 1–20.

21 Shapiro AM, Lakey JR, Ryan EA *et al.* Islet transplantation in seven patients with type 1 diabetes mellitus using a glucocorticoid-free immunosuppressive regimen. *N Engl J Med* 2000; 343: 230–8.

Other management issues

15: Should there be driving and employment restrictions for people with diabetes?

Kenneth M. MacLeod and Raymond V. Johnston

Introduction

This chapter will discuss the issue of whether there should be restrictions on driving and employment for those with diabetes mellitus. The debate is largely centred around those on insulin treatment, and the associated hypoglycaemic risk. Issues of concentration also particularly occur with the driving of large and/or passenger vehicles, and with potentially hazardous employments (e.g. fire fighting, armed forces, etc.). Though the two issues of driving and employment are each discussed separately here, it should be remembered that the issues are very similar, and in a number of cases employment and driving are identical problems to the individual—for example lorry driving, the ambulance service, bus and train driving, some postal and delivery jobs, etc. For this reason, driving will be dealt with in more detail. Finally, the 'evidence base' (or lack of it!) for current restrictions and legislation for driving and employment will be critically examined, as well as the potential for more logical regulations based on risk assessment and individualized decision making.

DRIVING AND DIABETES

Multiple factors contribute to road traffic accidents

The potential for multiple factors to combine, independent of any medical effects, to significantly and tragically increase road traffic accidents (RTAs) is vividly illustrated in the article describing the carnage wrought by major economic change following the dramatic political upheaval in Germany [1]. After reunification, East Germany suddenly experienced temporary affluence and a concomitant fourfold increase in death rates for car occupants. Death

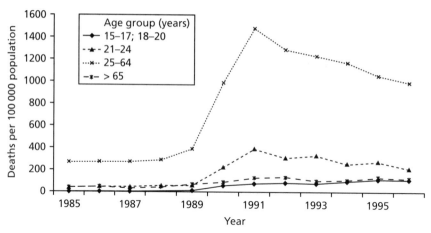

Fig. 15.1 Death rates per 100 000 population for car occupants by age in the former East Germany. Adapted from Winston *et al.* [1] with permission.

rates increased in all age groups but young adults (aged 18–24 years) were most severely affected. Between 1989 and 1994, the death rate increased 11-fold for those aged 18–20 years and eightfold for those aged 21–24 years. Sudden economic change and the availability of cars resulted in both a rise in vehicle ownership and an increase in the number of inexperienced drivers, driving on roads that were ill prepared for the traffic increase [1]. The combination of traffic congestion, young age of drivers and driver inexperience was deadly (Fig. 15.1). A simplistic approach to the multifaceted problem of road safety is therefore inappropriate, and the targeting of those most easily identifiable as posing a potential risk (e.g. all those with defined medical conditions) is unjust and unlikely to prove successful.

What is the available evidence that medical conditions contribute significantly to road traffic accidents?

Surveys in the UK and the USA have suggested that approximately 95% of RTAs involve an error by a road user and that one in 250 resulting in hospital admission is attributable to a preaccident medical condition [2,3]. The World Health Organization (WHO) have concluded that 'all forms of sudden illness are probably responsible for about one accident per thousand involving injury', but these figures must be a crude estimate at best and are now considerably out of date [4].

In a UK survey of 2000 road accidents in the early 1980s involving collapse at the wheel, grand mal (tonic–clonic) epilepsy was the commonest cause accounting for 39% of the collapses. Insulin-treated diabetes was a factor in 17% of cases and acute myocardial infarction in 10%. The most up-to-date UK estimate of the figure for insulin-treated diabetes available is for the year 1995 and is remarkably consistent at 16.5% (27 of 163 collapses at the wheel). The fact that insulin-treated diabetes is responsible for approximately one-fifth of all medical collapses at the wheel does not allow an assessment of how important a contributor to RTAs these 'collapses' are. For this we need the denominator figure of all accidents and we need to know whether the number of 'collapses' among insulin-treated patients are greater or fewer than the number among a matched group of non-diabetic controls. This data is not readily available.

How does diabetes and its treatment impact on driving performance?

Diabetes is associated with the potential to impair driving performance. Vision is a critically important sensory function required for driving and the visual standards applied to diabetes are those applied to the general population. The legal requirement is a combined visual acuity of 6/12 or better. Widespread ablative retinal photocoagulation, used in the treatment of proliferative retinopathy, may of itself reduce peripheral vision to a significant extent and lead to unfitness to drive [5]. In a recent study from the UK, Pearson and colleagues estimated that although there is a high risk of significant uniocular field loss following panretinal photocoagulation (PRP) for proliferative retinopathy (42%), this figure is reduced to 12% if both eyes are treated. In other words, 88% of patients will pass a binocular field of vision test even if both eyes have received PRP. Of note, the risk of failure was significantly greater in patients with type 2 diabetes [6].

Peripheral vascular disease and peripheral neuropathy can result in ulceration and amputation of extremities and limb weakness, making driving for some of those affected difficult, potentially dangerous and inappropriate. These visual, vascular and neuropathic complications of diabetes are long-term problems which often come announced and, at least where diabetes supervision is adequate, with a long lag-phase and a history of intervention in an attempt to retard progression. In these circumstances, if the complications do develop the patient often has appreciated the need for lifestyle change and the need for driving and employment restriction is understood, perceived as legitimate and accepted. The imposition of a blanket ban on insulin-treated drivers because of the potential for hypoglycaemia to suddenly and unpredictably affect driving performance is a different matter, particularly if the individual has never had an RTA, never had a severe episode of hypoglycaemia and retains normal awareness of hypoglycaemia.

Does hypoglycaemia have predictable effects on driving performance?

Unrecognized hypoglycaemia represents a significant driving hazard. In a well conducted study of driving performance using a sophisticated driving stimulator, 27 insulin-treated diabetic patients were assessed at plasma glucose concentrations of 6.3 mmol/l (euglycaemia), 3.6 mmol/l (mild hypoglycaemia) and 2.6 mmol/l (moderate hypoglycaemia) [7]. The 27 subjects studied were volunteers with type 1 diabetes and were selected to have no significant diabetic complications, no history of hypoglycaemia unawareness (though this was not defined) and no history of substance abuse. Moderate but not mild hypoglycaemia was associated with disrupted steering, causing significantly more swerving, spinning, time over the midline and time off the road. It also resulted in an apparent compensatory slowing. At a blood glucose concentration of 2.6 mmol/l, nine of the 27 patients (33%) experienced significant deterioration in their driving performance. Of greater concern was the fact that four of the nine (44%) remained unaware of the deterioration in their driving performance and said they would continue to drive. This study confirms that hypoglycaemia impairs driving performance and raises several important additional questions—what was it about the other 65% of drivers that allowed them to continue to drive safely and competently despite ambient blood glucose concentrations of 2.6 mmol/l? Was it metabolic, neurological or driving related factors (skill, training and experience)? Differential sensitivity to the disruptive effects of acute hypoglycaemia on speed of cognitive and motor performance has been shown experimentally and it is unwise to assume that all patients with type 1 diabetes suffer equivalent cognitive motor deficits at moderate hypoglycaemia [8].

In an extension of this study, Weinger and colleagues examined hypoglycaemic awareness (symptoms, intensity and type), cognitive performance and self-reported ability to drive safely, during a stepwise hypoglycaemic clamp [9]. The proportion of patients reporting that they could drive safely fell in parallel with fall in plasma glucose (from 70% at a glycaemic plateau of 4.4 mmol/l to 22% at a glycaemic plateau of 2.2 mmol/l). Men were more likely to judge that they could drive safely than women, especially during mild hypoglycaemia (3.3 mmol/l), and middle-aged patients with type 1 diabetes were more likely to report that they could drive safely at any given glucose level. This contrasts with the data from studies of the general population, where young men report the highest prevalence of high-risk behaviour. The authors propose three possible explanations for this apparent discrepancy. First, that age may be a proxy for driving experience, and that the more experienced driver may have been more confident of their driving ability, even during hypoglycaemia. Second, that medical staff are aware of the risks of RTAs, and dangerous driving violations in male drivers, and therefore place more emphasis on driving safety when counselling young people with type 1 diabetes. Third, that older people with long-duration diabetes and more prevalent neuropathy may have more cognitive impairment with consequent impairment of hypoglycaemia awareness and assessment of driving performance. Actual glucose level, cognitive index score, error in glucose estimation, intensity of symptoms, patients' age and sex were associated with perceiving safe driving ability, but self rating of driving experience, the number of RTAs, and the duration of diabetes were not [9].

Kovastchev and colleagues applied a stochastic model to explore the variations in possible outcome that occur at each step in the sequence from physiological change, to symptom perception, appraisal, and final decision making, with respect to hypoglycaemia and driving [10]. They provide mathematical support for the concept that symptom perception, appraisal and response are complex processes that can be altered by any number of cognitive, affective, social and environmental factors. There is not a one-to-one relationship (or 100% transition probability) between (i) physiological changes and symptom perception, (ii) symptom perception and accurate symptom appraisal and (iii) accurate symptom appraisal and appropriate self regulation. Hypoglycaemia can occur without symptoms, and did so 21% of the time in this data-set. This may have been a consequence of physiological variables, for example reduced neuroendocrine response, or psychological variables, such as attention mechanisms and competing motivations [11]. In the absence of symptoms the probability of recognizing hypoglycaemia is low (9%) but, even when symptom scores are high, hypoglycaemia is not always reported [10]. This failure to recognize symptoms occurs as a result of cognitive factors such as misattribution of symptoms and inaccurate symptom beliefs [11]. Even when hypoglycaemia is recognized the probability of appropriate decision making is not 100%. When hypoglycaemia was correctly identified, the probability of deciding to drive was 31%, and of deciding not to treat was 18%. This suggests these decisions are modified by personality, as well as cognitive factors that influence processes of risk appraisal [10]. Education and intervention need to target high-risk groups (perhaps middle-aged men, especially those with a history of cognitive impairment associated with hypoglycaemia), and focus on improving hypoglycaemic awareness, emphasize the need for regular glucose monitoring, and encourage good judgement and accurate risk appraisal to guide decision making during complex tasks such as driving (see case history 2).

Case history 1

A 56-year-old Hackney Carriage driver employed in the metropolitan area of London had type 2 diabetes of 6 years duration and experienced progressive deterioration of his glycaemic control. He was essentially asymptomatic but the HbA_{1c} confirmed chronic hyperglycaemia at 9.0% (normal range 4.1–6.5%) despite maximum doses of sulphonylurea, metformin and acarbose. The addition of a low-dose basal intermediate-acting (isophane) insulin at night significantly improved glycaemic control, with the HbA_{1c} falling to 6.8%. The diabetes was uncomplicated and there was no history of preceding hypoglycaemia, but despite this his vocational driving licence permitting him to drive taxis was revoked by the Public Carriage Office. On the first stage of a two-stage appeal the decision of the Assistant Commissioner of the Metropolitan Police Authority (the Licensing Authority) was to confirm the decision of the Public Carriage Office and the taxi-driving ban was upheld. On further appeal to the Magistrates' court after hearing lengthy medical evidence and legal opinion, the Magistrate accepted that there was no clear evidence of excess risk of RTAs in patients with insulin-treated diabetes and that this particular individual was in a low-risk group for unrecognized severe hypoglycaemia. He instructed the authority to restore the licence.

These data confirm that patients with diabetes, and particularly those treated with insulin, are at increased risk of hypoglycaemia, and that hypoglycaemia can result in RTAs. Hypoglycaemia can be considered a relatively specific acute metabolic complication of diabetes therapy. In questionnaire surveys, hypoglycaemia was consistently reported among diabetic populations as a cause for somewhere between 5% and 16% of the accidents they were involved in.

What is the risk of a road traffic accident for patients with insulin-treated diabetes?

Several published reports attempt to compare the driving performance of people with diabetes and those without. Despite a profusion of studies, there is no consensus in the literature as to whether or not the risk of RTA for the diabetic driver in general and the insulin-treated diabetic driver in particular is increased or reduced. There are numerous deficiencies in the evidence base. All of the studies conducted in this area are retrospective. They often fail to distinguish between types of diabetes, they rely on patient recall, they vary in definition of the terminology used (e.g. definitions of accident, injury and hypoglycaemia), are highly selective in their recruitment of the 'study population', and suffer from inherent ascertainment bias. Little objective information is provided in any of these reports regarding the impact of duration of diabetes, presence of hypoglycaemia unawareness, presence of diabetic complications or quality of metabolic control. Despite these many deficiencies, the studies are remarkably consistent in that they indicate little if any increased risk of RTAs (Table 15.1).

The studies are summarized in Fig. 15.1, and considered in more detail in a recent review article [12]. The studies taken together suggest that the insulin-treated diabetic driver does not pose a significant risk to road safety. Hansotia and Broste have suggested that given the very low rates of relative risk in the diabetic driving population (13 per 5665 accidents) in the 14-year period of their study, a blanket restriction will not significantly improve road safety [22]. By contrast, drivers under the age of 25 had significantly more (1508) accidents when compared with all older drivers combined, and men had 1586 more accidents than women. They make the point that a ban on all young or all male drivers would clearly be more productive in terms of improving road safety, but represent a totally unacceptable restriction of the freedom of individuals. Songer has commented further that despite all the debate over hypoglycaemia, it still remains only part of the accident puzzle and probably only a very minor component. Many more important factors have been shown to be related to truck and automobile accidents. These include young age, male sex, mileage driven, alcohol ingestion and previous accident history [13].

If the total accident risk is not excessive, but patients with diabetes treated with insulin are exposed to the significant and peculiar additional risk of hypoglycaemia, then other risk factors for RTAs must be of less consequence and reduced significance in these patients. It may be that heightened awareness of the potential problems result in many self-imposed driving restrictions. Both Songer *et al.* [16] and Eadington and Frier [17] found that most diabetic drivers who stopped driving did so voluntarily rather than as a consequence of revocation of their driving licence. Indeed, several authors have suggested that diabetes exerts a 'prophylactic effect on diabetes driving', and

Table 15.1 Road traffic accidents in diabetic patients and control groups. Modified from Cox *et al.* [14].

	Patients	Controls	*P*
Songer et al. [16]			
Number	121	121	
Crashes per 1000 000 miles	10.4	3.9	NS
Crashes for males	17.6	8.1	NS
Crashes for females	32.4	6.6	P < 0.01
Stevens et al. [18]			
Noumber	354	302	
Crashes per 1000 000 miles	4.9	4.8	
Eadington et al. [17]			
Number	140		
Crashes per 1000 000 miles	5.4	9.5–10	NS
Crashes for males	4.4		
Crashes for females	6.3		
Ysander [15]			
Number	219	219	
Crash frequency per 10 yr (%) 3.7	6.4	NS	
Traffic offences per 10 yr (%)11.9	12.3	NS	
Davis et al. [19]			
Number	108	1 651 245	
Crashes/100 drivers	7.4	7.1	NS
For males	9.2	8.7	NS
For females	4.9	4.8	NS
Waller [20]			
Number	287	922	
Crashes per 1000 000 miles	15.1	11.0	NS
Violations per 1000 000 miles	4.6	4.9	NS
Hansotia and Broste [21]			
Number	714	289 969	
Standardized moving violation ratios	1.14	1.00	NS
Standardized crash ratios	1.32	1.00	P < 0.01

that responsible patient behaviour may be the biggest factor contributing to the risk reduction. Eadington and Frier [17] suggest that self regulation by diabetic drivers, who cease driving because of declining health and driving skills, may offset the potential increase in risk of RTAs from hypoglycaemia. They conclude that diabetic drivers in general have the common sense and social responsibility to stop driving voluntarily as their health declines and complications develop. Other factors may also be contributing. For example, the 3-year licence restriction ensures that adequate visual and other explicit standards for driving are continually met. This may in fact be removing a vulnerable group from the study, i.e. those with the insidious onset of reduced visual acuity who are not being similarly identified from the general driving population.

Accepting the inherent limitations of the evidence base, the weight of informed opinion in this field has consistently concluded that further restrictions of motor vehicle licensing for patients with insulin-treated diabetes is unjustified [16–25].

The legal position

The legal position varies widely around the world with respect to driving restriction. This extent of the variation is illustrated by the data collected by the WHO as part of the DiaMond project [26,27]. Information was obtained between December 1990 and March 1991 regarding the rulings with respect to commercial vehicle driving licenses for patients with type 1 diabetes. The data is summarized in Table 15.2, and it is of interest to note that even within countries (e.g. the USA) opinion varied from state to state. While European governments have progressively restricted driving permits for insulin-treated diabetic drivers [28], in the USA the restrictions on motor vehicle driving have been relaxed [29–31]. Also in the USA, the Federal Aviation Administration have overturned the indiscriminate ban on recreational pilots with insulin-treated diabetes, and in the light of evidence, have begun to issue licenses on a case-by-case basis [25].

Table 15.2 Licensing regulations for diabetic lorry drivers treated with insulin [27].

Licensing permitted with no restriction	Licensing permitted with restrictions	Licensing not permitted
Argentina	Australia	Belgium
Brazil	Austria	Canada
Finland	Chile	Greece
Japan	Israel	Italy
Libya	New Zealand	Mexico
Puerto Rico		Poland
Tanzania		Romania
Thailand		Sweden
USA (70% of states)		USA (30% of states)

In the UK, it has been a legal requirement since 1975 to notify the Driving and Vehicle Licensing Agency of the diagnosis of diabetes. The driving licence issued to subjects with diabetes requiring insulin has been restricted to a maximum period of 3 years in place of the standard driving licence, which is valid until the age of 70 years. Renewal of the restricted license is subject to a satisfactory assessment of fitness to drive. For large goods vehicles (LGV) and other vehicles considered to require 'Group 2' entitlement, new applicants on insulin or existing drivers becoming insulin treated were barred in law from April 1991. Drivers licensed before this and treated with insulin are dealt with individually and may continue to drive heavy goods vehicles (HGV) subject to annual medical certification. Drivers of emergency vehicles, ambulances, police vehicles and fire engines are not explicitly dealt with in driver licensing legislation, and taxi drivers are licensed by local authorities under local government legislation. The Medical Commission on Accident Prevention recommends that Group 2 standards should be applied to drivers of all these groups. Group 2 licenses normally expire after the 45th birthday and are renewable up to age 65 years. Insulin-treated diabetic drivers are not eligible for Group 2 entitlement. With effect from January 1997, when the second European Union (EU) driver licensing directive came into force in the UK, insulin-treated diabetic drivers lost their entitlement to drive lighter goods vehicles (those weighing between 3.5 and 7.5 tonnes), and smaller passenger-carrying vehicles. The British Diabetic Association (now known as Diabetes UK) has campaigned vigorously against the blanket extension of restrictions with limited success, and has constantly pleaded that a policy of individual consideration now be adopted. The case for this approach will be discussed in the final section.

The case for individual assessment and independent decision making

It is evident from the above that while hypoglycaemia contributes to impaired driving performance, the overall contribution of hypoglycaemia is very small and there is a widely differing view as to how the data should be applied in practice. It appears that selective restriction of the small proportion of patients who account for the greatest increase in risk is the most effective and discriminating way to impose restrictions on insulin-treated diabetic drivers. Patients with tight glycaemic control are at increased risk, but in most studies the strongest predictors of risk of hypoglycaemia are a history of unawareness of hypoglycaemia, experience of frequent severe hypoglycaemia and previous experience of hypoglycaemic-related injury or accident

[32]. In a structural equation-modelling exercise, 18% of the variance of severe hypoglycaemia was accounted for by a history of previous severe hypoglycaemia, state of awareness of hypoglycaemia and the autonomic function score [33]. Present knowledge does not allow prediction with certainty, but it is possible to use a number of recognized clinical, historical and biochemical criteria to identify the subset of diabetic patients who are potentially at greatest risk from unrecognized severe hypoglycaemia.

The extant literature suggests that restricting those at greatest risk would make a significant contribution to a further reduction in accident rates in patients with diabetes. In a study modelling accident distribution in a large sample of Quebecois drivers [34], in all of the models Class 3 (straight truck) drivers with diabetes had an increased relative risk of accidents when compared with those in good health. By contrast, the Class 1 (articulated truck) drivers had a relative risk of RTA that was not increased (0.51). They suggest that a more rigorous selection criteria may have been applied for Class 1 drivers. Two companion papers predict that licensing people with insulin-treated diabetes to drive commercial motor vehicles would result in 42 additional crashes per year, and that the annual crash rate would consequently increase from 0.000785 to 0.0032 for non-insulin-dependent and 0.048 for insulin-dependent people [13,23]. The increase in relative risk is estimated to vary considerably between different categories of drivers with diabetes, and is calculated at 4.7 for all insulin-using drivers but 19.8 for drivers with a history of severe hypoglycaemia. The authors conclude that this increase in risk is well within the current accepted range of risk [13,23]. In Eadington and Frier's study a substantial proportion (16%) of the RTAs were attributed retrospectively by the patients to hypoglycaemia, but several of these patients not only reported a higher frequency of hypoglycaemic episodes, but had hypoglycaemia unawareness [17]. Identifying and disqualifying this vulnerable group from driving (temporarily or permanently) would be more effective in reducing the contribution of hypoglycaemia to the causation of RTAs. More liberal glycaemic control may be appropriate in individuals for whom driving is an essential vocational activity, to allow greater hypoglycaemic warning and reduced risk. Goals of glycaemic control and treatment regimens should be individualized and tailored to the specific needs and circumstances of the person with diabetes. The insulin analogues with their more favourable time–action characteristics may assist significantly [35]. Others have suggested that intensive education programmes such as blood glucose awareness training allow patients to more accurately estimate their blood glucose concentrations and to detect hypoglycaemia at an early stage [7]. The preliminary studies suggest that after such training the incidence of hypoglycaemia decreases and patients are less frequently involved in RTAs (crash rate per 10^6 miles driven 42% vs 15%) [36]. Even patients with hypoglycaemia unawareness, for whom a temporary driving ban is entirely appropriate, can regain symptomatic warning of impending hypoglycaemia and improve hypoglycaemia awareness by meticulous avoidance of hypoglycaemia [37] (case history 2).

Case history 2

A 27-year-old woman with a 15-year history of type 1 diabetes complicated by background retinopathy had a rear collision with another vehicle in 1994. There was no clear evidence to incriminate hypoglycaemia. The patient denied symptoms and the episode occurred mid-afternoon. No blood glucose testing was performed and no action was taken. Eighteen months later she was found slumped over the wheel of her car, which was parked in a lay-by. On this occasion the patient reported recognizing the onset of hypoglycaemia with typical symptoms (warmth, sweating, impaired cognition). She drove off the road and lapsed into unconsciousness before being able to ingest refined carbohydrate. The incident occurred on the way back from dropping her children off at school and she admitted having had her insulin without breakfast. Her glycaemic control was excellent with an HbA_{1c} level of 6.2% (normal range 4–6%) and review of her diary of home blood glucose tests confirmed frequent asymptomatic hypoglycaemia. A diagnosis of severe hypoglycaemia in someone with hypoglycaemia unawareness was made and a temporary driving ban imposed. Strategies to reduce the frequency of hypoglycaemia and improve awareness were adopted and following relaxation of the glycaemic targets, reduction in insulin therapy, 12 months without severe hypoglycaemia and restoration of hypoglycaemia awareness her driving license was restored. Three years later there has been no further history of RTA.

The case for individual assessment is thus strong. Additionally, a more structured approach to driving research should be encouraged—in particular, the assessment of quantitative risk, as used by at least some workers in the field [13,23].

EMPLOYMENT AND DIABETES

Introduction

Despite many advances in the treatment of diabetes and robust evidence that good control may prevent complications [38,39], there is poor understanding of the condition in the workplace—both in the minds of employers and the doctors who advise them. When reviewing employment issues in those with diabetes, or indeed any other disease, it is valuable to distinguish between employability on the one hand, and employment/unemployment on the other. The first category would refer to those whose diabetes may limit opportunities to enter the labour market, the second involves the issues of whether diabetes leads to premature withdrawal from the labour market.

The data on the experience of diabetes in the workplace and on that of discrimination therein is conflicting. Several studies have shown no evidence of employment discrimination [40–42]. By contrast Songer et al. [43] found higher job refusal rates among diabetic patients compared with a control group of siblings. This study has, however, been criticized for bias. Songer and colleagues asked patients whether diabetes was a reason for job refusal and it is possible that the answers could have been influenced by both recall and attributional bias, factors not compensated for in the study design. Matsushima et al. [44], however, in a case–control study also reported increased job refusal and lower income in young people with diabetes, although they found no significant differences in unemployment or employment. By contrast, Fritis and Nanjundapa [45] found a relationship between diabetes and unemployment, with a significantly higher unemployment rate in those people with diabetes compared to controls. They postulated that depression was the intervening mechanism. Despite the conflicting data in the literature, the wider representation of diabetic people in the workforce [46] may indicate less prejudice against employment or non-declaration of their diabetes.

The issue of prejudice in the working environment may fall foul of disability discrimination laws. In the UK, for example, the Disability Discrimination Act 1995 dictates that where impairment is being treated or corrected, the impairment is to be regarded as having the effect it would have without the intervention. This remains valid even if that intervention results in the effects of the disease being so well controlled that they are not apparent. The Act also provides for an individual with a progressive condition to be assumed to have an impairment which produces a significant adverse effect on their ability to carry out day-to-day activities before it actually does so. Diabetes (type 1 and type 2) is covered by the Act, and thus not employing an individual for a job which involves shift work because the employer (or indeed their medical adviser) feels that diabetic persons on insulin cannot undertake shift work, may contravene the Act. The Act provides for the employer to make *reasonable adjustment* to the working environment to accommodate an individual with a disability, and therefore a reasonable adjustment may be showing flexibility in meal breaks during a night shift for an employee with type 1 diabetes. However, it is better to assess the employee's fitness for shift work in the first instance, by obtaining a report from their diabetic physician, in order that the occupational physician advising the employer may make a equitable assessment.

One potential source of employment bias is the view held by many employers and their medical advisers, that the sickness absence rate of diabetic employees is higher than that of non-diabetic people. However, in well controlled studies the excess sickness absence is minimal or not significant, especially in those not treated with insulin [47]. A second source of bias is the feeling by many employers that diabetic employees may be at 'risk' in the working environment. This will be discussed in detail in the following section. An example of diabetes-related employment difficulties based on unreasonable criteria is shown in case history 3.

Case history 3

A 28-year-old man was a qualified chef and also had type 1 diabetes of 10 years' duration. He had no complications, was well controlled, attended clinic regularly and had no hypoglycaemia. With excellent work and medical references, he applied for a job as the senior chef on a luxury cruise liner; but was refused on the grounds of his insulin-treated diabetes. An appeal was lodged with full support from his general practitioner and hospital diabetologist, but was unsuccessful. The decision rested on British maritime law, which requires that all offshore personnel, no matter what their jobs, are considered as 'operative seafarers', since in an emergency they may be called upon to undertake direct seafaring tasks (lifeboat drill, ship evacuation, etc). Blanket health rules are therefore applied, and as personnel involved in steering, navigation and towering of ships are banned if they have diabetes that requires insulin treatment, the chef in this case was treated similarly. The British Diabetic Association took up the case, and against other arguments, pointed out that many airlines allow the employment of flight attendants with diabetics on insulin, and such staff clearly have potential emergency evacuation duties. Again, however, the appeal was unsuccessful.

Employment and risk

The basic questions an occupational physician should ask in any employment decision are:

1 Will the condition interfere with the safe conduct of the tasks required in the job?

2 Will the task required have an adverse effect on the medical condition?

In making the decision, an understanding of the concepts of hazard and risk are helpful. The terms are often used interchangeably by employers, but they are not synonymous. Hazard may be defined as the potential to do harm. Risk is the likelihood of that harm occurring, i.e. it can be quantified. A risk-free employment environment is an unattainable Utopia, and it is therefore logical to develop the concept of 'acceptable risk'. This may be based on 'target accident rates' and the maximum 'incapacitation' rate which will not result in any change in those rates. The UK Civil Aviation Authority, for example, sets the target accident rate for flying accidents. It is suggested that a reasonable target is 0.1 per million flying hours (1 in 10^7 hours). It is further suggested that no single cause (hydraulics, powerplant, flightcrew) should contribute more than 10% of the total number of fatal accidents. Therefore, flightdeck crew failure should not be responsible for more than 10% of the total (1 in 10^8 hours). Incapacitation only accounts for 10% of all flightcrew failures and thus this results in a fatal accident rate due to incapacitation of 1 in 10^9 hours.

The average annual cardiovascular mortality in a 65-year-old male is 1%, and this rate was thus suggested as the 'acceptable' level of incapacitation [43]. This approach makes three assumptions:

1 The pilot operates a multicrew aircraft.

2 Only 10% of the flight time (take-off and landing) is critical.

3 If incapacitation occurs during this time the other pilot will take over in 99% of cases.

The rate of 1% per annum is 1 in 10^6 hours and assumption 2 results in a further reduction of 1/10 to 1 in 10^7 hours. The incapacitation described in assumption 3 results in a reduction in risk of 1/100 to 1 in 10^9 hours. The end result is that an incapacitation rate of 1% or less in a multicrew situation will not affect the target accident rate [48].

The acceptable incapacitation rate of 1% per annum has initially been used in cardiovascular disease. This model has now been applied to diabetic aircrew [49,50]. The main incapacitation risk in diabetic people is hypoglycaemia, and the rate even in the best series exceeds 1% per annum, and thus they are not acceptable for professional or private flying. Even mild hypoglycaemia may affect cognitive function, and has obvious safety implications in the flying environment. The hypoglycaemic rate in sulphonylurea-treated diabetic persons does not quite reach the 1% per annum rate and therefore they are not acceptable for professional flying but may fly privately accompanied by a 'safety pilot'. Diet-controlled diabetics, and those on metformin and/or acabose, may fly both professionally and privately. This is subject to a satisfactory annual report from the diabetic specialist physician. The employment decision is thus a joint decision by the relevant specialists in both diabetes and aviation medicine—an important concept. The British Diabetic Association has published a *Diabetes Employment Handbook* [51], which gives full details of the employment implications of diabetes in aviation and a wide range of other occupations. This is a more 'evidence-based' approach than the somewhat 'anecdote-based' policy used to produce blanket bans on diabetic people being employed. Any employment restrictions should be based on a risk assessment applied to the specific working environment, and thus a job description should be examined or a visit to the workplace carried out—as suggested by Ramazzini [52], one of the founding fathers of occupational medicine.

Employment guidelines

The British Diabetic Association has published comprehensive guidelines for both employers and occupational health physicians based upon this logical risk-based approach. The lowest risk is in those individuals controlled on diet alone, and the highest in those treated with insulin. It is therefore logical to only apply restrictions which help to reduce risk. This approach has been used by Waclawski and Gill [47] and is shown below.
1 Diabetic people who are treated with diet alone should be able to undertake any employment without restriction, assuming they have no complications.
2 Those who are treated with oral agents can undertake most occupations again assuming no complications. Most employment regulations do not differentiate between sulphonylureas with their risk of hypoglycaemia and metformin and acarbose which do not carry this risk. Current regulations do not permit recruitment to the armed forces or emergency services. the use of sulpho-nylureas precludes recruitment to air traffic control and professional flying. The criteria relating to mainline train driving have recently been relaxed. This occupation is now permitted to diabetic employees who are on oral agents but are well controlled, are under regular specialist supervision, who self monitor blood glucose and do not suffer from hypoglycaemia. They must be free of significant complications. Vocational drivers

with uncomplicated diabetes, which is well controlled by diet alone or with oral agents, are usually permitted to continue driving large goods and passenger carrying vehicles, assuming they have no significant complications. Merchant seafarers and deep-sea fishermen are allowed to remain at sea subject to regular medical review.

3 Those persons whose diabetes is treated with insulin should not work in situations where sudden onset of hypoglycaemia poses a risk to themselves or others. For this reason they are not permitted to drive LGVs or public service vehicles (PSVs), enter the armed forces and emergency services, fly aeroplanes, drive trains or continue as seafarers or divers. It may be unwise for them to work in other severely hazardous environments. They may also be barred from certain occupations such as railway signal operators because of the possible risks to others.

Specific guidelines for insulin-treated diabetic persons in potentially hazardous occupations have been formulated by the British Diabetic Association Working Party on Driving and Employment [53] and are summarized in Table 15.3. These guidelines facilitated partially a major change in British health regulations for fire fighting, in relation to insulin-treated diabetics (case history 4).

Case history 4

A 30-year-old man was a fully qualified and operational London firefighter, and developed type 1 diabetes. The British Home Office, who are responsible for firefighting services nationally, operated a 'blanket' ban on insulin-requiring diabetic persons working as qualified firefighters, and he was taken off active duties. He undertook teaching and training work in the Fire Service, but ultimate dismissal on health grounds seemed likely. His diabetic control and motivation were exemplary, however, and he made vigorous appeals, supported by his diabetic clinic. Two years after diagnosis he was returned to full duties, and 9 years later remains operational with no diabetes-related problems at work. Following his reinstatement, other similar cases arose around the UK which were dealt with variably by their local Fire Services. The British Diabetic Association took up the case, and after vigorous campaigning the Home Office reversed their blanket ban in 1994 and allowed a policy of individual consideration for such cases, depending on expert evidence from both occupational physicians and diabetologists. There are currently at least 60 fully operational insulin-treated firefighters in the UK, and there have been no recorded episodes of hypoglycaemia in hazardous situations.

Table 15.3 Summary of the specific guidelines, formulated by the British Diabetic Association Working Party on Driving and Employment [53], for insulin-treated diabetic persons in potentially hazardous occupations.

1 People should be physically and mentally fit in accordance with non-diabetic standards
2 Diabetes should be under regular (at least annual) specialist review
3 Diabetes should be under stable control
4 People should self monitor their blood glucose and be well educated and motivated in diabetes self care
5 There should be no disabling hypoglycaemia and normal awareness of individual hypoglycaemic symptoms
6 There should be no advanced retinopathy or nephropathy, nor severe peripheral or autonomic neuropathy
7 There should be no significant coronary heart disease, peripheral vascular disease or cerebrovascular disease
8 Suitability for employment should be re-assessed annually by both an occupational and diabetic specialist physician, and should be based on the criteria outlined above

Employment decisions made on diabetic persons should follow the basic guidelines used in non-diabetic persons, which should be based on the two issues mentioned earlier.

1 Are they fit to carry out their tasks within the acceptable risk parameters?
2 Will the job adversely affect their health?

To make this decision in an equitable manner it is essential to have all the relevant evidence available. The most effective way to do this is for an occupational physician to assess each case on its merits with the appropriate information from the individual's diabetic specialist. Any restrictions applied should be based on evidence that they will decrease the risk of adverse events either in the workplace or to the diabetic person.

Charles Turner Thackrah [54], an eminent occupational physician in the nineteenth century who had an interest in diabetes in his early career, wrote: 'I lay claim to fairness of intention and honesty of detail. Unbiased by prejudice, unshackled by preconceived notions it has been my aim rather to ascertain facts than to support opinions.' This approach to employment decisions on diabetic persons still has a great deal to commend it.

References

1 Winston FK, Rineer C, Menon R, Baker S. The carnage wrought by major economic change: ecological study of traffic related mortality and the reunification of Germany. *BMJ* 1999; 318: 1647–50.
2 Taylor JF, ed. *Medical Aspects of Fitness to Drive. A Guide for Medical*

Practitioners, 5th edn. Indianapolis: Medical Commission on Accident Prevention, 1995.

3 Grattan E, Jeffcoate GO. Medical factors and road accidents. *BMJ* 1968; 1: 75.

4 World Health Organization. Report of inter-regional seminar on epidemiology control and prevention of road traffic accidents. *WHO/Accident Prevention* 1966; 66: 6.

5 Hulbert MF, Vernon SA. Passing the DVLC field regulations following bilateral pan-retinal photocoagulation in diabetes. *Eye* 1992; 6: 456–60.

6 Pearson AR, Tannner V, Keightley SJ, Casswell AG. What effect does photocoagulation have on driving visual fields in diabetes? *Eye*, 1998; 12: 64–8.

7 Cox DJ, Gonder-Frederick LA, Clarke WL. Driving decrements in type 1 diabetes during moderate hypoglycaemia. *Diabetes* 1993; 42: 239–43.

8 Gonder-Frederick LA, Cox DJ, Driesen NR, Ryan C, Clarke WL. Individual differences in neurobehavioural disruption during mild and moderate hypoglycemia in adults with IDDDM. *Diabetes* 1994; 43: 1407–12.

9 Weinger K, Kinsely BT, Levy CJ *et al.* The perception of safe driving ability during hypoglycaemia in patients with type 1 diabetes mellitus. *Am J Med* 1999; 107: 246–53.

10 Gonder-Frederick LA, Cox DJ, Kovatchev BP, Schlundt D, Clarke WL. A psychobehavioural model of risk of severe hypoglycaemia. *Diabetes Care* 1997; 20: 661–9.

11 Kovatchev B, Cox D, Gonder-Frederick L. Stochastic model of self-regulation decision making exemplified by decisions concerning hypoglycaemia. *Health Psychol* 1998; 17: 277–84.

12 MacLeod KM. Diabetes and driving: towards equitable, evidence-based decision-making. *Diabet Med* 1999; 16: 282–90.

13 Songer TJ, Lave LB, La Porte RE. The risks of licensing persons with diabetes to drive trucks. *Risk Analysis* 1993; 13: 319–26.

14 Cox DJ, Gonder-Frederick LA, Schroeder DB, Cryer PE, Clarke WL. Disruptive effects of acute hypoglycaemia on speed of cognitive and motor performance. *Diabetes Care* 1993; 16: 1391–411.

15 Ysander L. Sick and handicapped drivers. *Acta Chir Scand* 1970; 409(1): 1–82.

16 Songer TJ, LaPorte RE, Dorman JS *et al.* Motor vehicle accidents and IDDM. *Diabetes Care* 1988; 11: 701–7.

17 Eadington DW, Frier BM. type 1 diabetes and driving experience: an eight-year cohort study. *Diabet Med* 1989; 6: 137–41.

18 Stevens AB, Roberts M, McKane R, Atkinson AB, Bell PM, Hayes JR. Motor vehicle driving among diabetics taking insulin and non-diabetics. *BMJ* 1989; 299: 591–5.

19 Davis TG, Wehling EH. Oklahoma's medically restricted drivers—a study of selected medical conditions. *Oklahoma State Medical Association Journal* 1973; 66: 323–7.

20 Waller JA. Chronic medical conditions and traffic safety. Review of the California experience. *N Engl J Med* 1965; 273: 1413.

21 Hansotia P, Broste SK. The effect of epilepsy or diabetes mellitus on the risk of automobile accidents [see comments]. *N Engl J Med*, 1991; 324: 22–6.

22 Langens FN, Bakker H, Erkelens DW. Diabetic patients: no danger on the road. *Ned Tijdschr Geneeskd* 1992; 136: 1712–16.

23 Lave LB, Songer TJ, LaPorte RE. Should persons with diabetes be licensed to drive trucks?—Risk management. *Risk Analysis* 1993; 13: 327–34.

24 Mathiesen B, Borch-Jensen K. Diabetes and accident insurance. A 3 year follow up of 7599 insured diabetic individuals. *Diabetes Care* 1997; 20: 1781–4.

25 Mawby M. Time for law to catch up with life [editorial]. *Diabetes Care* 1997; 20: 1640.

26 DiaMond Project Group on Social Issues. Global regulation on diabetes treated with insulin and their operation of commercial motor vehicles. *BMJ* 1993; 307: 250–3.

27 Distiller LA, Kramer BD. Driving and diabetics on insulin. *S African Med J* 1996; 86: 1018–20.

28 Anonymous. *Council Directives on Driving Licences 91/439/EEC OJ-L237 of 24/8/91*. Publications of the European Communities, 1991.

29 Sullivan P. Court human-rights rulings change in CMA advice on diabetic drivers. *Can Med Assoc J* 1991; 144: 1042–3.

30 Ratner RE, Whitehouse FW. Motor vehicles, hypoglycemia and diabetic drivers. *Diabetes Care* 1989; 12: 217–22.

31 Department of Transportation Federal Highway Administration. Quantification of drivers: waivers; diabetes (49 CFR Part 391). *Fed Reg* 1992; 57: 48011–15.

32 MacLeod KM, Hepburn DA, Frier BM. Frequency and morbidity of severe hypoglycaemia in insulin-treated diabetic patients. *Diabet Med* 1993; 10: 238–45.

33 Gold AE, Frier BM, MacLeod KM. A structural equation model for predictors of severe hypoglycaemia in patients with insulin-dependent diabetes mellitus. *Diabet Med* 1997; 14: 309–15.

34 Dionne G, Desjardins D, Laberge-Nadeau C, Maag U. Medical conditions, risk exposure, and truck drivers' accidents: an analysis with count data regression models. *Acid Analysis Prev* 1995; 27: 295–305.

35 Holleman F, Schmitt H, Rottiers R *et al.* Reduced frequency of severe hypogly- caemia and coma in well-controlled IDDM patients treated with insulin lispro. *Diabetes Care* 1997; 20: 1827–32.

36 Veneman TF. Diabetes mellitus and traffic incidents. *Neth J Med* 1996; 48: 24–8.

37 Cranston I, Lomas J, Maran A *et al.* Restoration of hypoglycaemia awareness in patients with long-duration insulin- dependent diabetes and a history of hypoglycaemia without warning. *Lancet* 1994; 344: 283–7.

38 The Diabetes Control, Complications Trial Research Group. The effect of intensive treatment of diabetes on the development and progression of long- term complications in insulin dependent diabetes mellitus. *N Engl J Med* 1993; 329: 977–86.

39 UK Prospective Diabetes Study Group. Intensive blood-glucose control with sulphonylureas or insulin compared with conventional treatment in patients with type 2 diabetes (UKPDS 33). *Lancet* 1998; 352: 837–53.

40 Baker J, Scragg R, Metcalf P, Dryson E. Diabetes and employment: is there discrimination in the workplace? *Diabet Med* 1993; 10: 362–5.

41 Baker J, Scragg R, Metcalf P, Dryson E. Diabetes mellitus and employment: survey of a New Zealand workforce. *Diabet Med* 1995; 10: 359–63.

42 Robinson N, Bush L, Protopapa L, Yateman N. Employers attitudes to diabetes. *Diabet Med* 1989; 6: 692–7.

43 Songer T, LaPorte R, Dorman T *et al.* Employment spectrum of IDDM. *Diabetes Care* 1989; 12: 615–22.

44 Matsushima M, Tajima N, Agata T *et al.* Social and economic impact of youth onset diabetes in Japan. *Diabetes Care* 1993; 16: 824–7.

45 Fritis R, Nanjundappa G. Diabetes, depression and employment status. *Soc Sci Med* 1986; 23: 471–5.

46 Waclawski ER. Employment and diabetes: a survey of the prevalence of diabetic workers known by occupational physicians and the restrictions placed on diabetic workers in employment. *Diabet Med* 1989; 6: 16–19.

47 Waclawksi ER, Gill GV. Diabetes mellitus and other endocrine disorders. In: Cox RAF, Edwards FC, Palmer K, eds. *Fitness for Work: The Medical Aspects*, 3rd edn. Oxford: Oxford University Press, 2000: 322–34.

48 Tunstall-Pedoe H. Acceptable cardiovascular risk in aircrew. *Eur Heart J* 1988; 9 (Suppl G): 9–11.

49 Johnston RV. *An assessment of the value of a risk orientated approach to the problem of diabetes mellitus in professional aircrew check*. MFOM Thesis, 1997.

50 Johnston RV. Metabolic and endocrine disorders. In: Ernsting J Nicholson AN Rainford DJ, eds. *Aviation Medicine*. Oxford: Butterworth-Heinemann, 1999: 303–11.

51 British Diabetic Association. *Diabetes Employment Handbook*. London: BDA, 1997.

52 Ramazzini B (trans Wright WC). *De Morbis Artificium Diatriba*. Chicago: University of Chicago Press, 1940.

53 British Diabetic Association. *Diabetes and Potentially Hazardous Occupations*. London: BDA, 1996.

54 Thackrah CT. *The Effect of Arts, Trades and Professions on Health and Longevity*. Philadelphia, 1831.

16: How should erectile dysfunction in diabetes be managed?

David E. Price

Introduction

Few areas in the management of diabetes have changed so dramatically in recent years as the treatment of erectile dysfunction. We can now offer simple and effective therapies that can transform lives. Change, has, however, been a long time in arriving. For decades, impotence was the neglected complication of diabetes—largely ignored by diabetes healthcare professionals even though it was widely recognized to affect over 35% of diabetic men [1]. As recently as 1990, the problem was not even mentioned in the British Diabetic Association's guidelines for the care a diabetic patient should expect [2].

Previously, erectile dysfunction was generally assumed to be due to psychogenic causes, even in diabetes. However, attitudes to erectile dysfunction in diabetes changed when simple and effective physical treatments such as intracavernosal injection therapy and vacuum devices became available in the 1980s. At the same time, medical practitioners realized that erectile dysfunction often had a physical contribution.

Prevalence of erectile dysfunction

The Massachusetts Male Aging Study is, perhaps, the best population-based survey of the frequency of erectile dysfunction. The prevalence of complete erectile failure in the general community was reported to be 5% in men aged 40 years, 9.6% in men aged 40–70 years and 15% in those over 70 years [3,4].

The prevalence of significant erectile failure among diabetic men is considerably higher, reported variously as 23% [1] and 59% [2] of all diabetic men over the age of 18 years. In a survey of 428 diabetic men from 10 general practices, Hackett reported a prevalence rate of 55%, of whom 39% suffered from the problem all of the time [5]. This was significantly higher than in a non-diabetic control group, among whom erectile difficulties were intermittent in 26% and permanent in 5%. As in the general population, the prevalence of impotence in diabetic men increases significantly with age. McCulloch *et al.* reported a prevalence of 6% in diabetic men aged 20–24 years, which rose to 52% in men aged 55–59 years [6].

Quality of life issues

Erectile dysfunction can significantly impact on quality of life. A survey by the Impotence Association found symptoms of lowered self esteem and depression in 62% of men; 40% expressed concern with either new or established relationships and 21% blamed it for the break up of a relationship [7]. In Hackett's series, 45% of diabetic men claimed to think about their erectile failure all or most of the time, while 23% felt that it severely affected their overall quality of life and 10% that it severely affected their relationship with their partner [5]. Cummings also found that erectile dysfunction can adversely affect a relationship, reporting that 38% of diabetic men with erectile failure felt their relationship had suffered 'moderately' and 19% 'severely' [8].

Pathophysiology of erectile dysfunction in diabetes

Physiology of normal penile erection

Penile erection is predominantly a vascular event under the control of the autonomic nervous system. Sexual stimulation results first in an increase in parasympathetic activity, leading to relaxation of the smooth muscle of the cavernous and helicine arteries and of the corpus cavernosum [9,10]. The relaxation of the corpus cavernosum leads to compression of the outflow venules against the inflexible tunica albuginea, reducing venous outflow (Fig. 16.1). The single phenomenon of smooth muscle relaxation thus produces both increased arterial inflow and reduced venous outflow from the erectile tissue, leading to tumescence [11].

The role of nitric oxide

For many years, the erectile tissue of the penis was described as being supplied by non-adrenergic, non-cholinergic nerve fibres because the neurotransmitter responsible was unknown. Several neurotransmitters and peptides,

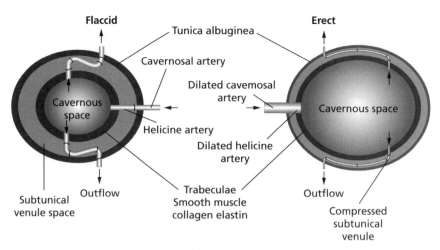

Fig. 16.1 Diagrammatic representation of the corpus cavernosum. During tumescence dilatation of the cavernosal and helicine arteries produces expansion of the cavernous space and compression of the outflow venules against the rigid tunica albuginea.

such as vasoactive intestinal polypeptide (VIP), acetylcholine and the pro-staglandins, may have a role in the physiology of erection, but it is now clear that nitric oxide (NO) produced by nitric oxide synthase (NOS) in the vascular endothelium and also released from the parasympathetic nerve ter-minals, is the central agent leading to the relaxation of smooth muscle in the erectile tissue (Fig. 16.2). NO from both neuronal and endothelial sources stimulates guanylate cyclase, leading to increased intracellular levels of cyclic GMP (cGMP). cGMP induces smooth muscle relaxation, probably by open-ing up calcium channels [12,13]; it is broken down by phosphodiesterase V, which is discussed below in the context of sildenafil.

The aetiology of erectile dysfunction in diabetes mellitus

Erectile dysfunction in diabetes has many potential causes, including specific diabetic complications of neuropathy and vascular disease, as well as condi-tions commonly associated with diabetes such as hypertension, various medications or psychogenic factors. Finally, it can be due to conditions un-related to diabetes, such as hypogonadism or spinal cord injury. In most diabetic men, erectile dysfunction is due predominantly to neuropathy or vascular disease.

The foundation for our present understanding of the pathophysiology of impotence in diabetes was the crucial study of Saenz de Tejada and colleagues

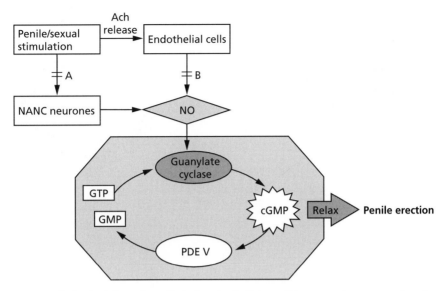

Fig. 16.2 Pathophysiology of erectile dysfunction in diabetes. Diagrammatic representation of pathways leading to relaxation of a corpus cavernosal smooth muscle cell. In diabetes, there are defects in nitric oxide smooth muscle relaxation due to neuropathy of the NANC fibres (A) and endothelial dysfunction (B). NANC, non-adrenergic, non-cholinergic neurones; NO, nitric oxide; PDE V, phosphodiesterase V, ACh, acetylcholine.

in 1989 [14]. Samples of corpus cavernosal smooth muscle taken from 21 diabetic and 42 non-diabetic men undergoing penile implant operations were induced to contract by noradrenaline (norepinephrine). Relaxation was then induced with either electrical-field stimulation, acetylcholine (which stimulates endothelial NO release), nitroprusside (an NO donor), or papaverine (which causes direct smooth muscle relaxation). The results suggested that smooth muscle relaxation and therefore tumescence is produced as a result of direct NO release from nerve terminals and from NO released from endothelial cells mediated by acetylcholine. In the diabetic subjects, both pathways were impaired compared with non-diabetics, implicating both autonomic neuropathy and endothelial dysfunction as contributors to impotence in diabetic men (Fig. 16.2). There is some suggestion that autonomic neuropathy may be the most important aetiological factor in type 1 diabetes whereas vascular dysfunction may predominate in type 2 diabetics [15].

Other factors contributing to erectile dysfunction in diabetes

Hypertension is a risk factor for erectile dysfunction [3] although the underlying risk is not known. The UK Prospective Diabetes Study (UKPDS) group

Antihypertensives	
Thiazide diuretics	
Beta-blockers	
Central sympatholytics (methyldopa, clonidine)	
Calcium channel blockers	} Low risk
ACE inhibitors	

Antidepressants
Tricyclics
Monoamine oxidase inhibitors
NB Selective serotonin re-uptake inhibitors can cause
ejaculatory problems

Major tranquillizers
Phenothiazines
Haloperidol

Hormones
Luteinizing hormone–releasing hormone (goserelin,
buserelin)
Oestrogens (stilboestrol)
Antiandrogens (cyproterone)

Miscellaneous
5α-reductase inhibitors (finasteride)
Statins (simvastatin, atorvastatin, pravastatin)
Cimetidine
Digoxin
Metoclopramide

Drugs of abuse
Alcohol
Tobacco
Marijuana
Amphetamines
Anabolic steroids
Barbiturates
Opiates

Table 16.1 Medications and drugs associated with sexual dysfunction.

showed that over 30% of diabetic men have hypertension at diagnosis [16]. Unfortunately, hypertension treatment itself is often implicated in causing erectile dysfunction, most notably beta-blockers and thiazide diuretics [17]. The least hazardous antihypertensives in this regard are calcium-channel blockers, angiotensin converting enzyme (ACE) inhibitors and, in particular, the alpha-blockers [18].

Table 16.2 Organic causes of erectile dysfunction.

Vascular	Cardiovascular disease
	Hypertension
	Arterio-occlusive disease
	Venous leakage
	Pelvic trauma
Neurological	Peripheral neuropathy
	Autonomic neuropathy
	Spinal and pelvic trauma
	Multiple sclerosis
Edocrinological	Hypogonadism
	Cushing's disease
	Hypopituitarism
	Hyperprolactinaemia
	Thyroid dysfunction
Abnormal anatomy	Penile curvature
	Hypospadias
	Micropenis
	Peyronie's disease
	Penile fibrosis
	Phimosis
Iatrogenic	Pelvic surgery
	Aorto-iliac surgery
	Renal transplantation
	Prostatectomy
	Drugs
Miscellaneous	Smoking
	Renal disease
	Hepatic disease

Many other drugs are associated with erectile dysfunction, and the commonest are listed in Table 16.1. Other conditions that may cause impotence are listed in Table 16.2.

Assessment and investigation of erectile dysfunction in diabetes

Clinical assessment

Many impotent men and their partners are anxious at the initial consultation and find it difficult to discuss the problem. A relaxed, matter-of-fact approach usually helps and once the subject has been broached, couples do not usually have a problem answering specific questions. A description of the nature of the erectile dysfunction should be obtained, not least to ensure the patient is complaining of impotence and not another related problem such as premature ejaculation. Erectile dysfunction in diabetic men is usually gradual in onset and progressive in nature. Often the earliest feature is the inability to sustain an erection long enough for satisfactory intercourse; this may be intermittent initially. Loss of erectile function of sudden onset is often taken to indicate a psychogenic cause, but there is little evidence to support this. Similarly, preservation of spontaneous and early morning erections does not necessarily indicate a psychogenic cause.

Loss of libido is consistent with hypogonadism but is not a reliable symptom. Many men will understate their sex drive for a variety of reasons, including guilt. Others suppress their libido as a defence mechanism to prevent the disappointment of failure. A history obtained from the partner without the patient present often reveals interesting and useful insight into the problem.

The physical examination of the patient's overall physical condition may provide clues about the aetiology of erectile dysfunction and also into the choice of treatment. Poor manual dexterity or a large protuberant abdomen may preclude the use of vacuum devices or self-injection therapy. The condition of the external genitalia should be assessed for the presence of a phimosis or Peyronie's disease. Examination should include an estimation of testicular volume and assessment of other features to suggest hypogonadism.

Investigation of erectile dysfunction in diabetes

In practical terms, hypogonadism is the only treatable cause of erectile dysfunction that needs to be considered when investigating an impotent diabetic man. There is evidence against a specific association between diabetes and hypogonadism; gonadal function should therefore only be assessed in a diabetic man with erectile dysfunction if coincidental hypogonadism is suspected. Serum testosterone and prolactin should be measured if there is loss of libido or any features of hypogonadism, but the usefulness of routine screening for these hormones in all diabetic men with erectile dysfunction remains controversial. Buvat and Lemaire reported that the serum testosterone was subnormal in 107 out of 1022 men with erectile dysfunction, but that 40% were normal on repeating the test; two pituitary tumours and one prolactinoma were discovered as a result [19]. They concluded that in the investigation of erectile dysfunction, serum testosterone should be measured routinely in all men over 50 years and in those under 50 who had reduced libido or abnormal physical examination.

General advice

Most diabetic men and their partners seeking treatment for impotence are middle aged and have been married for many years. Like all patients, they should be treated with respect and dignity. The couple should be told their problem is largely due to diabetes and that they should not blame themselves.

Some couples will seek treatment for erectile dysfunction in an attempt to save a failing relationship. Restoring a man's potency in this situation is rarely successful and is more likely to make things worse as it introduces a new tension into the relationship; the assistance of a suitably qualified psychosexual counsellor should be considered. Referral to a counsellor should also be considered if there is any suggestion of depression, severe anxiety, loss of attraction between partners, fear of intimacy or marked performance anxiety. However, psychosexual counsellors are not a prerequisite to offering an impotence service: several published series have suggested that diabetologists can offer treatment for erectile dysfunction with good results without the assistance of counsellors [20–24].

Spontaneous return of erectile function in diabetes occurs only rarely [25]. It is therefore probably wise to advise that natural erections are unlikely to return, and that treatment will be long term.

Health advice

Erectile dysfunction is an independent risk factor for cardiovascular disease. Therefore, when a man presents with erectile dysfunction his physician should consider taking the opportunity to assess his general health and offer lifestyle advice. Clearly if there are other medical problems they must be addressed. Improving poor metabolic control may help general well-being and may increase the likelihood of successful treatment. However, poor control should not be used as a reason to refuse treatment. There is an association between smoking and erectile dysfunction; therefore all patients who smoke should be advised to stop for reasons of general health, although there is no good evidence that stopping smoking will improve erectile function in an impotent diabetic man. Similarly, it is not clear whether reducing alcohol intake is beneficial.

If the patient is taking a medication known to cause erectile dysfunction, it may be tempting to change this in the hope of improving sexual function. However, this is usually a fruitless activity in diabetic men and is not advisable unless there is a convincing temporal relationship between starting treatment and the onset of erectile dysfunction.

Treatment options

Several options are now available for the treatment of erectile dysfunction. The choice of treatment will depend on local circumstances, personal experience and, most importantly, the patient's own preference.

Vacuum therapy

Vacuum devices became available in the 1970s and, apart from self-injection therapy, were the only effective treatment for erectile dysfunction for several years. Many early trials of vacuum devices were done by enthusiastic investigators on selected patients; perhaps not surprisingly, the reported results were excellent and rather better than more recent experience would suggest [26]. Several subsequent series of vacuum therapy in men with impotence of mixed aetiology have reported success rates of 50–90% [27–32]. None of these trials were controlled; nonetheless, the results left little doubt that vacuum devices are an effective treatment for impotence due to various causes.

Trials of vacuum therapy in diabetic men have shown similarly good results [21–24], even in the presence of extensive vascular disease or severe autonomic neuropathy [22].

Complications and contraindications

Vacuum therapy would appear to be remarkably safe; very few serious adverse events have been reported. Single cases have been reported case of skin necrosis [33] and penile gangrene [34]. Subcutaneous bruising is relatively common but is usually self limiting; most manufacturers advise that bleeding diatheses or anticoagulation therapy are contraindications to the use of vacuum therapy.

Most other side-effects are minor. Discomfort or pain due to the constriction band or during pumping is relatively common and can be the reason for discontinuing treatment. Failure to ejaculate can occur in up to one-third of men but anorgasmia is rare [24–27]. Female partners often report that the penis feels cold; intriguingly, one small study claimed this to be a bonus, not a problem! [35].

Intracavernosal injection therapy

The technique of intracavernosal self injection was first described by the French urologist Virag in 1982 [36]. He used papaverine, a non-selective phosphodiesterase inhibitor that acts as a smooth muscle relaxant and vasodilator. Papaverine is not licensed for this indication and has largely been superseded by alprostadil (prostaglandin E), which has been licensed for the treatment of erectile dysfunction since 1996. The principle of self-injection therapy is straightforward. Before intercourse, the drug is drawn up into a syringe and injected into the corpus cavernosum. The penis is massaged, and tumescence should occur within a few minutes. Initial studies of intra-cavernosal injection therapy were small and uncontrolled, but it was rapidly adopted across the world and soon became the treatment of choice amongst most diabetologists in the UK. In a large controlled trial in 1996, Linet showed alprostadil to be a highly effective means of treating erectile dysfunction [37]. In one of the few studies done exclusively in impotent diabetic men, Alexander reported that it was perfectly feasible for a physician to offer self-injection treatment for erectile dysfunction within a routine diabetic clinic [20].

This remains a popular treatment, although most studies show a disappointingly high long-term discontinuation rate [38–41], which mostly appears to stem from loss of interest [40,41].

Complications

Self-injection therapy using papaverine was soon found to carry a low but definite risk of priapism (a sustained unwanted erection) [42–44]. A meta-analysis of 10 published studies suggested the median probability of priapism (per person) was about 9% with papaverine and 3% with alprostadil [45].

Younger men with psychogenic or neurogenic impotence with better baseline erectile function appear to be at greater risk of developing priapism, while those with vasculogenic impotence have the least risk [43]. Although rare, this is clearly an important complication. Any man contemplating self-injection treatment must be warned of the risk and given specific instructions as to what to do should it occur.

Prompt treatment of priapism is important because it is painful and if untreated may lead to damage to the erectile tissue which makes successful treatment of the ED much more difficult. If the erection persists for more than 2 hours, then several manoeuvres can be undertaken that may terminate the erection, including vigorous leg exercises such as pedalling an exercise bicycle or running up and down stairs [46]. If these manoeuvres fail and the erection persists for more than 6 hours, urgent medical attention should be sought, as aspiration of blood from the corpora cavernosa may be required. This is made considerably easier if the patient already has written instructions to take to the nearest hospital emergency department.

Local adverse reactions, such as penile pain, are relatively common with self-injection therapy. Prolonged papaverine use may lead to fibrosis in the penis, but this has been reported only rarely with alprostadil [45].

Other injectable agents

Moxisylyte

Moxisylyte is an α_2-adrenoceptor blocker given by intercavernosal injection, which acts selectively to relax the smooth muscle of the corpus cavernosum. In a group of men with impotence of mixed aetiology, it appeared slightly less effective than alprostadil but was rather better tolerated [47]. It causes fewer local problems but can provoke systemic effects such as dizziness. An important advantage of moxisylyte is that it comes in a simple and easy to use autoinjector. However, in 1998 moxisylyte was withdrawn from the market in most countries due to poor sales, although it is still available in France.

Vasoactive intestinal polypeptide

Vasoactive intestinal polypeptide (VIP) is a vasodilator which has a role in the development of erection. When injected alone into the corpus cavernosum it has only modest effects and produces a limp erection; however, it is more impressive when given in combination with phentolamine [48]. In a study of 52 men with erectile dysfunction of mixed aetiology this combination produced an erection sufficient for intercourse in all cases, and 80% of the men were still using it 6 months later [49]. In a more recent study, injection of VIP with phentolamine succeeded in 67% of men who had failed with other vasoactive agents [50]. At the time of writing, however, there have been no studies published on this treatment in diabetic men and it is not yet licensed for the treatment of erectile dysfunction.

Transurethral alprostadil

The principle of transurethral therapy is quite simple. A slender applicator is inserted into the urethra to deposit a pellet containing alprostadil in polyethylene glycol (PEG). This gradually dissolves allowing the prostaglandin to diffuse into the corpus cavernosum. This preparation has been marketed with the acronym MUSE (Medicated Urethral System for Erection). The applicator is neat and simple to use and most men find it preferable to an intracavernosal injection. In a placebo-controlled study of 1511 men with erectile dysfunction of mixed aetiology, 65% were able to have intercourse after using MUSE [51]; the results in the subset of 240 diabetic men were similar [52]. The most common side-effect was penile pain, reported in 10.8% of applications. Hypotension occurred in 3.3% of men receiving alprostadil. Priapism and penile fibrosis were not described.

Transurethral alprostadil is best administered after emptying the bladder to improve lubrication. After administration the penis should be massaged to enhance adsorption of the drug: erection is maximal after approximately 30 minutes, during which time the man is advised to remain standing. No comparative studies have been done, but transurethral alprostadil appears to produce comparable penile rigidity to self-injection treatment: long-term usage has also been disappointing [53].

Oral agents

Several drugs have been tried as oral treatments for erectile dysfunction, including yohimbine, phentolamine, apomorphine and trazodone. Data on all of these are limited and none have stood the test of time. Androgens are indicated for the treatment of erectile dysfunction only in men with confirmed hypogonadism.

Phosphodiesterase V inhibitors

In the early 1990s a potential new cardiovascular drug, UK 92,480, was undergoing phase I and II testing by Pfizer UK. Investigators were surprised that many of the trial subjects refused to return their unused tablets. It turned out that many of the men who took the new agent found that their previous erectile dysfunction had resolved. The drug, later named sildenafil (Viagra), was to transform the management of erectile dysfunction, although history does not record how effective it was in its original indication.

Mechanism of action. Sildenafil is a selective inhibitor of phosphodiesterase type V (PDE V), an enzyme found in smooth muscle, platelets and the corpus cavernosum. The mechanism of action is shown in Fig. 16.2. Under conditions of sexual stimulation, intracellular NO concentrations increase and act via the second messenger cGMP to produce smooth muscle relaxation (see above). This is broken down in turn by PDE V. As sildenafil inhibits the actions of PDE V, it has the potential to enhance erections under conditions of sexual stimulation; in theory, sildenafil should only enhance an erection if the man is sexually aroused. Conversely, as the process of erection requires the presence of NO, sildenafil might not be expected to work in the absence of NO tone.

Evidence to support this mode of action of sildenafil comes from work done on human corpus cavernosal tissue *in vitro*. Sildenafil produced a dose-dependent increase in smooth muscle relaxation under conditions of electrical field stimulation; by contrast, electrical stimulation alone produced only modest relaxation [54].

Clinical trial data. In the first study of sildenafil, there was an increase in penile rigidity during visual sexual stimulation in 12 men with erectile dysfunction of unidentified cause [55]. A second similar study in diabetic men showed that sildenafil significantly improved both penile rigidity and sexual function [56]. The pivotal study was published in 1998. Five hundred and thirty-two men with erectile dysfunction of mixed aetiology were studied. In the group given sildenafil, 69% of all attempts at intercourse were successful compared with 22% in those given placebo [57]. Other studies in men with erectile dysfunction of mixed aetiology have shown similar results, with success rates of 65–77% [58,59]. Studies of sildenafil in other patient groups have reported success rates varying from 70% in men with hypertension [60], 76% in spinal cord injury [61], 63% in spina bifida [62] to 40% following radical prostatectomy [63].

In diabetic men the success rates for sildenafil have been reported to be between 56% and 59% [56,64]. Sildenafil has not been available long enough for any study of long-term usage, but in the experience of the author there was no loss of efficacy in seven diabetic men using sildenafil for 6 years.

Adverse effects. The adverse events from a subanalysis of 10 trials of sildenafil in diabetic men are given in Table 16.3 [60]. Headache and flushing might be expected as sildenafil is a vasodilator. The dyspepsia associated with sildenafil is usually mild and may be due to relaxation of the cardiac sphincter of the stomach. Abnormal vision is experienced by about 6% of men taking sildenafil; this may be because the drug also has some activity against phosphodiesterase VI which is a retinal enzyme. There have been no reports of sildenafil causing any permanent effects on vision.

Table 16.3 Adverse effects of sildenafil.

Adverse effect	Placebo ($n = 274$)	Sildenafil ($n = 418$)
Headache	3%	13%
Dyspepsia	0	11%
Flushing	1%	7%
Respiratory tract infection	4%	6%
Abnormal vision	0.4%	6%

Sildenafil and cardiovascular disease. Within weeks of the launch of sildenafil many adverse cardiovascular events—including myocardial infarction and death—were reported following use of the drug. These received wide media coverage, causing considerable concern amongst patients and some doctors, obliging the Food and Drug Administration (FDA) in the USA to open an Internet web site to inform the public about sildenafil. Adverse events associated with the use of sildenafil have been closely monitored by the regulatory authorities in the USA and Europe, and all the available evidence suggests that sildenafil *per se* is not associated with an increased risk of cardiovascular events [65], although there is a serious and potentially fatal interaction with nitrates and other drugs that enhance NO production or action (see below).

Sexual activity is usually no more strenuous than many ordinary activities such as playing golf or walking a mile in 20 minutes, although the estimated relative risk of myocardial infarction increases 2.5-fold in the 2 hours after intercourse in a patient without a cardiovascular history and 3-fold in a patient with a previous myocardial infarction [66]. Restoration of sexual activity may be associated with increased risk, and cardiovascular status should be assessed in all patients seeking treatment for erectile dysfunction. It has been suggested that men requiring treatment for erectile dysfunction should be classified according to their cardiovascular risk, and that those with the highest risk should be referred for a specialist cardiac evaluation; others could effectively be treated for erectile dysfunction in primary care [65].

Sildenafil and nitrates. Sildenafil is absolutely contraindicated in the presence of any form of nitrate therapy. Both agents act via the NO–cGMP pathway, and the combination can produce profound hypotension. Other drugs such as nicorandil and nebivolol that also act via NO should probably not be used concomitantly with sildenafil. Patients taking nitrate therapy who seek treatment for erectile dysfunction can be offered an alternative such as injection therapy or a vacuum device; alternatively, the nitrates could be stopped or replaced (a decision best taken in consultation with a cardiologist). It has been suggested that a nitrate can be safely given 24 hours after a sildenafil dose [67] and that a long-acting nitrate should be stopped 1 week before using sildenafil [65].

How to use sildenafil. Sildenafil should be taken orally about 1 hour before sexual activity (30 minutes is adequate if the stomach is empty). There follows a window of opportunity of about 4 hours for sexual activity. The recommended starting dose is 50 mg, although most diabetic men require 100 mg. Patients should be reminded that the drug only works in conjunction with sexual stimulation.

Given the choice of the available treatments, almost all men will choose an oral agent unless there is a contraindication. There is evidence that sildenafil is less likely to work in men with longstanding and severe erectile dysfunction, but no single factor precludes a successful outcome [68].

Social and political aspects. The advent of sildenafil was greeted with a reaction from the media that was unparalleled for most drug or medical advances. Much of the coverage focused on the potential health service cost of treating erectile dysfunction with this new agent. Few health services pay for erectile dysfunction treatment; indeed only Sweden offers full reimbursement. In the UK, the advent of sildenafil provoked a change in the law that for the first time prevented doctors from prescribing a licensed drug on the National Health Service. At present, National Health Service support is only available when erectile dysfunction is due to certain conditions (listed in Table 16.4): men with impotence from another cause have to pay for a private prescription.

Diabetes
Multiple sclerosis
Spinal cord injury
Prostate cancer
Treatment for renal failure
Radical pelvic surgery
Single-gene neurological disease
Prostactectomy
Poliomyelitis
Spina bifida
Parkinson's disease
Severe pelvic injury

Table 16.4 Conditions for which treatment for erectile dysfunction can be prescribed on the UK National Health Service.

The practical management of erectile dysfunction in a diabetic clinic

The recent advances in the management of erectile dysfunction have considerably eased the task of diabetologists attempting to offer an impotence treatment service for their patients. Until the 1980s few diabetes services offered treatment for erectile dysfunction: now few do not. It was previously common practice to establish a separate erectile dysfunction clinic, because of the time needed to start treatment with vacuum devices or self-injection therapy; with newer treatments such as sildenafil, there is now no reason why any interested diabetologist or general practitioner should not manage erectile dysfunction in a routine clinic.

Organizing an impotence clinic

An impotence service can be set up in various ways. The approach to history, examination and investigation are discussed above, which will depend on local circumstances. An outline plan can include the following measures.

Visit 1

- See the patient, with his partner if possible.
- History, examination and appropriate investigations.
- Ensure that the couple have a satisfactory relationship.
- Explanation of the problem; provide leaflet and videos outlining available treatments.
- Ask the couple to consider treatment options.

Visit 2 (2–4 weeks later)

- Couple decide which treatment.
- Provide information sheet on sildenafil and prescription, *or*
- Loan vacuum device with explanatory video, *or*
- Arrange separate appointment for couple to be shown self-injection treatment or transurethral alprostadil.

Visit 3 (2–3 months later)

- Assess outcome.
- Offer alternative if necessary.

Little equipment is needed in the management of erectile dysfunction. It is useful, however, to have a ready supply of educational material available in the clinic.

The following are particularly helpful:

• A pamphlet giving general information on erectile dysfunction in diabetes (e.g. 'Impotence and diabetes' published by the British Diabetic Association [now Diabetes UK]).

• Leaflets and videos about all the treatment modalities (available from the manufacturers and mostly free).

• A demonstration vacuum device, self-injection kit and transurethral applicator.

• If self-injection treatment is to be offered, there should be written instructions on how to increase the dose and on what to do in the event of priapism.

Screening for erectile dysfunction

Many impotent diabetic men would like help for their problem but are reluctant to seek it [1]. There is a certain logic, therefore, in suggesting that we should routinely ask all men attending a diabetic clinic about sexual function. Unfortunately, resources are limited and many diabetologists struggle to manage those impotent men who spontaneously ask for help. Furthermore, there is evidence that men whose impotence is picked up on screening respond less well to treatment [20]. Any decision to routinely ask about erectile dysfunction in the diabetic clinic should be made after considering the local resources available for treatment.

Summary

The problem of impotence has been long neglected by diabetologists but there is now widespread recognition that it is a common and distressing complication of diabetes. All diabetes care services should offer treatment for erectile dysfunction, especially as recently introduced treatments are effective and easy to use.

References

1 Price D, O'Malley BP, James MA, Roshan M, Hearnshaw JR. Why are impotent diabetic men not being treated? *Pract Diabetes* 1991; 8: 10–11.

2 British Diabetic Association. What diabetic care to expect. *Diabet Med* 1990; 7: 554.

3 Feldman HA, Goldstein I, Hatzichristou DG, Krane RJ, McKinlay JB. Impotence

and its medical and psychosocial correlates: results of the Massachusetts Male Aging Study. *J Urol* 1994; 151: 54–61.

4 Eardley I, Gale E, Kirby RS, Carson CC, Webster GD, eds. Diabetic impotence. In: *Impotence Diagnosis and Management of Erectile Dysfunction*. Oxford: Butterworth Heinmann, 1991.

5 Hackett GI. Impotence—the most neglected complication of diabetes. *Diabetic Res* 1995; 28: 75–83.

6 McCulloch DK, Campbell IW, Wu FC, Prescott RJ, Clarke BF. The prevalence of diabetic impotence. *Diabetologia* 1980; 18: 279–83.

7 Craig A. *Impotence Association Survey. One in Ten*. London: Impotence Association, 1997.

8 Cummings MH, Meeking D, Warburton F, Alexander W. The diabetic male's perception of erectile dysfunction. *Pract Diabetes* 1997; 14: 100–2.

9 Newman HF, Northup JD. Mechanism of human penile erection: an overview. *Urology* 1981; 17: 399–408.

10 Aboseif SR, Lue TF. Hemodynamics of penile erection. *Urol Clin North Am* 1988; 15: 1–7.

11 Krane RJ, Goldstein I, Saenz dTI. Impotence. *N Engl J Med* 1989; 321: 1648–59.

12 Bush PA, Aronson WJ, Buga GM, Rajfer J, Ignarro LJ. Nitric oxide is a potent relaxant of human and rabbit corpus cavernosum. *J Urol* 1992; 147: 1650–5.

13 Rajfer J, Aronson WJ, Bush PA, Dorey FJ, Ignarro LJ. Nitric oxide as a mediator of relaxation of the corpus cavernosum in response to nonadrenergic, non-cholinergic neurotransmission. *N Engl J Med* 1992; 326: 90–4.

14 Saenz de Tejada, Goldstein I, Azadzoi K, Krane RJ, Cohen RA. Impaired neurogenic and endothelium-mediated relaxation of penile smooth muscle from diabetic men with impotence. *N Engl J Med* 1989; 320: 1025–30.

15 Yamaguchi Y, Kumamoto Y. [Etiological analysis of male diabetic erectile dysfunction with particular emphasis on findings of vascular and neurological examinations.] *Nippon Hinyokika Gakkai Zasshi* 1994; 85: 1474–83.

16 UK Prospective Diabetes Study Group. Tight blood pressure control and risk of macrovascular and microvascular complications in type 2 diabetes. UKPDS 38. *BMJ* 1998; 317: 703–13.

17 Hogan MJ, Wallin JD, Baer RM. Antihypertensive therapy and male sexual dysfunction. *Psychosomatics* 1980; 234: 236–7.

18 Kochar MS, Zeller JR, Itskovitz HD. Prazosin in hypertension with and without methyldopa. *Clin Pharmacol Ther* 1979; 25 (2): 143–8.

19 Buvat J, Lemaire A. Endocrine screening in 1022 men with erectile dysfunction: clinical significance and cost–effective strategy. *J Urol* 1997; 58: 1764–7.

20 Alexander WD. The diabetes physician and an assessment and treatment programme for male erectile impotence. *Diabet Med* 1990; 7: 540–3.

21 Bodansky HJ. Treatment of male erectile dysfunction using the active vacuum assist device. *Diabet Med* 1994; 11: 410–12.

22 Price DE, Cooksey G, Jehu D, Bentley S, Hearnshaw JR, Osborn DE. The management of impotence in diabetic men by vacuum tumescence therapy. *Diabet Med* 1991; 8: 964–7.

23 Ryder RE, Close CF, Moriarty KT, Moore KT, Hardisty CA. Impotence in diabetes: aetiology, implications for treatment and preferred vacuum device. *Diabet Med* 1992; 9: 893–8.

24 Wiles PG. Successful non-invasive management of erectile impotence in diabetic men. *BMJ [Clin Res Educ]* 1988; 296: 161–2.

25 McCulloch DK, Young RJ, Prescott RJ, Campbell IW, Clarke BF. The natural history of impotence in diabetic men. *Diabetologia* 1984; 26: 437–40.

26 Nadig PW, Ware JC, Blumoff R. Noninvasive device to produce and maintain an erection-like state. *Urology* 1986; 27: 126–31.

27 Baltaci S, Aydos K, Kosar A, Anafarta K. Treating erectile dysfunction with a vacuum tumescence device: a retrospective analysis of acceptance and satisfaction. *Br J Urol* 1995; 76: 757–60.

28 Vrijhof HJ, Delaere KP. Vacuum constriction devices in erectile dysfunction: acceptance and effectiveness in patients with impotence of organic or mixed aetiology. *Br J Urol* 1994; 74: 102–5.

29 Sidi AA, Lewis JH. Clinical trial of a simplified vacuum erection device for impotence treatment. *Urology* 1992; 39: 526–8.

30 Korenman SG, Viosca SP, Kaiser FE, Mooradian AD, Morley JE. Use of a vacuum tumescence device in the management of impotence. *J Am Geriatr Soc* 1990; 38: 217–20.

31 Witherington R. Vacuum constriction device for management of erectile impotence. *J Urol* 1989; 141: 320–2.

32 Cooper AJ. Preliminary experience with a vacuum constriction device (VCD) as a treatment for impotence. *J Psychosom Research* 1987; 31: 413–18.

33 Kaye T, Guay AT. Skin necrosis caused by use of negative pressure device for erectile impotence. *J Urol* 1991; 146: 1618–19.

34 Rivas DA, Chancellor MB. Complications associated with the use of vacuum constriction devices for erectile dysfunction in the spinal cord injured population. *J Am Paraplegia Soc* 1994; 17: 136–9.

35 Maddison W, Roland JM. Vacuum tumescence: the female perspective [abstract]. *Diabet Med* 1995; 12 (Suppl 2): S3.

36 Virag R. Intracavernous injection of papaverine for erectile failure [letter]. *Lancet* 1982; ii: 938.

37 Linet OI, Ogrinc FG. Efficacy and safety of intracavernosal alprostadil in men with erectile dysfunction. The Alprostadil Study Group. *N Engl J Med* 1996; 334: 873–7.

38 Pagliarulo A, Ludovico GM, Cirillo-Marucco E, Corvasce A, Pagliarulo G. Compliance to longterm vasoactive intracavernous therapy. *Int J Impotence Res* 1996; 8: 63–4.

39 Flynn RJ, Williams G. Long-term follow-up of patients with erectile dysfunction commenced on self injection with intracavernosal papaverine with or without phentolamine. *Br J Urol* 1996; 78: 628–31.

40 Weiss JN, Badlani GH, Ravalli R, Brettschneider N. Reasons for high drop-out rate with self-injection therapy for impotence. *Int J Impotence Res* 1994; 6: 171–4.

41 Armstrong DK, Convery AG, Dinsmore WW. Reasons for patient drop-out from an intracavernous auto-injection programme for erectile dysfunction. *Br J Urol* 1994; 74: 99–101.

42 Padma-Nathan H, Goldstein I, Krane RJ. Treatment of prolonged or priapistic erections following intracavernosal papaverine therapy. *Semin Urol* 1986; 4: 236–8.

43 Lomas GM, Jarow JP. Risk factors for papaverine-induced priapism. *J Urol* 1992; 147: 1280–1.

44 Levine SB, Althof SE, Turner LA *et al.* Side effects of self-administration of intracavernous papaverine and phentolamine for the treatment of impotence. *J Urol* 1989; 141: 54–7.

45 Montague DK, Barada JH, Belker AM *et al.* Clinical Guidelines Panel on Erectile Dysfunction: summary report on the treatment of organic erectile dysfunction. *J Urol* 1996; 156: 2007–11.

46 Alexander W. Detumescence by exercise bicycle [letter]. *Lancet* 1989; i: 735.

47 Buvat J, Lemaire A, Herbaut-Buvat M. Intracavernous pharmacotherapy: comparison of Moxisylyte and prostaglandin E_1. *Int J Impotence Res* 1996; 8: 41–6.

48 Kiely EA, Bloom SR, Williams G. Penile response to vasoactive intestinal polypeptide alone and in combination with other vasoactive agents. *Br J Urol* 1989; 64: 191–4.

49 Gerstenberg TC, Metz P, Ottesen B, Fahrenkrug J. Intracavernous self-injection with vasoactive intestinal polypeptide and phentolamine in the management of erectile failure. *J Urol* 1992; 147: 1277–9.

50 Dinsmore W, Alderdice DK. Vasoactive intestinal polypeptide and phentolamine mesylate administered by autoinjector in the treatment of patients with erectile

dyfunction resistant to other intracavernosal agents. *Br J Urol* 1998; 81: 437–40.

51 Padma-Nathan H, Hellstrom WJ *et al.* Treatment of men with erectile dysfunction with transurethral alprostadil. Medicated Urethral System for Erection (MUSE) Study Group. *N Engl J Med* 1997; 336: 1–7.

52 Nolten WE, Billington CJ, Chiu KC *et al.* Treatment of Erectile Dysfunction (Impotence) with a Novel Transurethral Drug Delivery System: Results from a Multicenter Placebo-controlled Trial [abstract]. 10th International Congress of Endocrinology, 1996.

53 Fulgham PF, Cochran JS, Denman JL *et al.* Disappointing initial results with transurethral alprostadil for erectile dysfunction in a urology practice setting. *J Urol* 1998; 160: 2041–6.

54 Ballard SA, Gingell CJ, Tang K, Turner LA, Price ME, Naylor AM. Effects of sildenafil on the relaxation of human corpus cavernosum tissue *in vitro* and on the activities of cyclic nucleotide phosphodiesterase isozymes. *J Urol* 1998; 159: 2164–71.

55 Boolell M, Gepi-Attee S, Gingell JC, Allen MJ. Sildenafil, a novel effective oral therapy for male erectile dysfunction. *Br J Urol* 1996; 78: 257–61.

56 Price DE, Gingell JC, Gepi-Attee S, Wareham K, Yates P, Boolell M. Sildenafil: study of a novel oral treatment for erectile dysfunction in diabetic men. *Diabet Med* 1998; 15: 821–5.

57 Goldstein I, Lue TF, Padma-Nathan H, Rosen RC, Steers WD, Wicker PA. Oral sildenafil in the treatment of erectile dysfunction. Sildenafil Study Group. *N Engl J Med* 1998; 338: 1397–404.

58 Marks LS, Duda C, Dorey FJ, Macairan ML, Santos PB. Treatment of erectile dysfunction with sildenafil. *Urology* 1999; 53: 19–24.

59 Padma-Nathan H, Steers WD, Wicker PA. Efficacy and safety of oral sildenafil in the treatment of erectile dysfunction: a double-blind, placebo-controlled study of 329 patients. *Sildenafil Study Group. Int J Clin Prac* 1998; 52: 375–9.

60 Price DE. Sildenafil citrate (Viagra) efficacy in the treatment of erectile dysfunction in patients with common concomitant conditions. *Int J Clin Prac Suppl* 1999; 102: 21–3.

61 Giuliano F, Hultling C, El Masry WS *et al.* Randomized trial of sildenafil for the treatment of erectile dysfunction in spinal cord injury. Sildenafil Study Group. *Ann Neurol* 1999; 46: 15–21.

62 Palmer JS, Kaplan WE, Firlit CF. Erectile dysfunction in spina bifida is treatable [letter]. *Lancet* 1999; 354: 125–6.

63 Lowentritt BH, Scardino PT, Miles BJ *et al.* Sildenafil citrate after radical retropubic prostatectomy. *J Urol* 1999; 162: 1614–17.

64 Rendell MS, Rajfer J, Wicker PA, Smith MD. Sildenafil for treatment of erectile dysfunction in men with diabetes: a randomized controlled trial. Sildenafil Diabetes Study Group. *JAMA* 1999; 281: 421–6.

65 Jackson G, Betteridge J, Dean J *et al.* A systematic approach to erectile dysfunction in the cardiovascular patient: a consensus statement. *Int J Clin Pract* 1999; 53: 445–51.

66 Muller JE, Mittleman A, Maclure M, Sherwood JB, Tofler GH. Triggering myocardial infarction by sexual activity. Low absolute risk and prevention by regular physical exertion. Determinants of Myocardial Infarction Onset Study Investigators. *JAMA* 1996; 275: 1405–9.

67 Cheitlin MD, Hutter AMJ, Brindis RG *et al.* ACC/AHA expert consensus document. Use of sildenafil (Viagra) in patients with cardiovascular disease. American College of Cardiology/American Heart Association. *J Am Coll Cardiol* 1999; 33: 273–82.

68 Jarow JP, Burnett AL, Geringer AM. Clinical efficacy of sildenafil citrate based on etiology and response to prior treatment. *J Urol* 1999; 162: 722–5.

17: How should hypertension be managed in diabetes?

Peter M. Nilsson

Introduction

Hypertension in association with type 2 diabetes is a common cardiovascular risk factor, well described as part of a metabolic syndrome by the Swedish physician Eskil Kylin as long ago as 1923 [1], and linked to insulin resistance in more recent papers [2,3]. There exist different subgroups of hypertension in diabetes (Table 17.1), but the most common form is 'essential' hypertension, followed by hypertension secondary to diabetic nephropathy and various degrees of albuminuria. Treatment of hypertension in diabetes has been critically debated for a considerable time, but during the last decade several new randomized controlled trials (RCTs) have added to our clinical knowledge as part of evidence-based medicine in diabetology. In this chapter, treatment goals and drug therapy options will be discussed, focusing on the potential benefits of tight blood pressure control. Therefore, the clinical investigation and diagnostic procedures associated with hypertension will not be discussed in detail, as this can be found in general textbooks [4]. It should, however, be mentioned that the diagnosis of hypertension can be further evaluated and supported by the use of 24-hour ambulatory blood pressure monitoring (ABPM). Patients with diabetic nephropathy, for example, usually do not

Table 17.1 Subgroups of hypertension in diabetes.

Essential hypertension
Hypertension associated with diabetic nephropathy
Non-dipping at night-time ambulatory blood pressure monitoring
Isolated systolic hypertension
White-coat hypertension (and hyperglycaemia)
Supine hypertension with orthostatic hypotension
Secondary hypertension (to endocrine disorders, e.g. Cushing's syndrome)

show a decrease in night-time blood pressure ('non-dippers'), which is normally found in patients without nephropathy. Complementary clinical investigations of potential target organ damage (retinal changes, nephropathy, left ventricular hypertrophy) enables the physician to separate hypertension into various WHO stages (I–III), with no (I), moderate (II) or severe (III) organ damage as a consequence of longstanding or severe hypertension.

Definitions of hypertension in diabetes

In younger age groups, relevant to type 1 diabetic patients, a diastolic blood pressure in the range of 85–90 mmHg, or an individual increase of 10 mmHg or more between visits, may be compatible with hypertension in need of treatment, especially if microalbuminuria is also present as a risk marker for the development of nephropathy.

In the middle-aged or elderly hypertensive patient with type 2 diabetes, it is more commonly found that the systolic blood pressure is elevated above 140 mmHg, often but not always accompanied by a diastolic blood pressure elevation above 85–90 mmHg. It is estimated that 40–50% of all type 2 diabetes patients are hypertensive when diabetes is diagnosed [5].

Hypertension in diabetes represents an increased risk of cardiovascular disease (two to three times the risk of non-diabetic people), retinopathy, nephropathy and end-stage renal disease (ESRD), but also higher overall health care costs for these patients. A large proportion of diabetic patients with hypertension show signs of target organ damage and cardiovascular complications [6]. Hypertension in diabetes is thus a public health problem of considerable magnitude, and should be carefully dealt with. Unfortunately, however, only a small number of all diabetic patients with hypertension have acceptable blood pressure control, as shown in population-based studies both in the UK [7] and in Sweden (Table 17.2).

Table 17.2 National Diabetes Register (NDR) of Sweden: primary health care data from a national screening survey (1996), based on a total of 6072 men and 5653 women with diabetes, 77% of whom developed diabetes after age 60 (hypertensive diabetics, $n = 4699$).

Age (years)	Blood pressure (mmHg)		
	<85 DBP	<140 SBP	<140 SBP + <85 DBP
30–59	51%	40%	29%
60+	65%	22%	19%
Total	62%	25%	21%

DBP, diastolic blood pressure; SBP, systolic blood pressure.

Why is hypertension in diabetes increasing?

Many observational studies have indicated an increase in the prevalence of hypertension associated with type 2 diabetes. This might be due to different factors, as listed below.

A common view includes:

• Ageing populations and patients with longer duration of diabetes.
• Increased prevalence of obesity/insulin resistance in the population.
• New definitions of hypertension (the Sixth Report of the Joint National Committee) [8] and diabetes (American Diabetes Association and WHO) [9] and increased patient numbers.
• Secondary finding to increased screening and detection/control efforts.

An alternative view includes:

• Iatrogenesis (some antihypertensive drugs might induce type 2 diabetes).
• Birth cohort phenomenon (fetal growth retardation) [10].

Probably several of these factors are relevant to explain why hypertension in diabetes is a growing public health problem, not only for diabetologists at the hospital level to deal with, but most of all for primary healthcare physicians.

Have treatment aims changed?

The treatment goals have changed during the 1990s towards lower blood pressure levels, both systolic and diastolic, as shown in a summary of current guidelines and recommendations from the last decade (Table 17.3). Today, the present blood pressure goal of antihypertensive treatment is a mean casual blood pressure less than 130–140/85 mmHg, for all patients who can tolerate this blood pressure reduction without offsetting side-effects, for example

Table 17.3 Summary of diagnostic levels (mmHg) and blood pressure goals from published hypertension guidelines for diabetic populations: 1989–99.

Guideline	Optimal	Fair/acceptable	Poor
Canadian Diabetes Advisory Board [61]	<140/90	<150/90	>150/90
European IDDM Policy Group [62]	140/85	—	—
American Diabetes Association [63]	<130/85	—	—
European NIDDM Policy Group [64]	<140/90	160/95	>160/95
ALFEDIAM (French Association) [65]	<140/90	<160/90	>150/90
USA: Joint National Committee VI [66]	<130/85	<140/90	>140/90
ECS/ESH/EAS [51]	<130/85	—	—
British Hypertension Society [67]	<140/90	—	>140/90
WHO/ISH [68]	<130/85	—	—

caused by orthostatic reactions or compromised arterial circulation in critical vascular beds. It is still unclear if ambulatory blood pressure definitions of normality could be used also for patients with diabetes [11], but the addition of ABPM is useful in many other ways, for example to show if 'non-dipping' during the night exists.

Aim and choice of antihypertensive drug therapy in general

Strict blood pressure control is the primary goal (<130–140/85 mmHg) of treatment. This implies drug combination treatment for the majority (two-thirds) of patients, according to the long-term results of both the UK Prospective Diabetes Study (UKPDS) [12] and the Hypertension Optimal Treatment (HOT) study [13]. Therefore, the clinician must be able to use a broad variety of antihypertensive drugs, and from these drugs frequently choose alternative combinations with pharmacological synergism. Drug combination therapy usually means that lower dosages of single drugs can be used, which reduces the risk of adverse effects with high-dose monotherapy (Table 17.4).

Table 17.4 Practical guidelines for treatment of hypertension in patients with type 2 diabetes.

Invite the patient to jointly define an individual blood pressure goal, normally <130–140/85 mm Hg for all patients who can tolerate this level without orthostatic reactions

Start with 3–6 months of lifestyle interventions, such as weight loss in the obese, improved diet, sodium and alcohol restriction, increase in physical exercise and smoking cessation, if the blood pressure level does not demand immediate drug therapy

Consider suitable antihypertensive drug therapy with regard to factors such as age, target-organ damage, tolerance and costs, as well as scientific evidence

Be aware of absolute or relative contraindications for certain drug treatment. These include old age, malignancy or drug-specific hypersensitivity reactions

Try different ways to reach the blood pressure goal. Normally this takes drug combination treatment with synergistic pharmacological properties

Be prepared to reconsider and adjust treatment if this fails to achieve the goal. Failure might be due to factors related to the physician (lack of time and interest), the patient (lack of compliance), the disease (biological resistance, secondary hypertension) or the drug (dosages, duration, effects, and tolerability)

Always consider blood pressure control as only one component of a general strategy of multiple cardiovascular risk factor control: do not neglect other relevant risk factors and their treatment

Optimize treatment and plan for more frequent visits if metabolic and/or blood pressure control is poor, or (micro)albuminuria is increasing

Specific antihypertensive agents

Diuretics

Diuretics are often effective antihypertensive agents in diabetes, in which the total body sodium load is increased and the extracellular fluid volume expanded [14]. However, diuretics that increase urinary potassium and magnesium losses can worsen glucose tolerance, as insulin secretion is impaired by potassium depletion. Additionally, insulin sensitivity in peripheral tissues may be impaired [15,16]. The use of high-dose thiazide diuretics has increased the risk of non-diabetic hypertensive patients developing diabetes by up to three times in observational studies [17], even if this view has also been disputed [18]. In a recent observational study, it was shown that use of diuretics increased cardiovascular mortality in hypertensive type 2 diabetics who were still hyperglycaemic in spite of treatment [19].

Potassium depletion is particularly severe with high-dose chlorthalidone, less with frusemide (furosemide) and bendrofluazide (bendroflumethiazide) and apparently trivial with indapamide [20]. This mechanism is irrelevant to C-peptide negative type 1 diabetes patients who are totally dependent on exogenous insulin. Diuretics may precipitate hyperosmolar, non-ketotic coma and should be avoided or used at the lowest effective dose in patients with a history of this complication.

Thiazides may aggravate dyslipidaemia [21], although low dosages probably carry a small risk. Thiazides have also been associated with impotence and should be avoided in diabetic men with erectile failure.

Diuretics suitable for use in diabetic hypertension include frusemide, bendrofluazide, hydrochlorothiazide, spironolactone and indapamide. Low dosages should be used, sometimes in combination with potassium supplements or potassium-sparing drugs like amiloride. If ineffective, diuretics should be combined with another first-line drug, for example an ACE inhibitor or an angiotensin-II-receptor antagonist, rather than given at increased dosage. Caution must, however, be exercised for the combination of spironolactone and ACE inhibitor, as this increases the risk of hyperkalaemia. Frusemide can be used instead in patients with renal impairment (serum creatinine > 150 µmol/l) or oedema. Serum urea, creatinine and potassium should be checked initially and every 3–6 months thereafter, as dangerous hyperkalaemia can develop, especially in diabetic patients with renal impairment.

β-Adrenergic blocking agents

β-Receptor blockers may significantly lower blood pressure levels in diabetic patients with hypertension, even though renin release (one of these agents' major targets) is commonly reduced in diabetes, due to fluid retention. The main mechanism of action is to reduce blood pressure, heart rate and cardiac output via interference with β_1 and β_2 receptors in the myocardium and in the vessel wall. These drugs are, however, often ineffective in Afro-Caribbean patients, who commonly have low-renin hypertension. Like diuretics, β-receptor blockers may aggravate both hyperglycaemia and dyslipidaemia [22]. This is dependent on dosage and degree of selectivity of the drug used. Their hyperglycaemic effect is attributed to inhibition of β_2-adrenergic-mediated insulin release as well as decreased insulin action in peripheral tissues [23], and has been estimated to increase the risks of a non-diabetic person developing the disease by six-fold in observational studies, and up to 15-fold if given together with thiazides [17]. However, recent studies suggest that the hazards of both hyperglycaemia and hyperlipidaemia have been exaggerated and may be both dose-dependent and secondary to weight gain. The metabolic side-effects of β-receptor blockers can be reduced by using low dosages combined with other agents, particularly the calcium antagonists from the dihydropyridine group, or non-pharmacological efforts to decrease weight and improve physical activity.

β-Receptor blockers have other side-effects relevant to diabetes. They may interfere with the counter-regulatory effects of catecholamines released during hypoglycaemia, thereby blunting manifestations such as tachycardia and tremor and thus delaying recovery from hypoglycaemia [24]. In clinical practice, however, this rarely presents a serious problem, especially when cardioselective β_1-receptor blockers are used. β-receptor blockers may also aggravate impotence, and are generally contraindicated in second- or third-degree atrioventricular heart block, peripheral vascular disease (intermittent claudication), asthma and chronic airway obstruction. Recent studies have shown that β-receptor blockers can also favourably be used in cardiac failure, but more studies are needed in patients with concomitant diabetes.

Atenolol is a useful drug as it is cardioselective, water soluble (which reduces central nervous system side-effects and renders its metabolism and dosage more predictable) and effective as a single daily dose, which probably encourages compliance. It was also tested in the UKPDS [12]. Metoprolol in moderate dosages is another useful alternative. In secondary prevention after myocardial infarction, however, both non-selective and selective β-receptor blockers have been effective in diabetic patients [25].

Calcium antagonists

These useful vasodilator agents do not normally worsen metabolic control when used at currently accepted dosages, but sporadic cases with decreased glucose tolerance developing after the initiation of a calcium antagonist of the dihydropyridine class have been described [26]. This may be due to the inhibitory effect on calcium-mediated insulin secretion in susceptible patients, or compensatory sympathetic nervous activation (with insulin antagonistic effects) following vasodilatation.

Calcium channel antagonists (calcium entry blockers) have a slight negative inotropic effect and are contraindicated in significant cardiac failure, although the mild ankle oedema often associated with their use is probably due to relaxation of the peripheral precapillary sphincters rather than to right ventricular failure. Because of their other cardiac actions, they are particularly indicated in hypertensive patients who also have angina (e.g. sustained-release nifedipine and diltiazem), or supraventricular tachycardia (e.g. verapamil). Their vasodilator properties may also be beneficial in peripheral vascular disease. Calcium antagonists are ideally combined with selective β₁-receptor blockers, but the specific combination of verapamil and β-receptor blockers (especially with concomitant use of digoxin) must be avoided because of the risk of conduction block and asystole.

Sustained-release nifedipine, given once daily, is a convenient preparation for general use if orthostatic hypotension is not present, but has no specific effect in reducing albuminuria. Felodipine, isradipine and amlodipine are other useful agents if orthostatic reactions are not expected. The most selective drug for the peripheral vasculature, felodipine, was tested in the large-scale HOT study [13], which included almost 1500 diabetic patients and showed a significant stepwise decrease in cardiovascular events and mortality rates with lower diastolic blood pressure treatment goals (<90, <85, <80 mmHg) in these patients.

Angiotensin-converting enzyme inhibitors

ACE inhibitors may be used in diabetic hypertension, even when the general renin-angiotensin-aldosterone system (RAS) is not activated. One reason for this may be interference with local tissue-specific RAS. When used alone, however, these agents have a limited hypotensive action in many black patients. ACE inhibitors have no adverse metabolic effects, and may even improve insulin sensitivity [15,16,27]. These drugs are particularly beneficial in diabetic nephropathy, by reducing albuminuria and possibly its progression [28]. Their antiproteinuric effect may be due specifically to relaxation of the efferent arterioles in the glomerulus (which is highly sensitive to vasoconstriction by angiotensin II), so reducing the intraglomerular hypertension that has been postulated to favour albumin filtration, although the importance of this mechanism remains controversial [29]. This selective effect is not shared by other antihypertensive drugs. ACE inhibitors are also indicated in cardiac failure, in combination with relatively low dosages of diuretics.

A dry cough is reported by 10–15% of patients treated with ACE inhibitors, possibly due to interference with bradykinin-mediated mechanisms in the bronchial epithelium. Changing to another ACE inhibitor or an angiotensin-II-receptor blocker may reduce or alleviate this adverse reaction. ACE inhibitors occasionally precipitate acute renal failure, particularly in the elderly, those taking non-steroidal anti-inflammatory agents (NSAIDs) and patients with bilateral renal artery stenosis. Other side-effects (rashes, neutropenia, taste disturbance) are unusual with the low dosages currently recommended but are more prominent in renal failure. Hypoglycaemia has occasionally been reported to occur associated with the use of ACE inhibitors in diabetic patients [30]. Because of their tendency to cause potassium retention, potassium-sparing diuretics (spironolactone and amiloride) or potassium supplements should not be taken concurrently. Serum creatinine and potassium levels should be monitored regularly, especially in patients with renal failure, in whom hyperkalaemia may occasionally reach dangerous levels.

Captopril, enalapril, lisinopril and ramipril are traditional ACE inhibitors and they are all suitable for use in diabetic patients; enalapril, lisinopril and ramipril are given once daily for hypertension. The first dose of an ACE inhibitor should be small (e.g. 6.25 mg of captopril) and given just before bedtime to minimize postural hypotension, which may be profound in subjects overtreated with diuretics or on a strict sodium-restricted diet. The same problem may arise in patients with autonomic neuropathy.

Angiotensin-II receptor antagonists

This promising new class of drugs acts on the angiotensin-II (AT_1) receptor, decreases blood pressure and is metabolically neutral [31]. Recently, several angiotensin-II-receptor antagonists (AIIRA), such as losartan, irbesartan, valsartan and candesartan, have been introduced with potential for the treatment of hypertension in diabetes, showing less cough symptoms as side-effects [31]. Several large-scale RCTs including AIIRAs in diabetic patients are currently under way.

α_1-Receptor blockers

These antihypertensive drugs can lower blood pressure but also improve dyslipidaemia and insulin sensitivity [27]. Doxazosin is normally well tolerated, especially in combination therapy, and improves insulin sensitivity. This has been well described in hypertriglyceridaemic subjects [32]. Side-effects include nasal congestion and postural hypotension.

Recent clinical trials

With this information on individual drug properties, how should the clinician make a best choice? There exists today a substantial body of intervention studies (RCTs) as a background for clinical judgement according to 'evidence-based medicine'.

UKPDS

Most notably, in a substudy of the UKPDS [12] 1148 newly detected type 2 diabetic patients with a mean blood pressure of 160/94 mmHg were randomized to either 'tight' blood pressure control ($n = 758$), or 'usual care' blood pressure control ($n = 390$). In the former group, patients were also randomized to treatment based on the ACE inhibitor captopril ($n = 400$) or the β_1-selective blocker atenolol ($n = 358$). In summary, this landmark study has shown that a difference in achieved blood pressure levels of 10/5 mmHg between the two randomized groups (144/82 vs 154/87 mmHg) resulted in a substantial net benefit for the 'tight' control group. This included a reduction in diabetes-related endpoints (–24%), diabetes-related deaths (–32%), stroke (–44%) and microvascular endpoints (–37%), the last predominantly due to a reduced risk of retinal photocoagulation. A beneficial effect was, however, not reported for myocardial infarction or all-cause mortality [12]. There were no significant outcome differences between the groups on captopril- or atenolol-based therapies in the tight-control arm [33]. It should, however, be kept in mind that significantly more patients remained on captopril (80%)

than atenolol (74%) at the end of the study, and that more patients needed additional antidiabetic medication in the atenolol group (81%) compared with the captopril group (71%). The latter finding may be due to more pronounced weight gain over 9 years in the atenolol group than in the captopril group (3.4 vs 1.6 kg), a factor well known to decrease insulin sensitivity.

Other trials of antihypertensive agents

In the Systolic Hypertension in the Elderly Program (SHEP) study, a diuretic-based therapy (chlorthalidone) was more effective in reducing non-fatal stroke and myocardial infarction than placebo in elderly patients with systolic hypertension [34]. The two smaller studies, Appropriate Blood Pressure Control (ABCD) [35] and Fosinopril versus Amlodipine Cardiovascular Events Trial (FACET) [36], both had another aim than to study effects on cardiovascular end-points, for example renal function and metabolic control. In spite of that shortcoming, the ABCD study showed that treatment with an ACE inhibitor (enalapril) was more effective in reducing myocardial infarction than treatment with a calcium antagonist (nisoldipine), while FACET showed that treatment with another ACE inhibitor (fosinopril) was more effective in reducing major cardiovascular events than treatment with a calcium antagonist (amlodipine). FACET also showed that the combination of the two drugs was the most effective treatment [36]. It is possible that the protective effects of ACE inhibitors, or added-on β-receptor blockers, were more important for the results obtained in both studies than any detrimental effect of a calcium antagonist [37].

The Multicentre Isradipine Diuretic Atherosclerosis Study (MIDAS) was a study in which patients with hyperglycaemia were excluded at baseline and therefore not relevant to discuss in this context [38], even if this has been cited by others in the so-called calcium antagonist controversy [39].

The Captopril Prevention Project (CAPPP) study showed that in hypertensive type 2 diabetes patients, a therapy based on an ACE inhibitor (captopril) was more successful in preventing all fatal (−46%) and all cardiac events (−33%) compared with conventional treatment (thiazide diuretic and β-receptor blocker), in spite of less optimal blood pressure control in the captopril group [40].

Finally, the Systolic Hypertension in Europe (SYST-EUR) study reported results in a large subgroup of type 2 diabetic patients with systolic hypertension, randomized to treatment with either the calcium antagonist nitrendipine or placebo [41]. In the diabetic subjects, treatment reduced overall mortality by 55%, cardiovascular events by 69% and strokes by 73%, compared with placebo. It was shown that treatment with nitrendipine prevented cardiovascular events even more effectively than was reported for active treatment in the SHEP study, which had a similar design [34,41].

How to judge the role of thiazide diuretics in view of the trials?

It is quite clear from the SHEP study that low-dose thiazide diuretics are useful and effective in both elderly non-diabetic and diabetic patients with systolic hypertension [34], but should these drugs also be recommended for the middle-aged diabetic patient? A counter-argument is that thiazides will increase hyperglycaemia and decrease insulin sensitivity [15,16], an effect dependent on dose and treatment duration. This metabolic adverse effect may be of greater importance for middle-aged patients, facing many years to come of antihypertensive treatment, than in the elderly for whom haemodynamic effects may be more important in the shorter term. An increased risk of gout and impotence are also well-known side-effects with thiazide diuretic use, both conditions being more common in type 2 diabetic patients than in non-diabetic subjects. However, if low-dose thiazide diuretics can be combined with an ACE inhibitor or an angiotensin-II-receptor blocker, the blood pressure lowering effect will be potentiated, but the metabolic adverse effects will improve.

Can calcium antagonists be safely used in type 2 diabetes?

Much debate and controversy has been provoked in recent years by the use of calcium antagonist in hypertension, and also in diabetes [39]. After the publication of the *post hoc* analysis in the SYST-EUR trial [41], it seems well documented that use of a long-acting calcium antagonist of the dihydropyridine class is safe and more effective in preventing cardiovascular endpoints than placebo. This may not be so surprising after all, as the haemodynamic effect of blood pressure lowering should be of special importance for this group of elderly patients, when it is well established that hypertension control is very effective also in elderly hypertensives without diabetes [42–44]. Three other drugs of the same class are currently being tested in ongoing randomized large-scale studies; nifedipine in the International Nifedipine GITS Study: Intervention as a Goal in Hypertensive Treatment (INSIGHT) [45], amlodipine in the Antihypertensive and Lipid Lowering Treatment to Prevent Heart Attack Trial (ALLHAT) [46] and isradipine in the Swedish Trial in Old

Patients with hypertension-2 (STOP-2) trial [47]. Another class of calcium antagonists, diltiazem, is currently tested in the Nordic Diltiazem (NORDIL) trial [48]. In the INSIGHT study a calcium antagonist is compared with a thiazide diuretic, in ALLHAT with a thiazide diuretic, ACE inhibitor and α-receptor blocker, in STOP-2 with an ACE inhibitor, thiazide diuretic or β-receptor blocker.

Normally, calcium antagonists of the dihydropyridine class are very effective in combination with $β_1$-receptor blockers, which can improve side-effects such as tachycardia.

Ethnic groups and their problems

Hypertension in diabetes represents a serious medical problem in many ethnic groups, such as African-Americans [49,50]. In non-Caucasian patients, β-receptor-blockers and ACE inhibitors should normally be avoided due to reduced efficacy. Diuretics and calcium antagonists are often drugs to be preferred, at least in African-Americans [8].

Conclusions

The diagnosis and treatment of established hypertension is an integral part of the clinical risk stratification of the diabetic patient, as discussed and out-lined in current guidelines [51–54]. Hypertension in type 2 diabetes rep-resents a well documented risk factor for cerebrovascular and cardiovascular disease [55,56], especially if combined with varying degrees of albumin-uria. Observational studies have shown that conventionally drug-treated hypertensive patients with diabetes and cardiovascular disease still run an increased risk compared with diet-treated patients [57]. Treatment should therefore aim at normalizing the blood pressure, in most patients to <130–140/85 mmHg, irrespective of means. However, in subgroups of patients the different treatment modalities are of specific importance and should be constantly evaluated according to efficacy, clinical documentation in RCTs, cost effectiveness, safety and quality of life for the diabetic patient.

Tight blood pressure control has been shown to provide a substantial benefit for hypertensive type 2 diabetes patients in preventing both microvas-cular and macrovascular complications. This has been most clearly shown in the UKPDS [12] and the HOT study [13]. Furthermore, this treatment strategy seems to be cost effective as concluded from the UKPDS analyses of health economics in hypertensive patients [58].

New treatment modalities for hypertension are constantly being introduced but have to prove themselves, sooner or later, for efficacy and tolerability. In the future we can expect that the application of cardiovascular genomics will substantially change the way we handle hypertension in diabetes [59,60], and will help to address the challenges in tailoring antihypertensive treatment to the genotype of the individual patient.

Note added in proof

The STOP-2 [69], NORDIL [70] and INSIGHT [71] studies have now been concluded and published. Overall, they show that treatment with a calcium antagonist is equally effective as other treatments in hypertensive patients with type 2 diabetes.

References

1 Kylin E. Studien über das Hypertoni-Hyperglykemie-Hyperurikemisyndrom. Z Innere Medizin 1923; 7: 105–12.
2 Reaven GM. Role of insulin resistance in human disease. Diabetes 1988; 37: 1595–607.
3 Meigs JB, D'Agostino RB, Wilson P, Cupples A, Nathan DM, Singer DE. Risk variable clustering in the Insulin Resistance Syndrome—The Framingham Offspring Study. Diabetes 1997; 46: 1594–600.
4 Nilsson P. Diabetes and hypertension. In: Pickup JC, Williams G, eds. Textbook of Diabetes, 2nd edn. Oxford: Blackwell Scientific Publications, 1997.
5 Hypertension in Diabetes Study (HDS). 1. Prevalence of hypertension in newly presenting type 2 diabetic patients and the association with risk factors for cardiovascular and diabetic complications. The Hypertension Diabetes Study Group. J Hypertens 1993; 11: 309–17.
6 Hypertension in Diabetes Study (HDS). II. Increased risk of cardiovascular complications in hypertensive type 2 diabetic patients. The Hypertension Diabetes Study Group. J Hypertens 1993; 11: 319–25.
7 Colhoun HM, Dong W, Barakat MT, Mather HM, Poulter NR. The scope for cardiovascular risk factor intervention among people with diabetes mellitus in England: a population-based analysis from Health Surveys for England 1991–94. Diabet Med 1993; 16: 35–40.
8 The Sixth Report of the Joint National Committee on prevention, detection evaluation, treatment of high blood pressure. Arch Intern Med 1997; 157: 2413–46.
9 Alberti KGMM, Zimmet P, for the WHO Consultation Group. Definition, diagnosis and classification of diabetes mellitus and its complications. Part 1: Diagnosis and classification of diabetes mellitus. Diabet Med 1998; 15: 539–53.
10 Barker DJP, ed. Fetal and Infant Origins of Adult Disease, 1st edn. London: BMJ Books, 1992.
11 Schernthaner G, Ritz E, Phillipp T, Bretzel R. The significance of 24-hour blood pressure monitoring in patients with diabetes mellitus. Dtsch Med Wochenschr 1999; 124: 393–5.
12 UK Prospective Diabetes Study. Tight blood pressure control, risk of macrovascular, microvascular

complications in type 2 diabetes: UKPDS 38. *BMJ* 1998; 317: 703–13.

13 Hansson L, Zanchetti A, Carruthers SG *et al.* Effects of intensive blood-pressure lowering and low-dose aspirin in patients with hypertension: principal results of the Hypertension Optimal Treatment (HOT) randomised trial. *Lancet* 1998; 351: 1755–62.

14 Weidman P, Beretta-Picolli C, Keusch G *et al.* Sodium-volume factor, cardiovascular reactivity and hypotensive mechanism of diuretic therapy in mild hypertension associated with diabetes mellitus. *Am J Med* 1979; 67: 779–84.

15 Pollare T, Lithell H, Berne C. A comparison of the effects of hydrochlothiazide and captopril on glucose and lipid metabolism in patients with hypertension. *N Engl J Med* 1989; 321: 868–73.

16 Hunter SJ, Wiggam MI, Ennis CN *et al.* Comparison of effects of captopril used either alone or in combination with a thiazide diuretic on insulin action in hypertensive Type 2 diabetic patients: a double-blind crossover study. *Diabet Med* 1999; 16: 482–7.

17 Bengtsson C, Blohmé G, Lapidus L *et al.* Do antihypertensive drugs precipitate diabetes? *BMJ* 1984; 289: 1495–7.

18 Berglund G, Andersson O, Widgren B. Low-dose antihypertensive treatment with a thiazide diuretic is not diabetogenic. A 10-year controlled trial with bendroflumethiazide. *Acta Med Scand* 1986; 220: 419–24.

19 Alderman MH, Cohen H, Madhavan S. Diabetes and cardiovascular events in diabetes patients. *Hypertension* 1999; 33: 1130–4.

20 Osei K, Holland G, Falko JM. Indapamide—effects on apoprotein, lipoprotein, and glucoregulation in ambulatory diabetic patients. *Arch Intern Med* 1986; 146: 1973–7.

21 MacMahon SW, Macdonald GJ. Antihypertensive treatment and plasma lipoprotein levels. The associations in data from a population study. *Am J Med* 1987; 80 (Suppl 2A): 40–7.

22 Pollare T, Lithell H, Selinus I, Berne C. Sensitivity to insulin during treatment with atenolol and metoprolol: a randomized, double blind study of effects on carbohydrate and lipoprotein metabolism in hypertensive patients. *BMJ* 1989; 198: 1152–7.

23 Struthers AD. The choice of antihypertensive therapy in the diabetic patient. *Postgrad Med J* 1985; 61: 563–9.

24 Lager I, Blohme G, Smith U. Effect of cardioselective and non selective beta-blockade on the hypoglycaemic response in insulin-dependent diabetics. *Lancet* 1979; i: 458–62.

25 Kjekshus J, Gilpin E, Cali G *et al.* Diabetic patients and beta-blockers after acute myocardial infarction. *Eur Heart J* 1990; 11: 43–50.

26 Chellingsworth MC, Kendall MJ, Wright AD, Singh BM, Pasi J. The effects of verapamil, diltiazem, nifedipine and propranolol on metabolic control in hypertensives with non-insulin-dependent diabetes mellitus. *J Hum Hypertens* 1989; 3: 35–9.

27 Lithell HO. Effects of antihypertensive drugs on insulin, glucose and lipid metabolism. *Diabetes Care* 1991; 14: 203–9.

28 Lewis EJ, Hunsickler LG, Bain RP, Rohde RD *et al.* The effect of angiotensin-converting-enzyme inhibition on diabetic nephropathy. *N Engl J Med* 1993; 329: 1456–62.

29 Bank N, Klose R, Aynedjan HS, Nguyen D, Sablay LB. Evidence against increased glomerular pressure initiating diabetic nephropathy. *Kidney Int* 1987; 31: 898–905.

30 Herings RM, de Boer A, Stricker BH, Leufkens HG, Porsius A. Hypoglycaemia associated with use of inhibitor of angiotensin converting enzyme. *Lancet* 1995; 345: 1195–8.

31 Goodfriend TL, Elliott ME, Catt KJ. Angiotensin receptors and their antagonists. *N Engl J Med* 1996; 334: 1649–54.

32 Andersson PE, Lithell H. Metabolic effects of doxazosin and enalapril in hypertriglyceridemic, hypertensive men. Relationship to changes in skeletal muscle

blood flow. *Am J Hypertens* 1996; 9: 323–33.

33 UK Prospective Diabetes Study Group. Efficacy of atenolol and captopril in reducing risk of macrovascular and microvascular complications in type 2 diabetes. UKPDS 39. *BMJ* 1998; 317: 713–20.

34 Curb JD, Pressel SL, Cutler JA, Savage PJ. Effect of diuretic-based anti-hypertensive treatment on cardiovascular disease risk in older diabetic patients with isolated systolic hypertension. *JAMA* 1996; 276: 1886–92.

35 Estacio RO, Jeffers BW, Hiatt WR, Biggerstaff SL, Gifford N, Schrier RW. The effect of nisoldipine as compared with enalapril on cardiovascular outcomes in patients with non-insulin-dependent diabetes and hypertension. *N Engl J Med* 1998; 338: 645–52.

36 Tatti P, Pahor M, Byington RP *et al.* Outcome results of the fosinopril versus amlodipine cardiovascular events randomized trial (FACET) in patients with hypertension and NIDDM. *Diabetes Care* 1998; 21: 597–603.

37 Malmberg K, Rydén L, Wedel H. Calcium antagonists, appropriate therapy for diabetic patients with hypertension? *Eur Heart J* 1998; 19: 1269–72.

38 Borhani NO, Mercuri M, Borhani PA *et al.* Final outcome results of the Multicenter Isradipine Diuretic Atherosclerosis Study (MIDAS). A randomized controlled trial. *JAMA* 1996; 276: 785–91.

39 Pahor M, Psaty BM, Furberg CD. Treatment of hypertensive patients with diabetes. *Lancet* 1998; 351: 689–90.

40 Hansson L, Lindholm LH, Niskanen L *et al.* Effect of angiotensin-converting-enzyme inhibition compared with conventional therapy on cardiovascular morbidity and mortality in hypertension: the Captopril Prevention Project (CAPPP). *Lancet* 1999; 353: 611–16.

41 Tuomilehto J, Rastenyte D, Birkenhäger WH *et al.* Effects of calcium-channel blockade in older patients with diabetes and systolic hypertension. *N Engl J Med* 1999; 340: 677–84.

42 Dahlöf B, Lindholm LH, Hansson L, Scherstén B, Ekbom T, Wester P-O. Morbidity and mortality in the Swedish Trial in Old Patients with Hypertension (STOP-Hypertension). *Lancet* 1991; 338: 1281–5.

43 MRC Working Party. Medical Research Council trial of treatment of hypertension in older adults: principal results. *BMJ* 1992; 304: 405–12.

44 Staessen JA, Fagard R, Thijs L *et al.* Randomised double-blind comparison of placebo and active treatment for older patients with isolated systolic hypertension. *Lancet* 1997; 350: 757–64.

45 Brown MJ, de Castaigne A, Leeuw PW, Macia G, Rosentahl T, Ruilope LM. Study population and treatment titration in the International Nifedipine GITS Study: Intervention as a Goal in Hypertensive Treatment (INSIGHT). *J Hypertens* 1998; 16: 2113–16.

46 Davis BR, Cutler JA, Gordon DJ *et al.* Rationale and design for the Antihypertensive and Lipid Lowering Treatment to Prevent Heart Attack Trial (ALLHAT). ALLHAT Res Group. *Am J Hypertens* 1996; 9: 342–60.

47 Lindholm LH, Hansson L, Dahlöf B *et al.* The Swedish Trial in Old Patients with hypertension-2 (STOP-hypertension-2): a progress report. *Blood Pressure* 1996; 5: 300–4.

48 The Nordic Diltiazem Study (NORDIL). A prospective intervention trial of calcium antagonist therapy in hypertension. *Blood Press* 1993; 2: 312–21.

49 Jamerson K, deQuattro V. The impact of ethnicity on response to antihypertensive therapy. *Am J Med* 1996; 101: 22S–32S.

50 Flack JM, Hamaty M. Difficult-to-treat hypertensive populations: focus on African-Americans and people with type 2 diabetes. *J Hypertens Suppl* 1999; 17: S19–24.

51 Prevention of coronary risk in clinical practice. Recommendations of the Second Joint Task Force of European and other Societies on Coronary Prevention. Summary recommendations. *Eur Heart J* 1998; 19: 1434–503.

52 Anonymous. WHO/ISH guidelines for the management of hypertension. *J Hypertens* 1999; 17: 151–83.

53 Yudkin JS, Chaturvedi N. Developing risk stratification charts for diabetic and non-diabetic patients. *Diabetic Med* 1999; 16: 219–27.

54 Joint British recommendations on prevention of coronary heart disease in clinical practice. *Heart* 1998; 80 (Suppl 2): S1–29.

55 Stamler J, Vaccaro O, Neaton JD, Wentworth D. Diabetes, other risk factors, and 12-yr cardiovascular mortality for men screened in the Multiple Risk Factor Intervention Trial. *Diabetes Care* 1993; 16: 434–44.

56 Turner RC, Millns H, Neil HAW Risk factors for coronary heart disease in non-insulin dependent diabetes mellitus: United Kingdom prospective diabetes study (UKPDS. 23). *BMJ* 1998; 316: 823–8.

57 Tenenbaum A, Fishman EZ, Boyko V *et al*. Hypertension in diet versus pharmacologically treated diabetes. *Hypertension* 1999; 33: 1002–7.

58 UK Prospective Diabetes Study Group. Cost effectiveness analysis of improved blood pressure control in hypertensive patients with type 2 diabetes. UKPDS 40. *BMJ* 1998; 317: 720–6.

59 Kennon B, Petrie JR, Small M, Connell JMC. Angiotensin-converting enzyme gene and diabetes mellitus. *Diabet Med* 1999; 16: 448–58.

60 Pratt RE, Dzau VJ. Genomics, hypertension. Concepts, potentials, and opportunities. *Hypertension* 1999; 33 (part II): 238–47.

61 Expert Committee of the Canadian Diabetes Advisory Boad. Clinical practice guidelines for the treatment of diabetes mellitus. *Can Med Assoc J* 1992; 147: 697–712.

62 European IDDM Policy Group. Consensus guidelines for the management of insulin dependent (type 1) diabetes. *Diabet Med* 1993; 10: 990–1005.

63 American Diabetes Association. Clinical practice recommendations 1992–93. Diabetes Care 1993; 16 (Suppl 2): 1–18.

64 European NIDDM Group. A desktop guide for the management of non-insulin-dependent diabetes mellitus (NIDDM.) *Diabetes Med* 1994; 11: 899–909.

65 Members of the Board of Directors, Scientific Directors of ALFEDAIM (French). Arterial hypertension and diabetes. *Diabetes Metab* 1996; 22: 64–76.

66 Joint National Committee on Detection, Evaluation and Treatment of High Blood Pressure. Sixth Report of the Joint Committee on Detection, Evaluation and Treatment of High Blood Pressure (JNC-VI). *Arch Intern Med* 1997; 157: 2413–46.

67 Ramsay L, Williams B, Johnston G, MacGregor G *et al*. Guidelines for management of hypertension. Report of the Third Working Party of the British Hypertension Society. *J Hum Hypertens* 1999; 13: 569–92.

68 The World Health Organisation/International Society of Hypertension Guidelines Subcommittee. 1999 guidelines for management of hypertension. *J Hypertens* 1999; 17: 151–85.

69 Hansson L, Lindholm LH, Ekbom T *et al*. Randomised trial of old and new antihypertensive drugs in elderly patients: cardiovascular mortality and morbidity in the Swedish Trial in Old Patients with hypertension-2. *Lancet* 1999; 354: 1751–6.

70 Hansson LH, Hedner T, Lund-Johansen P *et al*. Randomised trial of effect of calcium antagonists compared with diuretics and β-blockers on cardiovascular morbidity and mortality in hypertension: the Nordic Diltiazem (NORDIL) Study. *Lancet* 2000; 356: 359–65.

71 Brown MJ, Palmer CR, Castaigne A, de Leeuw PW, Mancia G, Rosenthal T, Ruilope LM. Morbidity and mortality in patients randomised to double-blind treatment with long-acting calcium-channel blocker or diuretic in the International Nifedipine GITS Study: Intervention as a goal in Hypertension Treatment (INSIGHT). *Lancet* 2000; 356: 366–72.

Index